Dieting, Overweight, and Obesity

Dieting, Overweight, and Obesity

Self-Regulation in a Food-Rich Environment

Wolfgang Stroebe

American Psychological Association • Washington, DC

Published by
American Psychological Association
750 First Street, NE
Washington, DC 20002
www.apa.org

To order
APA Order Department
P.O. Box 92984
Washington, DC 20090-2984
Tel: (800) 374-2721; Direct: (202) 336-5510
Fax: (202) 336-5502; TDD/TTY: (202) 336-6123
Online: www.apa.org/books/
E-mail: order@apa.org

In the U.K., Europe, Africa, and the Middle East, copies may be ordered from
American Psychological Association
3 Henrietta Street
Covent Garden, London
WC2E 8LU England

Typeset in Goudy by Circle Graphics, Columbia, MD

Printer: Book-Mart Press, North Bergen, NJ
Cover Designer: Mercury Publishing Services, Rockville, MD
Technical/Production Editor: Harriet Kaplan

The opinions and statements published are the responsibility of the authors, and such opinions and statements do not necessarily represent the policies of the American Psychological Association.

Library of Congress Cataloging-in-Publication Data

Stroebe, Wolfgang.
  Dieting, overweight, and obesity : self-regulation in a food-rich environment / Wolfgang Stroebe. — 1st ed.
    p. ; cm.
  Includes bibliographical references and indexes.
  ISBN-13: 978-1-4338-0335-2
  ISBN-10: 1-4338-0335-6
  1. Obesity. 2. Obesity—Psychological aspects. 3. Reducing diets. 4. Weight loss. 5. Self-control. I. American Psychological Association. II. Title.
  [DNLM: 1. Obesity—psychology. 2. Diet, Reducing—psychology. 3. Obesity—diet therapy. 4. Weight Loss. WD 210 S919d 2008]

  RC628.S829 2008
  362.196'398—dc22
                              2007047666

British Library Cataloguing-in-Publication Data

A CIP record is available from the British Library.

Printed in the United States of America
First Edition

To Maggie and Katherine, of course

CONTENTS

PREFACE

It is one of the great paradoxes of our time that people are getting fatter and fatter, even though everybody seems to be dieting. The prevalence of overweight and obesity is increasing at such a dramatic rate all around the world that the World Health Organization (2000) has declared it a global epidemic. This situation is made worse by the fact that people seem to be unable to lose substantial amounts of weight or at least to keep from regaining the weight they have managed to lose. Nearly half the people on weight loss programs are likely to weigh more 4 years after their diet than they did before (Mann et al., 2007).

Why is self-regulation of weight so difficult? This is the central question addressed in this volume. Psychologists have developed a number of theories to answer this question. Most of these theories share the assumption that the world is populated by two kinds of people. The lucky ones eat when they feel hungry and stop when they feel full. By responding automatically to internal cues signaling bodily needs, they regulate their body weight perfectly and are never at risk of weight gain. The unlucky ones are unable to recognize these bodily cues either because they have never acquired this skill (e.g., Bruch, 1961) or because they have lost it (Herman & Polivy, 1984). Their eating is (mis)guided by signals that are unrelated to bodily needs. They eat because they mistake emotions for hunger (e.g., Bruch, 1961) or because their eating is triggered by eating-relevant external cues such as the sight or smell of palatable food (e.g., Schachter, 1971). A third theory assumes that chronic dieters regulate their eating according to diet rules of permissible daily calorie intake (Herman & Polivy, 1984), a strategy that is successful only as long as people are motivated and able to concentrate on their dieting.

Although all of these theories provide important insights into the regulation of eating and body weight, they all seem to miss one important aspect, namely the positive incentive value of palatable food: People often overeat because they enjoy food. To correct this oversight, my colleagues at Utrecht University (Utrecht, the Netherlands), Esther Papies and Henk Aarts, and I developed our own theory: the goal conflict theory of eating. Our theory assumes that chronic dieters (i.e., restrained eaters) who have difficulty controlling their weight often disregard bodily cues of hunger and satiety not because they are unable to recognize them but because they do not want to recognize them. According to our theory, the eating behavior of chronic dieters is dominated by a conflict between two incompatible goals, namely the goal of enjoying palatable food (i.e., eating enjoyment) and the goal of losing (or at least not gaining) weight (i.e., weight control). We assume that weight control is normally the dominant goal for chronic dieters and that they attach greater importance to this goal than to the goal of eating enjoyment. Even though the eating enjoyment goal is more desirable than the goal of dieting, the dieting goal is in the forefront of their minds (i.e., more cognitively accessible). Thus, chronic dieters can operate for a long time without ever thinking about eating enjoyment (e.g., when focusing on some involving task at work). Unfortunately, however, the environment is rich in stimuli symbolizing or signaling palatable food, and chronic dieters are very sensitive to such stimulation. Thus, walking past the window of a bakery displaying delicious-looking pastry or inhaling appetizing smells of cooking wafting out of a house window will inadvertently bring the goal of eating enjoyment to their minds (i.e., increase its cognitive accessibility). It is likely that initially these temptations will activate automatic attempts to shield the goal of weight control by inhibiting thoughts about the pleasures of eating. However, continued exposure to palatable food (or symbols representing or signaling palatable food) is likely to continue to bring to mind the goal of eating enjoyment to an extent that it gains dominance over the goal of weight control. Once this happens, all thoughts about eating control will temporarily be "forgotten" (i.e., inhibited), and people are likely to overeat.

One effective dieting strategy would therefore be to remain in an environment devoid of food cues and where food is not available. Unfortunately, such environments are hard to come by and even harder to live in. As Schachter (1971) once showed in one of his ingenious studies, religious Jews who were overweight and who wanted to observe the Jewish day of fasting (Yom Kippur) suffered less the more time they spent in the synagogue. Although one should not complain about living in a food-rich environment, because for most people palatable food is always within easy reach and advertising offers continual reminders of this fact, long-term dieting is difficult. Scientists have therefore called the developed world's food-rich environment "obsogenic," or even "toxic," and identified it as one of the major causes of the obesity epidemic.

Like all books on dieting and obesity, this volume focuses on people with weight problems. After all, these are the individuals who have been studied most extensively and about whom most is known. However, even though more than half of the population in the United States is overweight, a considerable percentage are normal weight, and little is known about how these individuals manage to control their weight. Some might do so by dieting, but others might not even feel the need to diet. There could be many reasons for this, but an important one is their genetic makeup. Body weight is strongly determined by genetic factors. However, it must be emphasized that unlike the genetic determination of eye color, the processes that mediate the impact of genetic factors on body weight are mostly under individual control, either directly (e.g., in the case of physical activity) or indirectly through decreased food intake and/or increased exercise (e.g., in the case of the genetic differences in the efficacy of people's metabolism). Overweight and obesity can therefore not be understood without some knowledge of the bodily processes by which food is converted into energy or stored as fat and the extent to which these processes are determined genetically.

It has often been claimed that psychologists study their own problems. Although this motive has, in my opinion, been overrated, it does apply to my interest in dieting and overweight. I cannot deny that my own experiences have influenced my scientific thinking about this topic. As long as I can remember, I have enjoyed good food, and this interest in food predates my weight concerns by decades. However, for the past 3 decades I have felt the need to keep to a calorie-controlled diet to avoid the physical consequences of my love for good food. In light of these experiences, it seemed plausible to me to conceptualize the dilemma of chronic dieters as a conflict between the goals of eating enjoyment and of eating control. Because cognitive goal theories have recently become a well-developed area of social psychology (e.g., Kruglanski et al.,

2002), I was able to draw on this work to develop this notion into a theoretical model of eating regulation. The findings of a series of experimental studies conducted to test hypotheses derived from our goal conflict theory have so far supported my basic assumption.

As mentioned earlier, my research on the goal conflict theory of eating has been conducted in collaboration with my colleagues Esther Papies and Henk Aarts. Without their insights and their input we could never have succeeded. I am also grateful for their comments on chapter 7 of this volume. Furthermore, I am indebted to an anonymous reviewer who reviewed the manuscript for the American Psychological Association and made many helpful comments. Finally, I am grateful to Genevieve Gill (development editor) and Harriet Kaplan (production editor). Both made substantial contributions to increase the readability of this book.

Dieting, Overweight, and Obesity

1

DIETING, OVERWEIGHT, AND OBESITY: AN INTRODUCTION

There has been a dramatic increase in the prevalence of overweight and obesity in Western industrialized countries. For example, obesity rates doubled in the United States and tripled in Great Britain from 1980 to 2000. These steep increases are a matter of grave concern, because obesity is associated with an increased risk of mortality and morbidity (World Health Organization [WHO], 2000). Furthermore, individuals who are overweight or obese are also the target of prejudice and discrimination (e.g., Brownell, Puhl, Schwartz, & Rudd, 2005). In light of these deleterious effects it is not surprising that individuals who are overweight or obese try to lose weight and that dieting has become popular. Recent data for a large sample of U.S. adults indicated that 24% of men and 38% of women were trying to lose weight (Kruger, Galuska, Serdula, & Jones, 2004). Such dieting efforts can result in substantial weight loss in the short run but are much less effective in the long run. Evidence from clinical weight-loss studies suggests that most participants fail to maintain their weight loss over extended periods and after a few years regain most of the weight they had lost (Jeffery et al., 2000; Mann et al., 2007).

Genetic factors contribute to the development of obesity, and some individuals are more at risk for gaining weight than are others at the same level of energy surplus (for a review, see Bouchard, Pérusse, Rice, & Rao, 2004).

3

However, because it is unlikely that the genetic makeup of the U.S. or British population has changed substantially since the 1980s, the rapid increases in obesity must have been due to environmental changes or most likely to an interaction of genetic dispositions with environmental and behavioral factors. Individuals ultimately become obese because they eat too much, particularly too much fatty food, and exercise too little.

This situation leads to the major questions addressed in this volume: Why do so many people become overweight and obese and why do individuals who are overweight or obese find it so difficult to lose weight? Because eating too much and exercising too little are failures of self-regulation, the psychological processes that are responsible for these self-regulatory problems need to be examined. For this reason, the main focus of this volume is on the psychology of dieting, overweight, and obesity, and psychological explanations of overweight and obesity are extensively reviewed and critically assessed. However, as with biological and genetic factors, it is unlikely that the psychological processes of self-regulation changed dramatically since the 1980s, and environmental changes promoting unhealthy eating and activity patterns are likely to have contributed to the dramatic increase in overweight and obesity observed during this period. Although it has become a truism that the increased popularity of fast food, snacks, and soft drinks is responsible for the obesity problem, a critical review of relevant scientific evidence suggests that some of these beliefs lack solid empirical foundation.

Can overweight and obesity be treated? What are the success rates of such weight-loss treatments? These are somewhat controversial topics, because over the past few decades, concerns have arisen that weight-reducing diets, aside from being of doubtful efficacy, may also have potentially harmful effects (e.g., Cogan & Ernsberger, 1999; Polivy & Herman, 1992). As a result of these concerns, the opposition to weight-loss interventions has been increasing over recent years, and a new paradigm that rejects dieting has emerged. However, although losing a significant amount of weight and keeping it off long-term is very difficult for people who are already seriously overweight, dieting has an important role in the weight regulation and the prevention of overweight in individuals with a disposition toward weight gain.

The National Task Force on the Prevention and Treatment of Obesity (2000b) defined dieting as "the intentional and sustained restriction of caloric intake for the purpose of reducing body weight or changing body shape, resulting in a significant negative energy balance" (p. 2582). I use the same definition for *dieting* in this volume. There is wide variation in the magnitude of the caloric restriction people use to attempt to lose weight and also in the kinds of behavior they engage in trying to achieve and to maintain this caloric restriction. Weight-loss attempts based on regular meals and consuming a balanced diet that contains fewer calories than the diet individuals consumed at their higher weight are unproblematic, particularly if they are combined with an increase in physical activity and exercise. What is unhealthy and further-more ineffective in terms of weight loss is for people to engage in extreme weight-control behaviors such as self-induced vomiting or use of laxatives, appetite suppressants, and diuretics.

PLAN OF THIS VOLUME

The central problem examined in this volume is why self-regulation of weight is so difficult for so many people. Rather than considering this as a purely psychological problem, the book takes the broader perspective that the self-regulation of weight is determined by an interplay of biological, environ-mental, and psychological factors. The book therefore examines genetic and environmental determinants of body weight as well as psychological theories of weight regulation. Chapter 2 sets the stage by addressing two important questions, namely how overweight and obesity are defined and why they are considered serious problems. To answer the first question, I review definitions of body-weight standards and the now widely accepted WHO classification of body weight (WHO, 2000). The second question is addressed in two sec-tions, one on the international prevalence of overweight and obesity and one on the social and health consequences associated with these weight problems. The review of prevalence of overweight and obesity in selected countries illustrates that the United States, although one of the world leaders, is not the only country experiencing a dramatic increase. In this section I also dis-cuss gender, social class, and race and ethnicity differences in the distribution of overweight and obesity. However, the steep increase in prevalence is not the only source of concern; the fact that individuals with obesity are stigma-tized and that obesity is associated with serious health impairment and a short-ened life span are also major issues. These are the reasons why the WHO declared obesity a global epidemic (WHO, 2000).

Having established overweight and obesity as behavioral health risks of global dimension, in chapters 3 through 7, I review and assess the biological, environmental, and psychological processes that could be responsible for the dramatic increase in obesity. To understand why people become overweight or obese, one needs a basic understanding of human metabolism and of the intricacies of human energy balance. Therefore, in the first two sections of chapter 3, I review physiological assumptions about the components of energy expenditure and energy input. In discussing energy expenditure, I show that the human body is an extremely efficient machine and that humans must engage in considerable amounts of physical exercise to work off even small amounts of food. The section on energy intake discusses the characteristics of the macronutrients carbohydrates, protein, fat, and alcohol that make up the energy sources the body uses. Every calorie consumed must be either used or stored, and in the long term, all unused calories end up in fat deposits. The third section on the genetic influence on body weight and obesity addresses the extent to which body weight is determined by genetic factors. Having established that there is a strong genetic disposition toward weight gain, the last section evaluates potential risk factors that might determine an individual's propensity toward overweight. This discussion does not result in the identification of a major culprit, a metabolic process that single-handedly is responsible for an increased risk of obesity, but in the recognition that the propensity to gain weight is the joint effect of several metabolic processes.

Genetic factors may determine who in a particular population is susceptible to gaining weight in a food-rich environment, but the number of people affected is determined by the features of this environment (Brownell, 2002). Chapter 4 therefore reviews aspects of the environment that are likely to have facilitated the increase in obesity rates in these countries. Because everybody "knows" that the increased popularity of fast food, snack food, and soft drinks, combined with the increased portion and container sizes, are responsible, I might have been tempted to shorten the book by omitting this chapter. However, proving that these factors are causally related to the obesity epidemic ultimately requires randomized controlled trials, and this evidence is frequently lacking. The last part of the chapter focuses on the role of the built environment in encouraging physical inactivity. I argue that urban sprawl, which is typical for U.S. communities, combined with high rates of car ownership, have contributed to the increase in overweight and obesity.

Even though a genetic disposition and environmental factors facilitate the development of overweight and obesity, weight gain is ultimately the result of an imbalance between food intake and energy expenditure. Chapters 5, 6, and 7 therefore discuss psychological explanations for why some people have difficulty controlling their weight. The psychosomatic theories and externality theory discussed in chapter 5 attribute obesity to a difference in the way individuals regulate their eating. Consumption by individuals of normal weight is assumed to be controlled by internal cues signaling satiety or hunger. In contrast, individuals with obesity are considered less responsive to internal cues. Their eating can be triggered by strong emotions or eating-relevant external cues such as the salience of palatable food or the fact that it is dinnertime.

Chapter 6 addresses restrained eating and the breakdown of self-regulation, and the focus of the discussion moves from obesity to chronic dieting. By studying restrained eaters (i.e., individuals who are chronic but unsuccessful dieters), one can gain insights into the processes that makes weight loss so difficult for individuals with obesity. Peter Herman and Janet Polivy (1984), two major figures in the area of eating research, integrated the concept of eating restraint into their boundary model of eating, which has dominated eating research since the 1980s. The boundary model proposes that the eating regulation of unrestrained eaters is guided by internal hunger and satiety cues. In contrast, restrained eaters are assumed to use dieting rules (i.e., diet boundary) to regulate their daily food intake. Because regulation via dieting rules and calorie limits is demanding of cognitive resources, it is liable to break down whenever restrained eaters are unable or unwilling to invest cognitive resources in their dieting attempts.

Although the boundary model is supported by a wealth of experimental evidence, a number of systematic inconsistencies motivated my colleagues and me to develop a goal conflict model of eating as an alternative theory of eating regulation. According to this model, which is described in chapter 7, the problem restrained eaters experience in controlling their diet is caused by a conflict between two incompatible goals, namely the goal of enjoying palatable food and the goal of losing (or at least not gaining) weight. Restrained eaters are normally able to focus on their weight control goal, but exposure to palatable food can increase the accessibility of the eating enjoyment goal and result in the suppression of thoughts about dieting. Unfortunately, a food-rich environment is full of stimuli that represent, symbolize, or signal palatable food, making it difficult for restrained eaters to stay focused on eating control. This is why restrained eaters find it difficult to abstain from eating palatable food once they have become aware of its availability.

What can individuals who are overweight or obese do to reduce their weight and what can societies do to slow down or stop the epidemic of weight gain? These are the questions addressed in chapter 8 on treatment and prevention of overweight and obesity. Strategies of weight-loss treatment range from highly structured behavioral programs and commercial weight-loss programs to the do-it-yourself diets the majority of people engage in when they want to lose weight. A review of the efficacy of these weight-loss attempts has indicated that people are able to lose substantial amounts of weight but that few are able to maintain their weight loss in the longer term. This is one reason for the development of nondieting approaches that focus on the psychological well-being of individuals who are overweight or obese and on reducing the risk of further weight gain rather than weight loss. The fact that weight loss is very difficult and maintaining weight loss even more so suggests that the only hope of conquering obesity is by primary prevention. The last part of chapter 8 therefore focuses on health education and environmental changes as the two strategies that have been used for primary prevention of overweight and obesity.

Readers who expect simple answers to the question of why self-regulation of weight is so difficult for so many people will be disappointed by this volume. There are no simple answers. The obesity epidemic is not due to a single cause, be it a "toxic environment," genetics, or an "obsogenic" lifestyle. Overweight and obesity are the result of an interplay of biological, environmental, and psychological factors. Thus, the major goal of this volume is to increase the reader's understanding of these different causes of overweight and obesity and of the processes by which they influence body weight and lead to weight gain. This understanding should help the reader to recognize that simple solutions are unlikely to address the problem. No wonder drug or wonder diet will "cure" obesity. Although substantial weight loss is feasible, it also appears to be exceedingly difficult to achieve and even more difficult to maintain. The major hope in conquering the obesity epidemic rests therefore in preventive measures that jointly address obsogenic lifestyles and the obsogenic environment.

2

PREVALENCE AND CONSEQUENCES
OF OVERWEIGHT AND OBESITY

When should somebody be considered merely overweight and when should somebody be categorized as obese? These are important questions not only for obesity researchers but also for the readers of their research. To study the causes and consequences of obesity, one needs a generally accepted system of categorizing body weight. Similarly, to interpret this research, one needs to understand the logic underlying this system. The first section of this chapter is therefore devoted to a discussion of body-weight standards. In the next section, I review epidemiological data on the prevalence of obesity in selected countries to illustrate the dramatic increase in obesity around the world. This rise in obesity obviously would not be a problem were it not for the serious social and health consequences experienced by individuals with obesity. To illustrate this, in the third section I review empirical evidence for the severity of these consequences. The evidence presented in this chapter should convince readers that the World Health Organization (WHO) is not exaggerating or alarmist in speaking of a global epidemic of obesity (WHO, 2000) and that developing interventions to fight this epidemic is an important task for health psychologists.

BODY-WEIGHT STANDARDS

The concepts of overweight and obesity imply a standard of normal or ideal weight against which a given weight is judged. Because height and weight are highly correlated, such a standard should be related to height. One way to do this would be to define ranges of normal or ideal weight for each height. This approach has been taken by U.S. life insurance companies, which understandably have an interest in identifying individuals who are at increased risk of dying young and thus are unprofitable to insure. The Metropolitan Desirable Weight Tables, published for 60 years by the Metropolitan Life Insurance Company (e.g., Metropolitan Life Insurance Company, 1959), compared individuals with an ideal weight standard for the age, sex, and height group to which they belonged.

A more convenient strategy, and one that has now been generally accepted, is to use an index of body weight, which is corrected for height, and then to define the range of normal or ideal weight for this index. The body mass index (BMI) provides such an index of weight corrected by height. The BMI is obtained by dividing weight in kilograms by height in meters squared (kg/m^2).[1] This index was suggested in the 19th century by the Belgian mathematician, astronomer, and statistician Adolphe Quetelet, who empirically studied the relation between weight and height in men and women. He originally reasoned that if "man increased equally in all his dimensions, his weight at different ages would be as the cube of his height" (Quetelet, 1842, p. 66). But after extensive empirical studies, he concluded that "the weight of developed persons, of different heights, is nearly as the square of the stature" (Quetelet, 1842, p. 66). Indeed, in adults not only is this index minimally correlated with height (Simopoulos, 1986), it has also been shown to correlate highly (<.90) with excess fat mass and abdominal obesity as evaluated by waist girth (Bouchard, in 2007b).

This still leaves open the question of how to define overweight and obesity. What should be used as the standard or point of reference for normal or desirable weight? For psychologists used to thinking in terms of test standardization, an obvious strategy would be to use the weight distribution based on a nationally representative database for a given population and then to define overweight and obesity in terms of a deviation from the population average. This approach has been taken by the U.S. National Center for Health Statistics (NCHS), which defined overweight as being above the 85th percentile of weight for height (Bray, Bouchard, & James, 1998). However, using population averages as a point of reference has serious dis-

---

[1]The equivalent formula for body weight measured in pounds and height measured in inches is weight × 703/height[2] (Bray, 2004).

advantages. First, there is no scientific basis for the assumption that the population average is in any way a healthy or ideal weight. The fact that population averages have been increasing steadily in most Western (and many non-Western) countries raises serious doubts about this assumption. Furthermore, if such statistical cutoff points were to be used to define obesity, then the continuous increase in BMI would necessitate frequent readjustments of obesity standards.

A preferable strategy for developing weight standards and one that has now been generally accepted is to use the BMI that is associated with the lowest overall risk to health as a point of reference. The classification of adult body weight suggested by WHO (2000) uses this approach (see Table 2.1). Obesity is further subdivided according to degrees of severity, with a BMI of 40 or greater reflecting very severe obesity requiring surgical treatment. These BMI values for adults are age independent and identical for both sexes. Because there is evidence that the BMI associated with the lowest mortality increases with age, an adjustment of BMI in relation to age may be desirable. In this volume, I use the term *overweight* to refer to the BMI range of 25 to 29.99 and *obesity* for the BMI range of 30 and above. Table 2.2 presents a categorization of different levels of body weight corresponding to BMI.

In children, BMI changes dramatically with age. It decreases over the 1st year of life in both males and females and reaches its lowest point between ages 4 and 5. After that, BMI begins to increase again (Dietz, 1998). Because of these changes, age-specific reference curves must be used in assessing BMI in children. Because there are few prospective data relating body weight in children to adult health outcomes, obesity in children has usually been defined in terms of deviation from an age-specific population average. The commonly used BMI-for-age cutoff point for obesity is at or greater than the 95th percentile of the age-specific weight distribution (Dietz, 1998).

TABLE 2.1
Classification of Adults According to Body Mass Index

Classification	Body mass index
Underweight	<18.50
Normal range	18.50–24.99
Overweight	25.00–29.99
Obesity	≥30.00
Mild (Class I)	30.00–34.99
Moderate (Class II)	35.00–39.99
Severe (Class III)	≥40.00

Note. From *Obesity: Preventing and Managing the Global Epidemic* (p. 9), by World Health Organization, 2000, Geneva, Switzerland: Author. Copyright 2000 by the World Health Organization. Adapted with permission.

TABLE 2.2
Body Mass Index (BMI) Table

	Normal						Overweight					Obese				
							BMI									
	19	20	21	22	23	24	25	26	27	28	29	30	31	32	33	34	35
Height (inches)							Body weight (pounds)									
58	91	96	100	105	110	115	119	124	129	134	138	143	148	153	158	162	167
59	94	99	104	109	114	119	124	128	133	138	143	148	153	158	163	168	173
60	97	102	107	112	118	123	128	133	138	143	148	153	158	163	168	174	179
61	100	106	111	116	122	127	132	137	143	148	153	158	164	169	174	180	185
62	104	109	115	120	126	131	136	142	147	153	158	164	169	175	180	186	191
63	107	113	118	124	130	135	141	146	152	158	163	169	175	180	186	191	197
64	110	116	122	128	134	140	145	151	157	163	169	174	180	186	192	197	204
65	114	120	126	132	138	144	150	156	162	168	174	180	186	192	198	204	210
66	118	124	130	136	142	148	155	161	167	173	179	186	192	198	204	210	216
67	121	127	134	140	146	153	159	166	172	178	185	191	198	204	211	217	223
68	125	131	138	144	151	158	164	171	177	184	190	197	203	210	216	223	230
69	128	135	142	149	155	162	169	176	182	189	196	203	209	216	223	230	236
70	132	139	146	153	160	167	174	181	188	195	202	209	216	222	229	236	243
71	136	143	150	157	165	172	179	186	193	200	208	215	222	229	236	243	250
72	140	147	154	162	169	177	184	191	199	206	213	221	228	235	242	250	258
73	144	151	159	166	174	182	189	197	204	212	219	227	235	242	250	257	265
74	148	155	163	171	179	186	194	202	210	218	225	233	241	249	256	264	272
75	152	160	168	176	184	192	200	208	216	224	232	240	248	256	264	272	279
76	156	164	172	180	189	197	205	213	221	230	238	246	254	263	271	279	287

Note. Adapted from *Body Mass Index Table,* by National Heart, Heart, Lung, and Blood Institute, n.d. Available at http://www.nhlbi.nih.gov/guidelines/obesity/bmi_tbl.pdf. In the public domain.

Despite the popularity of the BMI as a measure of body fat and obesity, the measure is not without limitations: It overestimates body fat among athletic or muscular persons and underestimates obesity in older adults (Garrow, 1999; Utz, 2004). Thus, heavily muscled athletes or body builders have a high BMI but are not obese. At the other extreme, older persons have a low lean body mass and may therefore have a high percentage of fat, even with a normal BMI.

A further limitation of the BMI is that it cannot describe where the fat is located around the body. As I discuss later, there is evidence that the health risk associated with obesity is affected by the distribution of body fat (e.g., Lapidus, Bengtsson, & Lissner, 1990). It appears that carrying excess abdominal fat increases one's risk of ill health and mortality even with BMI held constant (Després & Krauss, 1998). This kind of fat distribution can be assessed with the ratio of waist-to-hip circumference or more simply by measuring waist circumference alone.

According to the clinical guidelines published in 1998 by the U.S. National Heart, Lung, and Blood Institute of the National Institutes of Health, men and women with waist circumferences greater than 102 centimeters (40 inches) and 88 centimeters (35 inches), respectively, are consid-

TABLE 2.2
Body Mass Index (BMI) Table (Continued)

	Extreme obesity																	
36	37	38	39	40	41	42	43	44	45	46	47	48	49	50	51	52	53	54
172	177	181	186	191	196	201	205	210	215	220	224	229	234	239	244	248	253	258
178	183	188	193	198	203	208	212	217	222	227	232	237	242	247	252	257	262	267
184	189	194	199	204	209	215	220	225	230	235	240	245	250	255	261	266	271	276
190	195	201	206	211	217	222	227	232	238	243	248	254	259	264	269	275	280	285
196	202	207	213	218	224	229	235	240	246	251	256	262	267	273	278	284	289	295
203	208	214	220	225	231	237	242	248	254	259	265	270	278	282	287	293	299	304
209	215	221	227	232	238	244	250	256	262	267	273	279	285	291	296	302	308	314
216	222	228	234	240	246	252	258	264	270	276	282	288	294	300	306	312	318	324
223	229	235	241	247	253	260	266	272	278	284	291	297	303	309	315	322	328	334
230	236	242	249	255	261	268	274	280	287	293	299	306	312	319	325	331	338	344
236	243	249	256	262	269	276	282	289	295	302	308	315	322	328	335	341	348	354
243	250	257	263	270	277	284	291	297	304	311	318	324	331	338	345	351	358	365
250	257	264	271	278	285	292	299	306	313	320	327	334	341	348	355	362	369	376
257	265	272	279	286	293	301	308	315	322	329	338	343	351	358	365	372	379	386
265	272	279	287	294	302	309	316	324	331	338	346	353	361	368	375	383	390	397
272	280	288	295	302	310	318	325	333	340	348	355	363	371	378	386	393	401	408
280	287	295	303	311	319	326	334	342	350	358	365	373	381	389	396	404	412	420
287	295	303	311	319	327	335	343	351	359	367	375	383	391	399	407	415	423	431
295	304	312	320	328	336	344	353	361	369	377	385	394	402	410	418	426	435	443

ered to have abnormally high waist circumferences, whereas waist circumferences below this limit were considered normal (National Heart, Lung, and Blood Institute, 1998).

THE EPIDEMIOLOGY OF OVERWEIGHT AND OBESITY

Overweight and obesity are worldwide problems (see Figure 2.1). They not only are widespread in industrialized countries but also are becoming problems in some developing countries, where they often coexist with malnutrition and underweight (WHO, 2000). There are marked differences in obesity rates among different countries within the same region. For example, obesity rates are considerably lower in Belgium and the Netherlands than in Germany or Great Britain (WHO, 2000). Similarly, in sub-Saharan Africa, overall obesity rates are low, but in South Africa, obesity rates are high, particularly among Black women (WHO, 2005). Within any given country, obesity rates vary substantially according to various sociodemographic characteristics. In the following sections, I discuss the variation in obesity according to three

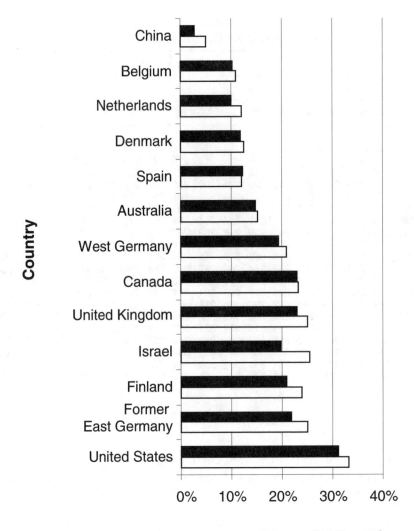

Figure 2.1. Prevalence of obesity in selected countries. Data for Australia, Belgium, China, Finland, Israel, and Spain from World Health Organization (2005); for Great Britain, from Rennie and Jebb (2005); for Canada, from Tjepkema (2006); for China, from Reynolds et al. (2007); for Denmark, from Bendixen et al. (2002); for West Germany and former East Germany, from Robert Koch Institut (2005); for the Netherlands, from Rijksinstituut voor Volksgezondheid en Milieu (2004); for the United States, from Ogden et al. (2006).

sociodemographic characteristics: gender, social class, and ethnicity. Finally, I review long-term trends in obesity.

Gender

As Figure 2.1 shows, in most countries obesity rates are higher for women than for men. This is especially true for minority women in the United States (C. L. Ogden et al., 2006), a difference that has remained stable, even though the gender gap in U.S. obesity has narrowed over the past 40 years (Utz, 2004). It is important to note, however, that the gender differences in weight are more complex than this global gender difference in obesity suggests. There is no significant gender difference in average BMI, and in the overweight category (BMI 25.0–29.9), rates have even been lower for women than for men (Fehily, 1999; NCHS, 2003; Utz, 2004). The fact that there is no difference in average BMI despite the difference in obesity could be due to a greater prevalence of underweight among women. However, even though *anorexia nervosa* (a disorder in which individuals try to achieve an abnormally low body weight) is mainly found in women, there are too few individuals with anorexia to account for this pattern. Furthermore, this fact would not explain the greater prevalence of overweight among men.

Social Class

Obesity also varies by social class. In the United States as well as in other industrialized countries, obesity has been more prevalent among the lower socioeconomic groups, and these effects are most prominent in women (e.g., Benecke & Vogel, 2005; Kuczmarski, Flegal, Campbell, & Johnson, 1994; Manios, Panagiotakos, Pitsavos, Polychronopoulos, & Stefanidis, 2005; Wardle & Griffith, 2001; for reviews, see Bray, 1998, Fehily, 1999; Sobal & Stunkard, 1989). This pattern was first demonstrated by Goldblatt, Moore, and Stunkard (1965), who found that among the highest socioeconomic groups, only 4% of women were overweight, whereas among the lowest socioeconomic groups, 36% were overweight.

In their classic review of this literature, Sobal and Stunkard (1989) reported that 28 of the 30 studies of the association of socioeconomic status (SES) and obesity in women conducted in Western industrialized countries found an inverse relationship, and none found a direct association. They offered a plausible normative explanation for this pattern: There is a strong norm for women to be slim, and this norm appears to be more closely observed among women of higher SES. Because men are under much less normative pressure to be slim, it is not surprising that the evidence for men was inconsistent, with an equal number of direct and inverse relationships being reported (Sobal & Stunkard, 1989).

In light of the plausibility of this pattern, it is puzzling that the disparity in obesity between different socioeconomic groups in the United States has been decreasing in recent years. Since 1971, the NCHS has conducted nationally representative surveys at regular intervals that assess body weight. These National Health and Nutrition Examination Surveys (NHANES) are representative for the whole (noninstitutionalized) U.S. population and provide information on measured body weight and size, categorized by gender, SES, and race or ethnic group. Using four waves of NHANES data collected between 1971 and 2000, Utz (2004) and Zhang and Wang (2004) found a significant decrease in the association between SES and obesity for the 1999 to 2000 period. This decrease is due to the fact that obesity rates have increased at a significantly faster rate in high compared with low socioeconomic groups during the past 4 decades. As Utz (2004) speculated, it seems as if "even those persons who traditionally bought or reasoned their way out of being obese . . . have become susceptible to the epidemic of obesity" (p. 152).

Because of the lack of appropriate longitudinal data for other countries, it is difficult to know whether this phenomenon is unique to the United States or is also happening elsewhere. All one can say is that even the most recent surveys reveal marked SES differences in Germany, Great Britain, and Greece. For example, on the basis of a survey conducted in 1998 in Germany, Benecke and Vogel (2005) reported higher levels of obesity in lower SES groups for both men and women, with the association being stronger for women than for men: 10% of women in the highest of three socioeconomic categories were obese compared with more than 30% in the lowest category. A similar pattern was reported for Greece by Manios et al. (2005). Finally, in Great Britain, Wardle and Griffith (2001) found obesity rates of 18.5% among women with the lowest SES, compared with 7.3% among their highest SES groups. No association was found for men. In recent years the inverse association between SES and obesity seemed to emerge even for women in non-Western, agricultural countries, which in the earlier studies reviewed by Sobal and Stunkard (1989) had shown a direct relationship (Monteiro, Moura, Conde, & Popkin, 2004).

Ethnicity and Race

In some countries, there is also ethnic variation in the prevalence of obesity. In the United States, racial–ethnic differences in obesity rates emerge and remain significant even after social class has been controlled for (Utz, 2004). Thus, according to the NHANES data collected in the United States in 1999 and 2000, 50% of the non-Hispanic Black women were obese compared with 40% of Mexican American women and 30% of non-Hispanic White women (NCHS, 2003). Although direction of cause and effect is unclear, it is nevertheless interesting that being overweight is much less stigmatized among

Black than among White women (Hebl & Heatherton, 1998). For men, there was practically no difference in obesity levels across these different ethnic and racial categories (NCHS, 2003). Black men used to have somewhat higher obesity rates than did White men before 1990, but unlike those for White men, the obesity rates for Black men have hardly changed since 1980 (Utz, 2004). Thus, for some reason, Black men appear to have been protected against the obesity epidemic. In the Netherlands, the few available data suggest that obesity rates are higher for both men and women of Turkish, Moroccan, and Surinam or Antillean origin than for the Dutch of European origin (Rijksinstituut voor Volksgezondheid en Milieu [RIVM], 2004).

Long-Term Trends

Most alarming are the long-term trends in obesity over the past few decades. Since 1980, obesity rates in the United States have doubled (see Figure 2.2) and in Great Britain nearly tripled. In 1976, 15.1% of the American population was obese; in 2003 to 2004, the average obesity rate was 32.3% (C. L. Ogden et al., 2006). Although there is some indication that the rate of increase has slowed for men since the turn of the century, it has continued to grow at the same rate for women. In Britain, rates have risen from 6% for men and 8% for women in 1980 to 23% and 25%, respectively, in 2002 (Rennie

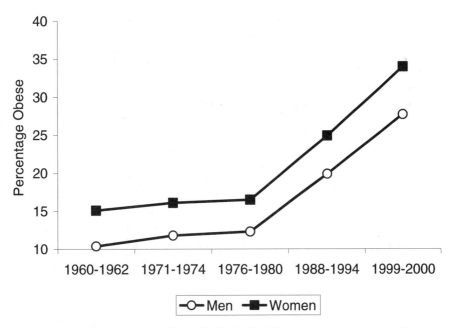

Figure 2.2. Adult obesity prevalence in the United States based on measured weight (National Center for Health Statistics, 2003).

& Jebb, 2005). In Canada, obesity increased from 9% in men and 8% in women in 1981 (M. S. Tremblay, Katzmarzyk, & Willms, 2002) to 20.9% in men and 23.2% in women in 2004 (Tjepkema, 2006). Even in the Netherlands, a European country that has enjoyed relatively low rates of obesity, rates have nearly doubled during the past few decades—from 6% for men and 8% for women in 1987 (WHO, 2000) to 10% and 12%, respectively, in 2003 (RIVM, 2004). In Germany, a country with already high levels of obesity, rates increased less steeply. Thus, between 1991 and 1998, rates for men increased from 17.4% to 19.4% in the regions that originally formed the Federal Republic and from 20.6% to 21.8% in the new (formerly East German) states. For women, rates increased from 19.6% to 20.9% in the old states and decreased from 25.8% to 24.2% in the new states (Benecke & Vogel, 2005).

Of particular concern is the fact that obesity rates are also increasing for children. In the United States, the percentage of children who are overweight (defined as BMI-for-age at or above the 95th percentile) has nearly quadrupled since the mid-1960s. Among children and teens aged 6 to 19, 16% are obese according to 1999–2000 NHANES data (NCHS, 2006). Similar trends can be observed in Canada (Tremblay et al., 2002), Great Britain (Bundred, Kitchiner, & Buchan, 2001), and the Netherlands (RIVM, 2004). These developments are worrisome because children with obesity are at an increased risk of becoming adults with obesity.

It is important to note, however, that the average weight of the U.S. population increased much less than one would expect given the change in obesity rates. Whereas the percentage of persons with obesity doubled between 1960 and 2002, the average BMI increased by only 10%.[2] At the same time, the standard deviation increased from 4.67 to 6.39 (Utz, 2004). Thus, the increase in obesity rates does not reflect a linear upward shift in population weight but a disproportional increase in the number of individuals in the U.S. population who are overweight (Utz, 2004).

THE CONSEQUENCES OF OVERWEIGHT AND OBESITY

Increased rates of obesity would be of little concern were it not for the fact that they are associated with social stigmatization and an increased risk of morbidity and mortality. The second half of this chapter reviews some of the major social and health consequences typically found to be associated with overweight and obesity.

---

[2]It is interesting to note that around 1990, when the prevalence of obesity in the United States was already much higher than in Britain and France, there was only a difference of 1 to 2 points in average BMI (Laurier, Guiguet, Chau, Well, & Valleron, 1992).

The Social Consequences

Individuals with obesity are likely to be the target of prejudice and discrimination, and these effects are particularly strong for women (Brownell, Puhl, Schwartz, & Rudd, 2005). Prejudice, as a negative attitude toward an outgroup, is based on the stereotypical beliefs that society shares about the members of this group. The stereotype that exists in Western culture about those who are overweight or obese is rather unflattering. They are perceived as less intelligent, less hardworking, less attractive, less popular, less successful, less athletic, and more weak willed and self-indulgent than are individuals of normal weight (Hebl & Mannix, 2003). Although the stereotypical view of individuals who are overweight or obese also contains positive traits—for example, that they are caring, friendly, humorous, and sympathetic (Bessenoff & Sherman, 2000)—the overall attitude toward individuals with obesity tends to be negative (Crandall & Biernat, 1990).

Weight discrimination against peers already can be found in children and adolescents (Puhl & Latner, 2007). For example, Cramer and Steinwert (1998) found that U.S. children as young as 3 to 5 years of age, regardless of their own body weight, perceived children who were overweight as mean and as undesirable playmates. Numerous studies also have shown that adolescents who are overweight or obese are more likely to be victims of bullying than are their peers who are of normal weight (Puhl & Latner, 2007). However, there is evidence for subcultural variation in antifat attitudes. A study of White and Black women found White women rating White targets who were overweight as lower in attractiveness, intelligence, popularity, happiness, relationship success, and job success than targets who were thinner. For Black women, there was little evidence of this type of stigmatization (Hebl & Heatherton, 1998).

Past research has demonstrated that stereotypical knowledge can be activated automatically (e.g., Devine, 1989). It often comes to mind automatically when the individual is exposed either to a member of the stereotyped group or to a stimulus (e.g., photo, word) symbolizing that group. Evidence for automatic activation of the obesity stereotype was provided in an experiment by Bessenoff and Sherman (2000), who used a subliminal priming task to test for automatic activation of the stereotype. Participants were exposed subliminally (i.e., very brief exposure seen only as a flash of light) to pictures of women who were fat, pictures of women who were thin, or neutral pictures. Previous research had demonstrated that subliminal exposure to stimuli representing stereotyped groups increased the mental accessibility of the relevant stereotype in people's minds (e.g., Wittenbrink, Judd, & Park, 1997). Accessibility was tested with a lexical decision task that had to be performed immediately after subliminal presentation of the prime. In a lexical decision task, respondents are presented with words or nonword letter strings and must decide as quickly as possible whether the stimulus represents a word or a nonword. The assumption is that the more accessible a word is in respondents' minds, the less time they should need to recognize it and the less time they should need to decide that they have seen a word rather than a nonword. The words used in Bessenoff and Sherman's study were stereotype relevant and stereotype irrelevant positive and negative trait words. Bessenoff and Sherman found that subliminal exposure to pictures of women who were fat rather than exposure to pictures of women who were thin decreased the time respondents needed to recognize negative trait words (i.e., response latency), regardless of whether these trait words were relevant or irrelevant to the fat stereotype. This finding suggests that the priming activated respondents' negative attitude (i.e., their overall evaluation) toward individuals who were obese rather than their stereotype.

It is unfortunate that the negative attitude toward obesity prevalent in Western society has important behavioral implications that pervade all walks of life. Given that individuals who are overweight or obese are perceived as less physically attractive and given that physical attractiveness is an important determinant of people's choice of a marriage partner, one would expect that individuals who are overweight or obese have greater difficulties finding a partner than do individuals who are of normal weight. There are also reasons to expect that this effect should be stronger for women than for men. Women more than men are judged on the basis of their appearance, and physical attractiveness has been found to have a greater influence on the marital choices of men than on those of women (Stroebe, Insko, Thompson, & Layton, 1971). Consistent with these expectations, a prospective study by Gortmaker, Must, Perrin, Sobol, and Dietz (1993) found that young women who were overweight at the beginning of the study were far less likely to marry during the subsequent 7-year period than were young women who differed from them in no way except for their body weight (see Figure 2.3). The women who were overweight who did finally marry were far more likely to move down in social class than were women who were not obese.

Discrimination against individuals with obesity is not limited to the interpersonal domain. A study conducted in 1964 and 1965 found that high school students who were obese were less frequently accepted into prestigious Ivy League colleges than were students who were not obese (Canning & Mayer, 1966). Again, the effects were more marked for women than for men. Thus, many more of the women who were not obese went to one of the high-prestige colleges, even though a comparison of application rates showed that women of both weight groups were equally interested in attending a high-ranking college (Canning & Mayer, 1966). Because these colleges require an interview before accepting students, the lower admission rates of women with obesity are likely to be due partly to the antifat stereotypes of the interviewers. However, there is also evidence that greater unwillingness of parents to pay college fees for more overweight children exacerbates this difference (Crandall, 1991).

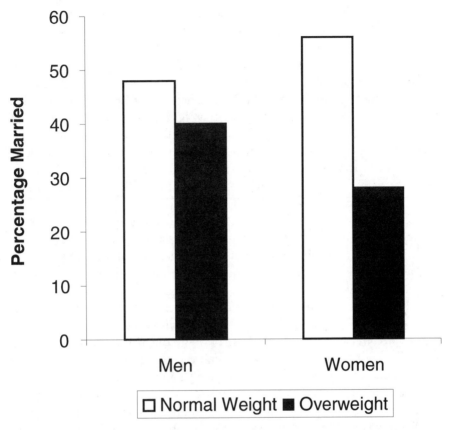

Figure 2.3. Percentage of normal-weight and overweight men and women who were married at the end of the study. Data from Gortmaker et al. (1993).

That these effects are not limited to the United States is demonstrated by a large-scale Swedish study that followed a cohort of more than 700,000 men for more than 30 years (Karnehed, Rasmussen, Hemmingsson, & Tynelius, 2006). Men who were obese at 18 had been doing worse in the educational system than their peers who were of normal weight, even when adjustments were made for intelligence and parental education. That antifat prejudice of teachers may have contributed to this association is suggested by the fact that at any given intelligence level, men with obesity had lower school marks in the ninth grade than did those who were of normal weight.

The authors of two longitudinal studies that found an inverse relationship between IQ in childhood or adolescence and later obesity also suggested that educational attainment could have mediated this relationship (Chandola, Deary, Blane, & Batty, 2006; Halkjoer, Holst, & Sorensen, 2003). In a population-based study of more than 17,000 men and women conducted in

Great Britain, Chandola et al. (2006) found that childhood IQ measured at age 11 was inversely related to obesity at age 43. Adjustment for paternal social class had little impact on this association. However, the association was markedly reduced when adjustments were made for participants' educational attainment, occupational social class, and diet. It was further found that education affected weight gain in adulthood independent of childhood IQ. The authors concluded that association between IQ and obesity was substantially mediated by education and healthy eating. Similarly, the findings of a smaller study, in which a cohort of Danish men who were of normal weight at age 19 was followed for nearly 40 years, also pointed to education as a likely mediator of the association between IQ at age 19 and the development of obesity in later life (Halkjoer et al., 2003).

Discrimination continues when individuals who are obese enter the job market. In a review of studies of weight-based discrimination in employment, Roehling (1999) concluded that evidence of discrimination is found at virtually every phase of the employment cycle, including selection, placement, compensation, and promotion. In one study, 16% of the employers surveyed said that they would not hire women who were obese under any circumstances (Stunkard & Sobal, 1995). When individuals with obesity do get jobs, their salaries are often lower than are those of their colleagues who are of normal weight (Frieze, Olson, & Good, 1990). However, even though there is evidence of discrimination against men with obesity, again the discrimination against women with obesity appears to be stronger even in the work environment. Using data from the U.S. National Longitudinal Survey of Youth, Register and Williams (1990) found that women who were overweight earned on average 12% less than did women of normal weight, a difference that was not observed for men. A recent review of studies on inequity in pay according to body weight by Fikkan and Rothblum (2005) indicated that this pattern is not unusual. Although weight discrimination in pay does occur for men, the evidence with regard to women is much more consistent.

Roehling (1999) discussed a number of processes that could mediate the impact of the obesity stereotype on employment decisions. One possibility is that weight might bias decisions through its influence on physical attractiveness. There is evidence that attractive individuals are favored over equally qualified people in hiring decisions, recommendations for promotion, and ratings of competence (Roehling, 1999). The bias against individuals who are overweight or obese could thus be part of the general bias against people who are less physically attractive. A second possibility is that decisions are influenced by the specific content of the stereotype toward those who are obese. If an employer subscribes to the stereotype that individuals with obesity are less intelligent and hardworking than are individuals of normal weight, these beliefs are likely to influence his or her decision. Because both of these processes are more likely to influence judgments when individuals are either unable or unwilling to think about the decision very deeply and to use the individuating information that might be available about the job candidate, the obesity stereotype should have less influence when decisions are important and when an employer has time to consider all the relevant information.

A third process, however, could affect decisions even when individuals are motivated and able to invest time and effort in their decision. An employer might decide against hiring an individual with obesity on purely rational grounds. Being aware of the societal prejudice against obesity, an employer might expect a person who is obese to perform less ably in jobs that require a great deal of contact with customers (e.g., sales). Because of the health problems associated with obesity (e.g., Garrow, 1999), those who are obese are likely to have more absences resulting from sickness. For example, a longitudinal study conducted with workers in Denmark found that obesity predicted a 57% higher sickness absence (Labriola, Lund, & Burr, 2006). An employer who is aware of the association between obesity and health might therefore decide against hiring an individual with obesity, fearing higher rates of absenteeism or greater health costs.

The Psychological Consequences

In light of this evidence of serious stigmatization of individuals who are overweight or obese, it is not surprising that BMI is positively related to body dissatisfaction (e.g., Vander Wal & Thelen, 2000; Wilson, Tripp, & Boland, 2005). A recent meta-analysis of studies of risk and maintenance factors of eating pathology confirmed body dissatisfaction as a major risk factor for the development and maintenance of disordered eating (Stice, 2002). At the same time, appearance is a powerful motivator of weight control and weight-loss attempts. Unless people are dissatisfied with their weight and their appearance, they are unlikely to try to do something about it. Even moderate weight loss is associated with positive health consequences for individuals who are overweight or obese (Institute of Medicine, 2002). Furthermore, the intervention studies discussed in chapter 8 (this volume) have demonstrated that dieting sensibly does not increase, and often even decreases, the risk of the development of eating pathology. Thus, it seems to be not body dissatisfaction per se that is problematic but rather the unhealthy strategies some individuals adopt to reduce their weight.

Overweight and obesity are also associated with lower levels of self-esteem. A meta-analysis of 71 studies of the association between body weight and self-esteem reported a correlation of $-.12$ between actual weight and self-esteem and of $-.33$ for self-perceived weight (C. T. Miller & Downey, 1999). The association was somewhat higher for women ($r = -.23$) than for men ($r = -.19$) and for samples containing mainly individuals of high SES rather than low SES (.31 vs. .16). All these associations as well as the differences between them were statistically significant. Effect sizes were also larger in White or predominantly White samples than in minority group samples, but this difference failed to reach acceptable levels of significance. These findings suggest that body weight, and particularly self-perceived body weight, has a substantial impact on the self-esteem of certain sections of the population such as women or individuals of high SES.

One would expect that the stigma attached to being obese should result in emotional damage. It is therefore surprising that the empirical evidence is less than clear. Thus, in a meta-analysis of early studies that compared individuals who were obese with individuals who were not obese with regard to levels of psychopathology, Friedman and Brownell (1995) failed to find differences with regard to depression and anxiety. As Friedman and Brownell noted, most of these studies did not use established diagnostic criteria in defining depression and also varied in their definition of obesity. Two recent studies that used clinical criteria for the diagnosis of depression and also used acceptable criteria for the definition of obesity found that those who are obese are at higher risk of depression. Onyike, Crum, Lee, Lyketsos, and Eaton (2003) used data collected in the context of NHANES III (1988–1994) to examine the association between obesity and past-month major depression. The NHANES study used the Diagnostic Interview Schedule (Helzer & Robins, 1988), a structured interview designed for use by trained interviewers, allowing diagnoses according to the operational criteria of the *Diagnostic and Statistical Manual of Mental Disorders* (3rd ed.; American Psychiatric Association, 1980). The diagnosis of a major depression requires the persistence of depressed mood for at least 2 weeks and the presence of at least four of eight other depressive symptoms. Obesity was found to be associated with a significant increase in the risk of past-month major depression, an effect that was particularly marked for individuals with extreme degrees of obesity (Class III). The association with past-year major depression and lifetime major depression was weaker but still significant.

As with all cross-sectional studies, the causal direction is unclear in the study by Onyike et al. (2003). Their findings could have been due to a greater tendency of individuals with depression to put on weight. However, this interpretation cannot account for the findings of a longitudinal study conducted by Roberts, Kaplan, Shema, and Strawbridge (2000). They used data from the 1994 and 1995 waves of the Alameda County Study, a longitudinal study in which a cohort of 6,928 individuals was followed for a 20-year period. Depression was assessed with the *Diagnostic and Statistical Manual for Mental Disorders* criteria for major depressive episodes. Excluding all participants who were diagnosed as having had a major depressive episode at baseline in 1994, individuals with obesity were found to be more depressed in 1995 than were individuals of normal weight. Thus, individuals who had been obese in 1994 had twice the risk than did individuals of normal weight of developing a major depressive episode in 1995. Because these are new depressive episodes, this finding is quite striking. Taken together, these studies do suggest that individuals who are obese are more likely than persons of normal weight to suffer from bouts of depression.

The Health Consequences: Mortality

Life insurance companies have a long-standing interest in identifying groups of individuals at an increased risk of dying young. As early as 1913, the American Society of Actuaries published cross-sectional analyses showing that being overweight was associated with decreased longevity (Garrow, 1999). Since then, the association between obesity and health has been well documented in longitudinal studies such as the Framingham Study (Dawber, 1980; Hubert, Feinleib, McNamara, & Castelli, 1983), the Harvard Alumni Study (C. D. Lee, Blair, & Jackson, 1999), the American Cancer Society Studies (Calle, Thun, Petrelli, Rodriguez, & Heath, 1999; Stevens, Cai, Evenson, & Thomas, 2002), the Nurses' Health Study (Manson et al., 1995), and the Health Professionals Follow-Up Study (Baik et al., 2000). By now, there can be no doubt about the negative relationship between obesity and longevity. It is less clear, however, whether being overweight (i.e., BMI 25.0–29.9) is also associated with increased mortality risk. Although most studies report a continuous increase in risk from normal weight through overweight to obesity (e.g., Manson et al., 1995; see Figure 2.4), a recent meta-analysis of the association between BMI and mortality based on data from 26 studies conducted in the United States and other countries found a significant increase for obesity but not for overweight (McGee, 2005).

The Shape of the Body Mass Index–Mortality Association

The controversial issue about the association of BMI and mortality is whether it is a linear one, with no specific lower threshold, or whether it is a J- or U-shaped function, implying that being underweight is also unhealthy. Proponents of the linear relationship between BMI and mortality argue that curvilinear findings result from two confounding variables, namely cigarette smoking and undetected illnesses. First, smokers weigh less than do nonsmokers and also have a higher mortality rate. Second, undetected illnesses at the time of entry into a longitudinal study might have the same effect.

The importance of controlling for these confounds has been illustrated in the Nurses' Health Study, a 16-year longitudinal study of a sample of 115,195 registered female (mainly White) nurses in the United States (Manson et al., 1995). An analysis adjusted only for age resulted in a J-shaped relation between BMI and overall mortality (see Figure 2.4), with mortality being lowest among women with a BMI from 19.0 to 26.9. Multivariate adjustment for

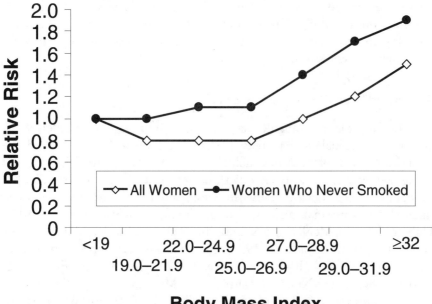

Figure 2.4. Relationship between body mass index and relative risk of mortality among women in the Nurses' Health Study. Data from Manson et al. (1995).

smoking and other risk factors strengthened the relationship but did not materially alter the shape of the curve. However, when women who had never smoked were examined separately, the apparent excess relative risk of mortality associated with leanness was eliminated. For former and current smokers, the association between BMI and mortality remained J-shaped. Similar results for men were reported in a study based on data from the Physician's Health Study, a prospective study of a large sample of male physicians in the United States (Ajani et al., 2004).

It is puzzling, though, that the BMI–mortality relationship in the Nurses' Health Study was not materially altered when smoking-related variables (e.g., number of cigarettes smoked per day, duration of smoking) were controlled for. Even control for length of time since stopping in former smokers did not make a difference. This is particularly surprising because the health risks of smoking have been shown to decline continuously after stopping (U.S. Department of Health and Human Services and the Department of Agriculture, 1990). Furthermore, even some of the studies of individuals who had never smoked failed to replicate the finding that a J- or U-shaped relationship between BMI and mortality is replaced by a linear association when former and current smokers are excluded from the analysis. For example, Calle et al. (1999), in a 14-year prospective study of more than 1 million adults conducted in the United States, found that the mortality risk among the leanest men and women (BMI < 18.5), although reduced, remained significantly elevated even after the analysis was limited to respondents who had never smoked and who had no history of disease at intake. Stevens et al. (1998) found some evidence for a curvilinear relationship between BMI and mortality in younger women who had never smoked but not in men. Iribarren, Sharp, Burchiviel, and Petrovitch (1995) found no increase but did find evidence for "a shallow J-shaped pattern" in men who were free of disease and who either had never smoked or had stopped smoking. Finally, two extensive meta-analyses of prospective cohort studies also found mortality risk to increase with low and high BMI (McGee, 2005; Troiano, Frongillo, Sobal, & Levitsky, 1996). The increased mortality risk for low BMI levels remained even after smoking was controlled for. In a recent expert statement, the National Task Force on the Prevention and Treatment of Obesity (2000a) drew the following conclusions:

> Most observational studies have shown a U- or J-shaped relationship between BMI and mortality, with individuals at very low and very high weights at increased risk. Such a relationship is found even after attempts are made to adjust for confounding factors, such as smoking or preexisting illness. (p. 901)

Should Weight Recommendations Be Age Specific?

Although the 1990 Dietary Guidelines for Americans recommended age-specific ranges of weight for height, with heavier weights indicated for people 35 years of age or older, the 1995 Dietary Guidelines for Americans omitted age-specific recommendations. Yet there is reason to believe that these new federal guideline standards for ideal weight (BMI 18.7 to <25) may be overly restrictive for older populations. Several studies found that the relative mortality risk associated with an increase in the BMI declined with age (e.g., Baik et al., 2000; Diehr et al., 1998; Stevens et al., 1998). However, Manson et al. (1995) observed no evidence of a modifying effect of age in their analyses of the data of the Nurses' Health Study. Acknowledging this inconsistency, Heiat, Vaccarino, and Krumholz (2001) concluded in their review of studies of the relationship between BMI and mortality in older individuals (65 years and older) that although there is some support for the assumption that obesity increases the mortality risk even in older persons, studies do not support overweight as a risk factor.

Are Weight Recommendations Equally Applicable to All Races?

Because many of the major longitudinal studies in the United States were based on nearly all-White samples, little is known about the extent to which these weight recommendations are also applicable to other racial–ethnic groups in the United States. The limited available evidence suggests that African American men and women with obesity run a slightly lower mortality risk than do Americans of European descent. The most reliable assessment of racial differences in the weight–mortality relationship is based on data from two large longitudinal studies of representative national population samples, namely the NHANES I Epidemiologic Follow-up Study and the NHIS Mortality Follow-up Study (Durazo-Arvizu et al., 1997). Durazo-Arvizu et al. (1997) found that despite great similarities in the weight–mortality association between Black and White respondents, the BMI associated with the lowest mortality risk was 1 to 3 BMI units higher among Blacks than Whites. However, this difference failed to reach significance in the multivariate analysis. Consistent with these findings, the National Task Force on the Prevention and Treatment of Obesity (2000a) concluded that the BMI associated with minimum mortality rate was 1 to 3 points higher in African American than in White respondents. Less information is available for Asian Americans, Hispanic Americans, and Pacific Islanders.

Health Consequences: Morbidity

Higher levels of body weight and fat are associated with medical complications that lead to an increased risk of morbidity. In particular, overweight and obesity are associated with an increased risk of cardiovascular diseases, diabetes mellitus, dyslipidemia, and certain cancers (Garrow, 1999; Pi-Sunyer, 2002). There is strong evidence that visceral body fat indicated by high waist circumference is an independent predictor of many of these complications (Després, 2002; Janssen, Katzmarzyk, & Ross, 2002).

Coronary Heart Disease

Coronary heart disease is the leading cause of death in the United States and in most industrialized countries. It is also a major cause of excess mortality among people with obesity. In the Framingham Study, relative weight at intake was an independent predictor of coronary heart disease for both men and women (Hubert et al., 1983). In the Nurses' Health Study (Manson et al., 1995), rates of death resulting from coronary heart disease among obese women (BMI > 29) were four times higher than those among the leanest women. A similarly strong association with obesity was observed in the Health Professionals Follow-up Study (Baik et al., 2000) and in the two Cancer Prevention studies (Calle et al., 1999; Stevens et al., 1998).

Stroke is the third leading cause of death in the United States. Most strokes are *ischemic*, that is, they are caused by reduced blood flow to the brain when blood vessels are blocked by a clot or have become too narrow for blood to pass through. Risk factors for stroke are high blood pressure, atherosclerosis, or history of diabetes. In the Nurses' Health Study, the risk of ischemic strokes was 75% higher in women with a BMI of greater than 27 and 137% higher in those with a BMI greater than 32 compared with women who had a BMI of less than 21 (Rexrode et al., 1997). Data from the Framingham Study indicated that risk of stroke increased linearly with body weight (Higgins, Kannel, Garrison, Pinsky, & Stokes, 1988).

Hypertension, a major risk factor for the development of coronary heart disease and for stroke, is positively associated with overweight and obesity. On the basis of epidemiological studies, it has been estimated that for every 10-kilogram rise in body weight over normal, there is an average increase of 3 mmHg in systolic and 2 mmHg in diastolic pressure (Pi-Sunyer, 2002). A 7.5 mmHg difference in diastolic pressure within the range of 70 to 110 mmHg is associated with a 29% difference in heart disease risk and a 46% difference in the risk of stroke (WHO, 2000). The comparison of the impact of BMI categories and waist circumference suggests that waist circumference is an independent predictor of hypertension (Janssen et al., 2002).

Diabetes Mellitus

An estimated 8% of U.S. men and women aged 20 years or older have diabetes (National Task Force, 2000a). Diabetes is a disorder of glucose metabolism. In diabetes, the body either produces too little insulin (Type 1) or is resistant to insulin (Type 2), causing excess levels of glucose in the blood. Type 2 (non-insulin-dependent) diabetes accounts for 90% to 95% of all cases of diabetes (National Task Force, 2000a). This form of diabetes, which used to develop so exclusively in adulthood as to be known as *adult-onset diabetes*, is now increasingly seen in children, particularly from minority populations (Rosenbloom, Joe, Young, & Winter, 1999).

There is a strong positive correlation between BMI and Type 2 diabetes. In an analysis based on data from the Women's Health Study, a prospective study of nearly 37,878 female health care professionals aged 45 years and older who were healthy at baseline, Weinstein et al. (2004) found the risk of having developed Type 2 diabetes 6.9 years later to be 4 times higher for women who were overweight and 14 times higher for women who were obese compared with women of normal weight. A recent analysis of the association between obesity and lifetime risk for developing diabetes estimated that lifetime risk at age 18 in the United States increased from 7.6% to 70.3% between men who were underweight and men who were very obese and from 12.2% to 74.4% for women (Narayan, Boyle, Thompson, Gregg, & Williamson, 2007). There is also evidence that abdominal body fat as indicated by high waist circumference is an independent predictor of Type 2 diabetes (Janssen, Katzmarzyk, & Ross, 2002). The reason for the relationship between obesity and Type 2 diabetes is not totally understood. However, there is clear evidence that excess fat accumulation is associated with increased insulin resistance, and insulin resistance is a predisposing factor for diabetes (Albu & Pi-Sunyer, 1998).

Dyslipidemia

Lipids are a broad category of substances including fats and fatlike matter such as cholesterol. Cholesterol is produced mainly by the liver. Contained in most tissues, they are also the main components of deposits in the lining of arteries. They are carried in the blood mainly by two proteins, namely low-density lipoproteins (LDLs) and high-density lipoproteins (HDLs). LDL cholesterol is considered bad cholesterol because at high levels it can be deposited on the walls of the blood vessels, thereby helping the formation of plaque. Plaque formation leads to a narrowing of the arteries and thus to atherosclerosis. Obesity is associated with three specific abnormalities of lipids in the bloodstream (Pi-Sunyer, 2002): elevation of triglyceride levels, depression of HDL cholesterol levels, and increased presence of small LDL cholesterol particles.

Cancer

Obesity increases the risk of many forms of cancer, including colon cancer, prostate cancer, endometrial cancer (a malignant growth of the uterus), postmenopausal (but not premenopausal) breast cancer, and pancreatic cancer (e.g., Baik et al., 2000; Manson et al., 1995; Michaud et al., 2002; Murphy, Calle, Rodriguez, Kahn, & Thun, 2000; National Task Force, 2000a). In the Nurses' Health Study, rates for cancer were twice as high among women who were obese as among the women who were the leanest, predominantly because of increased mortality caused by colon, breast, and endometrial cancers (Manson et al., 1995). In the Health Professionals Follow-Up Study, the risk of cancer was one and a half times as great for men under age 65 who were obese as for men under age 65 who were of normal weight (Baik et al., 2000). Calle et al. (1999) reported a 40% to 80% increase in risk of dying from cancer in their heaviest group of men and women (BMI > 35).

Musculoskeletal Disease

Osteoarthritis is a condition caused by wear and tear on the joints and an erosion of their lubricated sliding surfaces. Increasing body weight causes increasing stress on the weight-bearing joints and is probably the main reason for the increased risk for osteoarthritis among those who are obese. However, dietary and metabolic factors have also been implicated (National Task Force, 2000a). On the positive side, increased body weight does offer protection against the development of osteoporosis, a bone disease that causes the bones to lose protein structure and mineral content.

Other Health Conditions

Overweight and obesity are associated with several other health conditions, such as respiratory disease, gall bladder disease, and liver disease in both sexes and, in women, menstrual irregularities.

PHYSICAL FITNESS, OBESITY, AND HEALTH

So far I have interpreted the association between obesity and health exclusively in terms of potential direct physiological effects of obesity. However, increasing evidence indicates that a substantial part of this association is due to the fact that individuals who are obese engage in less physical exercise than do individuals of normal weight and have lower levels of cardiorespiratory fitness (Blair & Leermakers, 2002). It is surprising that until recently, studies of the association of obesity and health did not control for levels of physical activity. After all, the inverse relationship between levels of physical exercise, respiratory fitness, and BMI has long been known, and a sedentary lifestyle and lack of fitness are well-known behavioral risk factors for cardiovascular disease and diabetes (U.S. Department of Health and Human Services, 1996).

The findings of several recent studies that controlled for cardiorespiratory fitness or levels of physical activity in their assessment of the association of obesity with morbidity or mortality leave no doubt that the low levels of respiratory fitness and physical activity of those who are obese contribute to their health problems. However, the extent to which this contribution accounts for the overall relationship between obesity and health is at present unclear. In a longitudinal study of a large sample of men, Barlow, Kohl, Gibbons, and Blair (1995) and C. D. Lee et al. (1999) found that mortality rates were determined mainly by cardiorespiratory fitness. With fitness controlled for, the association between BMI and mortality became nonsignificant. Their analysis was based on the Aerobics Center Longitudinal Study, a cohort study of more than 25,000 men whose cardiorespiratory fitness was assessed with a maximal treadmill exercise at baseline and whose vital status was followed for 8 to 10 years. However, Stevens et al. (2002), who used data from the Lipid Research Clinics Study, reported independent effects of both respiratory fitness and obesity on all-cause mortality and mortality resulting from cardiovascular diseases, even though the effects of BMI were often not significant. The Lipid Research Clinics Study, a multicenter study conducted in geographically diverse centers in the United States, gathered data from 2,506 women and

2,860 men whose fitness was measured at baseline in 1972 to 1976 with a treadmill test and whose vital status was followed through 1998. Finally, Hu et al. (2004), in an analysis based on data from the Nurses' Health Study, found a significant association between BMI, all-cause mortality, and cardiovascular mortality, even after they controlled for levels of physical activity. Physical activity was assessed repeatedly during several waves with a physical activity questionnaire. With regard to morbidity, findings are similarly inconsistent (e.g., Weinstein et al., 2004; Wessel et al., 2004).

The issue of physical activity as it relates to obesity definitely needs to be attended to in future research. Even now, the majority of studies show that regular physical activity has health benefits at any weight, despite the fact that physical exercise is not a very effective method of losing weight, particularly for women (e.g., Donnelly et al., 2003; Garrow & Summerbell, 1995). Thus, the important message implied by this research is that increased physical exercise and cardiorespiratory fitness have significant benefits for individuals who are obese or overweight, benefits that extend beyond the contribution of exercise to weight loss and weight maintenance.

CONCLUSIONS

Since 1980, obesity rates have been increasing dramatically in most industrialized countries. This development is a matter of concern because obesity is not only highly stigmatized, it also is associated with an increased risk of morbidity and mortality. Obese individuals and particularly obese women are targets of prejudice and discrimination, which affects all aspects of their lives. They find it more difficult to get married, to get accepted to college, and to get a job. If they do find employment, their salaries are likely to be lower than those of individuals of normal weight and equal competence. In light of this pervasive prejudice against individuals who are overweight or obese, it is not surprising that the stigma attached to being obese is associated with increased levels of depression and with decreased levels of self-esteem. Because appearance is a more important factor in women than in men, it is plausible that both the prejudice and the impact on self-esteem are stronger for women than for men. However, not all societal groups appear to pursue the goal of thinness with equal rigor. In particular, Black women in the United States appear to be less concerned about being slim. Although the cause–effect relationship is unclear, they are also the group with the highest obesity rate.

In addition to these social consequences, obesity also has been linked to serious health impairment. Numerous cross-sectional and longitudinal studies have demonstrated that obesity is associated with an increased risk of morbidity and mortality. However, despite intensive research efforts devoted to the weight–health relationship, a number of issues are still controversial. Thus, it is not yet clear whether the mortality risk also increases with underweight. A second issue of contention concerns the interpretation of the mechanisms responsible for the association between body weight and health. It is unclear to what extent these health impairments are due to direct physiological effects of obesity or to the fact that individuals who are obese engage in less physical exercise than normal weight individuals. Having established in this chapter that there is a substantial increase in the prevalence of overweight and obesity in most developed and even some developing countries and that because of the physical and social consequences of obesity this increase is a matter of concern, chapter 3 is the first of five chapters that focus on potential causes of this increase.

3

ENERGY BALANCE AND THE
GENETICS OF BODY WEIGHT

As discussed in chapter 2, the prevalence of overweight and obesity is increasing around the world, and the consequences of these conditions can be severe. It is therefore important to consider what makes someone become overweight and obese in the first place. Even if one accepts that obesity ultimately results from a chronic imbalance between energy intake and energy expenditure, there are likely to be individual differences in susceptibility to weight gain that are genetically determined. In this chapter I review some basic principles of the energy balance equation that are relevant to the development of obesity and discuss the extent to which genetic factors affect this balance.

The first section of this chapter reviews the basic physiological assumptions about the components of energy expenditure (i.e., resting metabolic rate, thermic effect of food, and physical activity). The second section addresses the input side, the components of energy intake. In this section, I introduce the concept of energy density of macronutrients and argue that as far as energy storage is concerned, not all calories are the same. In the third section, I discuss the extent to which weight and obesity are genetically determined. Having established that there is a strong genetic influence on body weight, in the fourth section I review evidence on some of the biological risk factors that predispose individuals to gain weight.

THE COMPONENTS OF ENERGY EXPENDITURE

The breakdown of nutrients frees energy, which the cells use to perform the various forms of biological work. According to the first law of thermodynamics, energy cannot be created or destroyed. It can only be converted from one form to another. The internal energy that results from the breakdown of organic nutrients can appear as heat, be used to perform work, or be stored in the body. *Metabolism* refers to the entire range of biochemical processes involved in the transformation of nutrients into internal energy. The total energy expenditure per unit time is called *metabolic rate*. It can be divided into three components: the resting metabolic rate (RMR), the thermic effect of food (TEF), and physical activity.

Resting Metabolic Rate

The RMR is the energy expended by an individual who is awake but resting in a fasting state (i.e., not actively digesting) and in a comfortable temperature. The RMR can be considered the metabolic cost of living. It reflects the costs of maintaining body functions, including temperature, at rest. Sleep results in a 10% decrease in metabolic rate below RMR, and starvation can decrease it by up to 30% (Ravussin, 2002). In sedentary adults, the RMR is responsible for 60% to 70% of daily energy expenditure (Ravussin, 2002; Schutz & Jéquier, 2004; Tataranni & Ravussin, 2002). Thus, we humans need most of our energy simply for keeping our body functioning. More than half of our energy is used up by organs with a high metabolic activity, such as the liver, the kidneys, the brain, and the heart, even though these organs account for only 5% of body weight (Schutz & Jéquier, 2004). The metabolic rate of muscles per unit of body weight is considerably lower than that of heart and kidneys but still higher than that of adipose tissue, which accounts for only 4% of the RMR in individuals who are not obese (Schutz & Jéquier, 2004). Fat-free mass (FFM) is therefore the major factor explaining interindividual variation in RMR. Because the aging process is associated with a decrease in muscle mass and an increase in adipose tissue, RMR declines with age from the 2nd to the 7th decade at a rate of 1% to 2% per decade (Tataranni & Ravussin, 2002).

RMR is positively correlated with body weight: Individuals who are obese or overweight have a higher RMR because not all the weight people gain when becoming overweight or obese consists of metabolically inactive fat cells (Prentice, 1999a). Increased heart and skeletal muscle are needed to support the increased weight, and the digestive tract and the liver are enlarged to process the increased food intake. Thus, an estimated 25% of the additional weight is metabolically more active lean tissue (Prentice, 1999a).

Thermic Effect of Food

The TEF (i.e., the increase in energy expenditure after a meal) is mainly due to the energy costs of nutrient absorption, processing, and storage. The TEF accounts for approximately 10% of daily energy expenditure (Ravussin, 2002; Schutz & Jéquier, 2004; Tataranni & Ravussin, 2002).

Physical Activity

Definitions of physical activity have varied a great deal over the years. In the past, the term was used synonymously with exercise, but now *physical activity* is used as an umbrella term describing any bodily movement produced by skeletal muscles that increases energy expenditure. There have been two ways of forming subcategories. One way has been to subdivide it according to the context in which it occurs (e.g., occupational, household, leisure time). It also has been subdivided into volitional exercise (e.g., sport and fitness-related activities) and nonexercise activities. Nonexercise activities reflect the whole range of activities of daily living, such as fidgeting, spontaneous muscle contraction, maintaining posture when not lying down, and also walking and shopping (Levine, Eberhardt, & Jensen, 1999; Levine et al., 2005; Levine, Vander Weg, & Klesges, 2006). Physical activity is the most variable component of daily energy expenditure and contributes substantially to both intrapersonal and interpersonal variability in energy expenditure. It accounts for 20% to 30% of the total energy expenditure in sedentary individuals and for 50% or more of the total energy expenditure in very active individuals (Hill, Saris, & Levine, 2004). With work-related physical activity becoming less important in most professions, more recent research on physical activity has focused on the effects of volitional exercise (e.g., U.S. Department of Health and Human Services, 1996). However, unless individuals are exceedingly athletic, the nonvolitional activities of daily living may be as important as volitional activities as a source of energy expenditure (Levine et al., 1999, 2005).

Individuals who are overweight or obese are physically less active than are persons of normal weight. This seems to be true for all ages, both genders, and in volitional as well as nonvolitional activities (Hill et al., 2004; Levine et al., 2005). As is discussed in chapter 4 (this volume), the causal direction of this association is not clear. On the one hand, a sedentary lifestyle is likely to contribute to the development of obesity. On the other hand, being obese is likely to make physical activity more strenuous and less enjoyable. The two processes are not mutually exclusive. It is plausible that they both contribute to the negative association between obesity and physical activity. The fact that those who are obese are physically less active does not mean, however, that they spend less energy on physical activities. After all, moving a large body requires more energy. The lower activity level of individuals with obesity is likely to

TABLE 3.1
Duration of Various Activities to Expend 150 Kilocalories
for an Average 70-Kilogram (154-Pound) Adult

Intensity	Activity	Approximate duration in minutes
Moderate	Volleyball, noncompetitive	43
Moderate	Walking, moderate pace (3 miles/hour, 20 minutes/mile)	37
Moderate	Walking, brisk pace (4 miles/hour, 15 minutes/mile	32
Moderate	Table tennis	32
Moderate	Raking leaves	32
Moderate	Social dancing	29
Moderate	Lawn mowing (powered push mower)	29
Hard	Jogging (5 miles/hour, 12 minutes/mile)	18
Hard	Field hockey	16
Very hard	Running (6 miles/hour, 10 minutes/mile)	13

Note. Data from U.S. Department of Health and Human Services (1996, p. 148, Table 4-10).

be compensated for by the greater energy costs involved in moving around with a greater body weight.

Implications for Weight Gain and Weight Loss

The human body is a very efficient machine. Table 3.1 lists how long one must do various activities to expend 150 kilocalories. As one can see, to work off the equivalent of eating a 150-gram (5.25-ounce)[1] serving of creamy fruit yogurt, 30 grams (1.05 ounces) of salami, or 200 milliliters (6.8 fluid ounces) of white wine, an adult who weighs 70 kilograms (154 pounds) has to walk at a moderate pace for 37 minutes, jog for 18 minutes, or dance for 29 minutes. From a perspective of weight control, working off these calories seems hardly worth the effort. However, a daily excess of 150 kilocalories amounts to 54,750 kilocalories per year. One kilogram (2.2 pounds) of weight gain represents 7,700 kilocalories of body energy (Hill, Wyatt, Reed, & Peters, 2003). Fortunately, not all these calories will be stored as weight gain, because the biochemical processes involved in absorbing, processing, and storing ingested nutrients also use energy. As a conservative estimate, Hill et al. (2003) suggested 50% efficiency; that is, for every 150 excess kilocalories consumed, at least 75 kilocalories will be deposited as energy stores. Thus, the daily excess

---

[1]The scientific literature uses the metric system for the expression of weight and length, and all research findings in the obesity literature are reported in terms of this system. Therefore, I use metric units of measurement throughout this book but add the conversion to U.S. measures for readers who are more familiar with that system.

consumption of one creamy yogurt could result in a weight gain of 3.5 kilograms (7.7 pounds) per year. Walking to work every day instead of driving could therefore be worth the effort, at least if one likes creamy yogurt.

Can formerly lean people become obese from eating one creamy fruit yogurt per day in excess of their energy requirements? Probably not, because as they gain weight, their total energy expenditure increases. Their metabolic rate goes up, because part of the weight gain is due to an increase in metabolically active lean tissue and because the weight gain will increase the energy they have to expend on physical activity. Thus, after a certain amount of weight gain, their daily energy requirements will have increased by 150 kilocalories, and unless they add another creamy yogurt to their diet, their weight will stabilize (Tataranni & Ravussin, 2002).

This is the good news. The bad news is that the reverse sequence unfolds as people lose weight. Total energy requirement decreases with weight loss, and unless people reduce their calorie intake even further (or become even more physically active), their weight will stabilize. They will stop losing weight, even if they are still faithful to their weight-reducing diet. This effect might be somewhat reduced if they convert part of the fat into muscle mass, not only because they lose less weight but because muscles are metabolically more active than fat.

THE COMPONENTS OF ENERGY INTAKE

All the energy needed by the body comes from the metabolism of four classes of nutrients, namely carbohydrates, protein, fat, and alcohol. They are typically referred to as *macronutrients*, because (with the exception of alcohol) they are required in relatively large amounts in the diet (Carr, 2003). The other essential nutrient classes, namely vitamins, minerals, and water, do not contain energy.

The different macronutrients differ in energy content: 1 gram (0.035 ounces) of carbohydrate or protein contains 4 kilocalories, 1 gram of alcohol contains 7 kilocalories, and 1 gram of fat contains 9 kilocalories. Thus carbohydrates and proteins are the macronutrients with the lowest energy density (i.e., amount of dietary energy per unit of weight), and fat has the highest energy density. The average Western diet consist of approximately 50% carbohydrates, 35% to 40% fat, and 10% to 15% proteins (e.g., Batterham et al., 2006). According to the dietary recommendations of the U.S. Department of Agriculture, dietary fat should be reduced to 30% and protein intake increased to 20% (Grilo, 2006; U.S. Department of Health and Human Services and the Department of Agriculture, 1995).

Carbohydrates are a diverse family of substances that includes sugar, starches, and fibers. Sugars and starches are sources of energy, whereas fibers are not. Fibers pass through the digestive tract without being absorbed (Carr, 2003). Potatoes, bread, noodles, fruits, and soft drinks are major sources of carbohydrates, although like most foods, they also contain other macro-nutrients. Foods high in proteins include meat, fish, cheese, eggs, and nuts. High-protein diets have been shown to result in the greatest hunger reduction and decrease of ad libitum calorie intake of all macronutrients (e.g., Batterham et al., 2006). Fats include not only the visible fats such as butter, margarine, and oil but also the "invisible" fats that form part of most of our food. The major sources of alcohol (ethanol) are so well known that they do not have to be listed here. It should be added, however, that in addition to ethanol and water, beer, cider, and white wine also contain carbohydrates (sugar).

Because diets high in fat are usually energy dense and palatable, high-fat diets increase the risk of the development of obesity through passive over-consumption. Thus, numerous studies show that when individuals are asked to eat freely from diets that covertly have been manipulated to vary in fat content, high-fat concentration will lead to overconsumption (e.g., Lissner, Levitsky, Strupp, Kalkwarf, & Roe, 1987; Stubbs, Harbron, Murgatroyd, & Prentice, 1995). Thus, Lissner et al. (1987) created three diets of similar foods and similar palatability, in which fat contributed either 15% to 20%, 30% to 35%, or 45% to 50% of the total caloric content. Under conditions of ad libitum food consumption, calorie intake was higher for the high-fat (2,714 kilo-calories) than the low-fat (2,087 kilocalories) diet (see Figure 3.1). Whereas participants lost some weight over the 14 days of a trial when consuming the low-fat diet, the high-fat diet resulted in weight gain (see Figure 3.2). These findings were replicated in a study conducted by Stubbs et al. (1995) that also covertly manipulated fat content (20%, 40%, and 60%).[2]

Several factors contribute to the impact of fat composition on energy intake. The main one is probably that people are used to eating a certain amount of food (i.e., weight or volume), and they do not compensate for the greater calorie density of the high-fat diet (Rolls, 2000). One reason for the lack of compensation is presumably the fact that the fat content was covertly manip-ulated. Had participants known about the high-fat content of the diet, they might have consciously reduced their intake. There is evidence that individ-uals compensate for variations in fat content if they are informed about these variations (Mela, 1995). However, in everyday life, people are also often unaware of the fat content of the food they eat. Furthermore, the fact that there was no compensation suggests a failure of bodily mechanisms to regulate over-consumption of high-fat foods.[3] In light of these findings, it is puzzling that

---

[2]Further evidence that fat-reduced diets result in weight loss comes from studies that show weight loss with diets that replace fat with the fat substitute Olestra (e.g., Bray et al., 2002).

[3]One reason for this could be that fat is less satiating than are carbohydrates. There is some evidence that individuals feel less hungry after a meal high in carbohydrates than after a high-fat meal with the same calorie content (Blundell, Burley, Cotton, & Lawton, 1993; but see also Raben, Agerholme-Larsen, Flint, Holst, & Astrup, 2003). However, as Rolls (2000) has argued, this difference in satiation could be due to differences in energy density rather than fat content.

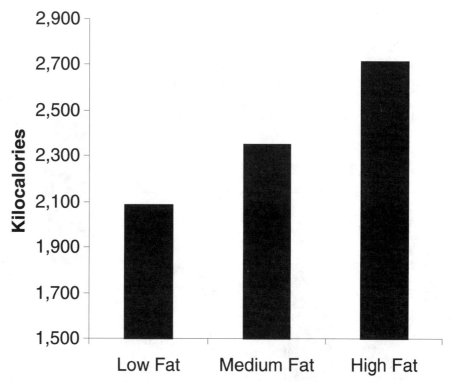

Figure 3.1. Mean daily energy intake by fat content of diet. From "Dietary Fat and the Regulation of Energy Intake in Human Subjects," by L. Lissner, D. A. Levitsky, B. J. Strupp, H. J. Kalkwarf, and D. A. Roe, 1987, *American Journal of Clinical Nutrition, 46,* p. 889. Copyright 1987 by the American Society for Nutrition. Adapted with permission.

neither cross-sectional nor longitudinal studies have been consistent in supporting the assumption that obesity is more prevalent among individuals whose fat intake is high (for reviews, see Lissner & Heitmann, 1995; Prentice, 1999a; Willett, 1998).

The most likely reason for this discrepancy is that food intake of free-living individuals is hard to measure. People tend to underreport their food consumption, and the degree of underreporting is positively correlated with body mass index (BMI; Black et al., 1991; Braam, Ocké, Bueno-de-Mesquita, & Seidell, 1998; Seidell, 1998). Individuals with obesity underreport their energy intake in general and their fat intake in particular (Goris, Westerterp-Platenga, & Westerterp, 2000). Consistent with this explanation, the few cross-sectional studies that used methods to measure food intake objectively outside the laboratory observed an association between obesity and intake of high-fat foods (Larson, Tataranni, Ferraro, & Ravussin, 1995) or purchase of high-fat foods (Ransley et al., 2003). Thus, Larson et al. (1995) showed that when

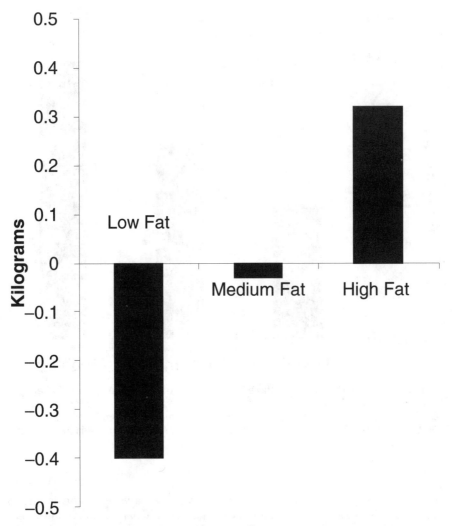

Figure 3.2. Mean change in body weight over 14-day treatment periods by fat content of diet. From "Dietary Fat and the Regulation of Energy Intake in Human Subjects," by L. Lissner, D. A. Levitsky, B. J. Strupp, H. J. Kalkwarf, and D. A. Roe, 1987, *American Journal of Clinical Nutrition, 46,* p. 889. Copyright 1987 by the American Society for Nutrition. Adapted with permission.

placed in a controlled environment in which fat intake could be measured precisely with an automated food selection system (two food-vending machines), women who were fatter selected items with higher fat content and ate more food than did women who were leaner. Ransley et al. (2003) used food purchases at a supermarket as their dependent measure. They found that households composed mainly of overweight individuals purchased food higher in fat than did households consisting mainly of individuals of normal weight.

ENERGY STORAGE AND MACRONUTRIENT BALANCE

The calories individuals consume have to be either used or stored. If more energy is used than is consumed, people lose weight. On the other hand, if the total energy intake exceeds energy expenditure, they gain weight. Until a few decades ago, researchers believed that all calories were the same and that all macronutrients formed a readily convertible energy currency within the body. Since then, it has been discovered that this view is overly simplistic and that fat synthesis from other macronutrients, particularly from carbohydrates, is relatively rare in humans (Hellerstein, Schwarz, & Neese, 1996; Prentice, 1999b; Tataranni & Ravussin, 2002). Thus, if macronutrients are being stored rather than oxidized (i.e., used as energy), they can be stored only in their own specific compartment.

Because humans have widely different storage capacities for different macronutrients, this fact has important implications. Whereas our storage capacity for fat is nearly unlimited, the capacity for protein storage as body protein and carbohydrate storage as glycogen is very limited, and alcohol cannot be stored at all. Alcohol calories are therefore sometimes referred to as "empty calories." This does not mean, however, that as far as weight is concerned, one can consume alcohol with impunity. Because alcohol cannot be stored (and is furthermore toxic), it immediately stimulates alcohol oxidation and forces the suppression of oxidation of other macronutrients, particularly fat (Sonko et al., 1994). The body runs on alcohol as fuel and saves the fuel metabolized from the other nutrients for later use. As a result, the calories contained in alcohol count toward total calorie intake. Thus, if a person's energy balance would have been neutral, except for the glass of white wine he or she drank with a meal, the wine calories will be used as fuel, forcing the retention of an equivalent in (now not burned) fat calories. This is bad news, because when alcohol is consumed during a meal, its energy content is not compensated for by an equivalent decrease in energy intake from other macronutrients (Mattes, 1996; A. Tremblay et al., 1995). Furthermore, alcohol seems to even stimulate appetite (e.g., Westerterp-Platenga & Verwegen, 1999). It is therefore puzzling that epidemiological evidence does not show a clear relation between daily alcohol intake and BMI (e.g., Colditz et al., 1991). However, alcohol consumption does seem to be associated with increased abdominal fat deposits (e.g., Wannamethee, Shaper, & Lennon, 2005).

Carbohydrates are metabolized into glucose, which is an essential fuel for the brain and also provides the main source of energy for muscles during strenuous exercise. Nevertheless, the capacity for carbohydrate storage is small, and carbohydrate storage is tightly regulated. Although some of the daily carbohydrate intake is stored as glycogen, a substantial proportion of average daily intake is utilized for energy as glucose, suppressing fat oxidation (Tataranni & Ravussin, 2002). Because protein stores are also limited and

tightly controlled, excess consumption of proteins stimulates protein oxidation and suppresses fat oxidation. Thus, because of the limited storage
capacity for carbohydrates and proteins, there is a tight autoregulatory link
between levels of intake and oxidation, with intake stimulating the use of
glucose and protein for energy and forcing fat retention. Because humans
have a virtually infinite capacity to store fat by expanding adipose tissue stores,
there is no need for the body to regulate fat oxidization. As noted by Prentice
(1999b), "fat oxidation is determined totally by the level of oxidation of the
other fuels; when oxidation levels are high, fat oxidation is suppressed, and
vice versa" (p. 70).

GENETIC INFLUENCE ON BODY WEIGHT AND OBESITY

Before I review epidemiological studies that assess the extent to which
body weight and obesity are determined by genetic factors, I would like to discuss two implications of such heritability estimates that are often misunder-
stood. First, if a trait is found to be largely genetically determined, it does not
necessarily mean that individuals are powerless to change it. Genetic determination of body weight does not have the same implications as does genetic
determination of eye color or blood type. Though people cannot change their
eye color or blood type, they can influence several of the processes that are
responsible for the genetic influence on body weight. For example, the extent
to which people are physically active is strongly determined by genetic factors
(Frederiksen & Christensen, 2003; Goran, 1997; Joosen, Gielen, Vlietinck,
& Westerterp, 2005), as is their daily calorie intake (Rankinen & Bouchard,
2006), both of which are under individual control.

The second source of frequent misunderstanding relates to the form in
which heritability is typically reported. Genetic studies report the proportion
of variance in a given trait in the population studied that is due to genetic
compared with environmental influences. For example, the most likely estimate of heritability of body weight is that between 60% and 70% of the body
weight variation is due to genetic factors (Bouchard, Pérusse, Rice, & Rao,
2004; Maes, Neale, & Eaves, 1997). Much of the remaining 30% to 40% of the
variance is due to environmental influences. It is important to note that any
estimate based on a particular study reflects a historical situation that existed
at the time that study was conducted. If the relevant environmental conditions became more homogeneous, the variance due to environmental factors
would decrease and genetic influence would gain in importance. Conversely,
however, if we were able to increase the variability of the environmental factors that are relevant for body weight, the proportion of variance accounted
for by genetic factors would decrease.

Estimates of Heritability

The most direct assessment of the genetic influence on body weight can be gained from studies of monozygotic (MZ) twins who have been reared apart. MZ twins are genetically identical. If they have been separated in childhood and have grown up in different environments, any similarity in their body weight would be purely a reflection of genetic influence. Thus, the correlation of the weight of MZ twin pairs reared apart reflects the proportion of variance in weight that is genetically determined. In a study of 93 male and female pairs of MZ twins reared apart, Stunkard, Harris, Pedersen, and McClearn (1990) reported a correlation between the BMI values of these twin pairs of .70 for men and .66 for women, suggesting that 66% to 70% of the variance in body weight is determined by genetic factors.

MZ twins who have been reared apart are rare specimens, and sample sizes are usually small in this type of study. It is therefore fortunate that heritability estimates can also be based on twins reared together, even though both MZ and DZ (dizygotic) twins are then needed to arrive at an estimate. Like ordinary siblings, DZ twins share only half of their genes. Therefore, if weight is partially determined genetically, DZ twins should be less similar in their BMI than are MZ twins, and this difference in similarity should reflect the impact of the 50% of genetic endowment. According to a widely used method originally suggested by Falconer (1981), heritability estimates can be derived from a comparison of the within-pair correlations in BMI for the two types of twin pairs. Because these twins grew up in the same environment, the difference between the two sets of correlations reflects 50% of heritability. Thus, multiplying this difference by two gives an estimate of heritability: $2 \times (r_{MZ} - r_{DZ})$.

Using a sample of 1,974 male MZ and 2,097 male DZ twins, Stunkard, Foch, and Hrubec (1986) estimated that approximately 80% of the variance in BMI is accounted for by genetic factors. The sample size of this study also allowed the researchers to check whether the genetic influence on BMI remains the same across the whole range of BMI values. They found that the similarity in BMI of MZ twins was consistently much greater than that of DZ twins across BMI values ranging from 15 to 40, suggesting that heritability is reasonably high across the whole BMI range from underweight to overweight.

Because siblings or parents and their children share 50% of their genes, heritability estimates can also be based on studies of the nuclear family. Finally, heritability can also be assessed in adoption studies. For example, siblings who have grown up in different environments share only genetic sources of variance, whereas two biologically unrelated individuals who have been raised in the same family share only environmental sources of variance. Bouchard et al. (2004) summarized the heritability estimates for BMI based on large numbers of twin, nuclear family, and adoption studies. The results were quite heterogeneous. The heritability estimates were highest with twin studies (50% to 80% of the variance), intermediate with nuclear family studies (30% to 50% of the variance), and lowest for adoption studies (10% to 30% of the variance). However, as Maes et al. (1997) pointed out, family and adoption studies share the disadvantage that children and parents or siblings are assessed at different ages, which could result in an underestimation of heritability if different genetic or environmental factors account for the variation in BMI at different ages. Using data from the Virginia 30,000, a huge study that included twins and their parents, siblings, spouses, and children, Maes et al. estimated genetic variance in BMI at 67%.

The Impact of the Environment

There can be no doubt that body weight is strongly determined by genetic factors. However, even the estimate of Maes et al. (1997) still allows for a substantial influence of environmental factors on body weight. Because meals are typically shared within families, one would expect the shared family influence to be the most important environmental influence on weight and obesity. One strategy to assess the impact of shared family environment has been to compare siblings who were reared together with siblings who grew up in different families. The study of Stunkard et al. (1990) of MZ twins reared apart, which I reviewed earlier, also included a sample of MZ twins who grew up in the same family. If the family environment exerted a strong influence on weight and obesity, one would expect that twins who grew up in the same family would be much more similar in their BMI than would twins who were reared apart. The surprising finding of this study was that there was hardly any difference in the BMI correlations between the two groups of twins. Shared family environment did not contribute to the variation in BMI. Evidence from adoption studies comparing adopted children with their biological and adoptive parents is consistent with this finding (for a review, see Grilo & Pogue-Geile, 1991). However, as Segal and Allison (2002) argued, in the classic twin design, nonadditive genetic effects (e.g., gene–environment interactions) and common environmental effects are confounded. Findings such as those reported by Stunkard et al. might therefore underestimate shared-environment effects. Similarly, in adoption studies, shared-environment effects might have been obscured by the age differences between parents and children or between siblings and by the fact that shared-environment effects are most likely to emerge in young children. In a study design that added virtual twins (same-age unrelated siblings reared together since infancy) to the classic twin design, Segal and Allison (2002) found evidence for a significant effect of shared environment.

Gene–Environment Interactions

Are some individuals more at risk for weight gain than are others? Is there a genetic predisposition toward overweight and obesity? In the terminology of genetic studies, such a genetic predisposition would be a gene–environment interaction, that is, a situation in which the response of a phenotype (e.g., amount of body fat) to environmental changes (e.g., dietary restrictions) depended on the genotype of the individual. Impressive demonstrations of the presence of gene–environment interactions in weight gain and weight loss have been reported by Bouchard and colleagues (Bouchard et al., 1990, 1994). In these studies MZ twin pairs were submitted either to positive energy balance induced by overfeeding or to negative energy balance induced by exercise training.

In the overfeeding study, 12 pairs of adult male MZ twins ate a 1,000-kilocalorie-per-day surplus for 84 days over a 100-day period (Bouchard et al., 1990). They were kept sedentary, except for a 30-minute walk every day. These twin pairs gained an average of 8.1 kilograms (17.8 pounds) over the 100-day period, but there was large interindividual variation in weight gain, with some individuals gaining relatively little weight and others gaining a lot (see Figure 3.3, left panel). Because all individuals were exposed to the same amount of excess calories, the differences observed in weight gain demonstrated that individuals differ in their propensity to gain weight when their energy intake is

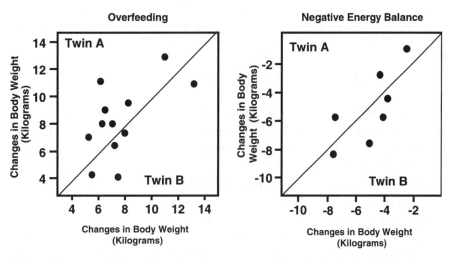

Figure 3.3. Intrapair resemblance in the response of identical twins to long-term changes in energy balance. Left panel: 12 pairs of identical twins were submitted to 84,000 kilocalories of energy intake surplus over 100 days. Right panel: 7 pairs were subjected to a negative energy balance protocol caused by exercise. The energy deficit was 58,000 kilocalories over 93 days. Left panel from "The Response to Long-Term Overfeeding in Identical Twins," by C. Bouchard, A. Tremblay, J. P. Després, G. Thériault, A. Nadeau, P. J. Lupien, J. Dussault, S. Moorjani, S. Pinault, and G. Fournier, 1990, *New England Journal of Medicine, 322,* p. 1479. Copyright 1990 by the Massachusetts Medical Society. Reprinted with permission. Right panel from "The Response to Exercise With Constant Energy Intake in Identical Twins," by C. Bouchard, A. Tremblay, J. P. Déspres, G. Thériault, A. Nadeau, P. J. Lupien, S. Moorjani, D. Prudhomme, and G. Fournier, 1994, *Obesity Research, 2,* p. 404. Copyright 1994 by NAASO—The Obesity Society. Reprinted with permission.

greater than their energy expenditure. More important, however, these findings also showed a strong genetic influence on the propensity to gain weight. If this differential sensitivity had been unrelated to genetic factors, then some members of MZ twin pairs should have gained little weight whereas others should have gained a lot. In fact, there was at least 3 times more variance in weight gain between than within pairs (the within-pairs correlation in weight gain was .55).[4]

In the experiment, which induced a negative energy balance, seven pairs of adult MZ twin pairs had to exercise on cycle ergometers twice a day, 9 out of 10 days for 93 days, while being kept on constant daily energy intake (Bouchard et al., 1994). Mean body weight loss was 5.0 kilograms (11.0 pounds), and again there was a great deal of variation in weight loss. However, as in the overfeeding study, there was more heterogeneity between twin pairs than within pairs (see Figure 3.3, right panel). In fact, the intraclass correlation for the weight changes of twin pairs was .74.

Although the heritability estimates for body weight and obesity from epidemiological studies of genetic influence are rather heterogeneous, the majority of studies suggest a strong genetic influence. The studies of Bouchard et al. (1990, 1994) provide further evidence of a gene–environment interaction, indicating not only that some individuals are more disposed to weight gain but also that this disposition appears to be at least partly determined by genetic factors.

RISK FACTORS FOR BODY WEIGHT GAIN

Now that the existence of a genetic disposition toward weight gain has been established, it is important to know the processes that underlie this genetic propensity in order to identify risk factors for body-weight gain. It is ironic that traits that are now considered risk factors must have bestowed a survival advantage on our hunter–gatherer forefathers—and mothers—in evolutionary times. Having an efficient metabolism that uses little energy in times of uncertain food supplies and allows the accumulation of fat stores during times of plenty must have increased chances of survival during periods of starvation. The "thrifty gene" hypothesis was originally suggested by Neel (1962), although his 1962 article did not specifically focus on energy balance and obesity (Bouchard, 2007a, 2007b). The most likely risk factors for body-weight gain are relevant behaviors (food intake and physical activity) and metabolic processes.

---

[4]When body mass and body composition were controlled for, the intrapair resemblance for changes in resting metabolic rate brought about by overfeeding was not significant. Furthermore, neither the resting metabolic rate nor the thermic response to a standardized meal correlated with the body mass and adiposity changes observed in the study. This finding could have been a power problem resulting from the small sample size, but it could also suggest that the differential weight gain was due to differences in nonexercise physical activity.

High Level of Food Intake

There is evidence from both family and twin studies that genetic factors account for a substantial proportion of the variance in food intake. On the basis of their recent review of family and twin studies of the genetics of food intake phenotypes, Rankinen and Bouchard (2006) concluded that the magnitude of effects was heterogeneous across studies but typically ranged from 20% to 40%. As Rankinen and Bouchard argued, this effect is not trivial and is of the same magnitude as that observed for metabolic processes such as blood pressure and plasma triglyceride level. The fact that food intake is both strongly genetically influenced and at the same time under volitional control supports the point made earlier that genetic determination of a trait does not always imply that individuals are powerless to change it.

Low Levels of Physical Activity

As mentioned earlier, energy spent on physical activity accounts for a sizable proportion of daily energy expenditure. There is also evidence that levels of physical activity are genetically influenced. A review of twin and family studies of genetic influence on leisure-time physical activity found heritability estimates to vary across studies from 29% to 62% of the total variance (Frederiksen & Christensen, 2003). A small twin study that assessed all body movements during daily living with a triaxial accelerometer placed on a belt at the lower back found genetic factors to explain 78% of the variance in physical activity over 17 consecutive days (Joosen et al., 2005). The study is particularly interesting because it also assessed activity-induced energy expenditure in daily life using the doubly labeled water method and found genetic factors to account for 72% of the variance in activity-induced energy expenditure.

Several longitudinal studies found low levels of physical activity associated with increased obesity risk (for reviews see chap. 4, this volume; Hill et al., 2004; U.S. Department of Health and Human Services, 1996). For example, in the Nurses' Health Study, sedentary occupations were significantly associated with obesity, whereas light activities such as standing or walking around at home and brisk walking were prospectively associated with significantly lower obesity risks (Hu, Li, Colditz, Willet, & Manson, 2003). However, the most direct evidence to indicate that physical inactivity is associated with an increased risk of weight gain comes from recent studies of Levine and colleagues (Levine, Eberhardt, & Jensen, 1999; Levine et al., 2005) of the association of nonexercise activity thermogenesis (NEAT) with obesity. To examine the role of NEAT in obesity, Levine et al. (2005) recruited 10 volunteers who were lean and sedentary and 10 volunteers who were mildly obese and sedentary and measured their body postures and movements for 10 days. They found that the participants who were obese were seated for 164 minutes longer per day than were the volunteers who were lean. Levine et al. (2005) calculated that if their participants who were obese had engaged in NEAT to the same extent as did their volunteers who were lean, they would have expended an additional 352 kilocalories per day. Levine et al. subsequently persuaded their participants who were obese to go on a weight-loss diet and their participants who were lean to undergo supervised overfeeding. As a result, those who were obese lost 8.0 kilograms (17.6 pounds), and those who were lean gained 4.0 kilograms (8.8 pounds). To their great surprise, when they studied posture allocation again, the researchers had to conclude that "both the obese subjects losing weight and the lean subjects gaining weight maintained their original posture allocation" (Levine et al., 2005, p. 585).

Further evidence for the importance of differences in habitual levels of NEAT comes from an earlier study of Levine et al. (1999) that assessed changes in NEAT of 16 individuals who were not obese and who were overfed for 8 weeks with 1,000 kilocalories per day. The amount of fat that participants gained varied greatly, ranging from a weight increase of only 0.36 kilograms (0.79 pounds) to a gain of 4.23 kilograms (9.33 pounds). Because participants had been instructed to keep volitional exercise at a very low level, changes in exercise-related thermogenesis over the course of the study could be attributed to changes in NEAT. Results showed that changes in NEAT directly predicted resistance to fat gain with overfeeding: The correlation between changes in NEAT and fat gain was .77. Levine et al. (1999) concluded that

> activation of NEAT can explain the variability in fat gain with over-eating. As humans overeat, those with effective activation of NEAT can dissipate the excess energy so that it is not available for storage as fat, whereas those with lesser degrees of NEAT activation will likely have great fat gain and be predisposed to develop obesity. (p. 213)

Low Resting Metabolic Rate

As was shown earlier, RMR is the one component that explains the largest proportion of total daily energy expenditure. Lower levels of RMR in individuals who will become obese would therefore offer a plausible explanation for the development of obesity. However, research on the role of RMR in the etiology of obesity has led to conflicting results. Bouchard et al. (1989) concluded on the basis of a study involving twins as well as parent–child pairs that even after adjusting for FFM, there was a strong genetic effect on RMR. It is less clear, however, to what extent differences in RMR contribute to obesity. A meta-analysis of 12 studies that compared the RMR of individuals who were formerly obese with that of people who had never been obese found that after differences in body size and body composition were controlled for, the individuals who were formerly obese had a 3% to 5% lower RMR than did individuals who had never been obese (Astrup et al., 1999).[5] In addition to a regular meta-analysis, Astrup et al. also obtained individual subject data from 124 individuals who were formerly obese and 121 individuals who were never obese from 15 studies included in their meta-analysis and analyzed the difference between these two groups. When RMR was adjusted for FFM and FM, this analysis resulted in only a marginally significant effect ($p < .10$). Furthermore, the lower RMR in the formerly obese group was entirely accounted for by the 15% of individuals who had particularly low RMR (> 1 standard deviation below the mean).

As discussed earlier, cross-sectional findings are ambiguous with regard to the cause–effect sequence. Though the findings of Astrup et al. (1999) might suggest the possibility that a low RMR constitutes a risk factor for weight gain, it is also possible that the low RMR is a consequence of weight loss. The body seems to go into an energy-saving mode when confronted with a substantial reduction in energy supply (i.e., adoptive thermogenesis). Ongoing fasting can therefore reduce RMR (e.g., Ravussin, Burnand, Schutz, & Jéquier, 1985). Although most of the studies selected for the meta-analysis took great care to include only participants who were weight stable, not all studies provided sufficient detail to rule out the possibility that effects could have been the result of ongoing fasting rather than stable weight loss (Astrup et al., 1999). Since the time period covered by Astrup et al. (1999) in their review, two studies have been published that made certain to include individuals who were formerly obese and who had stabilized their weight loss (Weinsier, Hunter, Zuckerman, & Darnell, 2003; Wyatt et al., 1999). Both studies failed to find significant differences between their samples of those who were formerly obese and of those were never obese.

One would have hoped that findings from longitudinal studies would help to resolve this inconsistency, but the picture that emerges from these studies is less than clear. A prospective study among Pima Indians showed that low relative RMR, adjusted for FFM, FM, age, and sex, was a risk factor for body gain. Compared with individuals with the highest RMR at baseline, those with the lowest RMR had an 8 times greater risk of gaining 10 kilograms (22 pounds) within the 4-year period (Ravussin et al., 1988). However, as Prentice (1999b) cautioned, the extent to which this finding can be generalized is unclear because the Pima Indians have very high rates of obesity for reasons other than metabolic rate. Furthermore, two other longitudinal studies failed to find that low levels of RMR were predictive of obesity. In their analysis of data from the Baltimore Longitudinal Study of Aging, Seidell, Muller, Sorkin, and

---

[5]It seems that not all studies in the traditional meta-analysis corrected RMR for fat mass (FM) as well as FFM. Because FM also contributes to RMR (Schutz & Jéquier, 2004) and because those who were formerly obese were heavier than those who were never obese, failure to control for FM might have contributed to the difference observed between the two groups.

Andres (1992) found no association between resting energy expenditure and weight change in 775 European American men over a period of 10 years. Similarly, Weinsier et al. (2000) observed a nonsignificant correlation between RMR (adjusted for body composition) and weight regain in a sample of women who had previously lost weight during a dietary intervention. Finally, Bouchard et al. (2004) reported from their study of controlled overfeeding that RMR did not correlate with body mass and adiposity changes.

What can be concluded from this pattern of findings? The one lesson learned since the use of box scores was replaced by meta-analyses is that if competently conducted research results in equivocal findings (i.e., some positive and some null findings), the reason is usually that there is an effect but it is weak. Thus, I tend to agree with the conclusion drawn some years ago by Weinsier, Hunter, Heini, Goran, and Sell (1998), namely that "available evidence suggests that such variations in resting energy expenditure have, at best, only a small impact on one's tendency to gain weight" (p. 146).

Food-Induced Thermogenesis

Bouchard et al. (1989) also found food-induced thermogenesis to be influenced by genetic factors. Furthermore, there is some evidence that food-induced thermogenesis is decreased in individuals with obesity (De Jonge & Bray, 1997; Jéquier & Schutz, 1988). However, the extent to which this effect plays any role in the development of obesity is less clear (Schutz & Jéquier, 2004). Prospective studies have failed to find an association between a low TEF and weight gain (e.g., Tataranni, Larson, Snitker, & Ravussin, 1995). Furthermore, Bouchard et al. (1990) found thermic response to a standardized meal to be unrelated to the changes in body mass and composition observed in their study of controlled overfeeding. Thus, as Ravussin (2002) concluded, "one could safely state that any decrease in the thermic effect of food amounts to only a small number of calories and that a minimal weight gain (and thus increased RMR) would be sufficient to offset this decreased energy expenditure" (p. 57).

Low Rates of Fat Oxidization

Differences between individuals in their tendency to store fat rather than oxidize it could also be a risk factor that predisposes individuals toward obesity. The nonprotein respiratory quotient measured over 24 hours and during sleep allows one to gain information about the source of fuel an organism is using because the relationship between the volume of carbon dioxide released and the volume of oxygen consumed depends on the type of macronutrient the organism is oxidizing. For glucose the respiratory quotient is 1.000; for saturated fat it is .667. Thus, higher respiratory quotients are an indication of greater reliance on carbohydrate rather than fat oxidization.

Studies based on respiratory quotient found some support for the assumption that a low rate of fat oxidization could be a risk factor for weight gain. Thus, Astrup, Beuman, Christensen, and Toubro (1995) and Larson, Ferraro, Robertson, and Ravussin (1995) found significantly higher respiratory quotients among weight-stable, formerly obese men and women than among comparable individuals who had never been obese. Furthermore, in a longitudinal study in Pima Indians, a relatively high respiratory quotient was found to predict weight gain (Zurlo et al., 1990). Individuals in the highest 10% for respiratory quotient values (i.e., "low fat oxidizers") had a 2.5 times greater risk of gaining 5 kilograms (11 pounds) or more body weight than did those in the lowest 10% (i.e., "high fat oxidizers"). Similar results were reported for the male lean participants in the Baltimore Longitudinal Study of Aging (Seidell et al., 1992). Finally, Froedevaux, Schutz, Christin, and Jéquier (1993) demonstrated that body-weight regain in a sample of 10 women who were moderately obese, after they had lost weight with a low-energy diet, was predicted by their respiratory quotient. Those who were able to maintain weight loss had a lower respiratory quotient than did those experiencing weight relapse.

In contrast to the findings reported so far, Weinsier et al. (1995) found no significant difference between the fasting respiratory quotients of 24 women who were formerly obese and those of comparable women who had never been obese. Furthermore, when those women were monitored over a 4-year period, the individuals who were formerly obese regained all the weight they had lost, whereas the women who had never been obese stayed within the range of normal weight. In neither group did the respiratory quotient predict weight gain. However, in light of the fact that all the differences observed in this study, though nonsignificant, were in the right direction, a meta-analysis of studies of the association between respiratory quotient and obesity risk would probably lead one to conclude that there was an association but that differences in the rate of fat oxidization accounted for only a small proportion of variance in obesity.

Low Serum Concentration of Leptin

Leptin is a hormone produced by the adipose tissue that provides information to the central nervous system about the amount of energy stored in fat cells (Considine & Caro, 1996). Administration of leptin to young lean rodents leads to dramatic fat and weight loss (Considine & Caro, 1996). Furthermore, treating mice that have a genetic mutation that results in profound obesity (*ob/ob* mice) with small doses of leptin markedly reduces their food intake, breaks down their fat stores, and results in weight loss (for a review, see Considine & Caro, 1996; Zhang & Scarpace, 2006).

At first, there was hope that leptin would provide the magic bullet for the treatment of obesity. If individuals with obesity suffered from a leptin deficiency, then treating them with leptin would provide a cure. However, studies that assessed serum leptin levels in individuals with obesity and individuals of normal weight indicated that the *ob* gene was functioning normally in individuals with obesity. Serum leptin concentrations were higher in individuals with obesity than in individuals of normal weight and also increased with increasing percentage of body fat (Campfield, Smith, & Jeanrenaud, 2004). Thus, as Campfield et al. (2004) concluded, "most obese humans are not deficient in leptin, but rather . . . have elevated circulating leptin concentrations" (p. 466).

It is therefore not surprising that the only large clinical trial of leptin with 54 individuals who were lean and 74 individuals who were obese led to somewhat disappointing findings (Heymsfield et al., 1999). Although the group of obese individuals treated for 24 weeks with the highest dose lost a significant amount of weight, the effects of the treatment were not substantial enough to justify further clinical trials. A more recent and much smaller study including 30 men with obesity treated with somewhat smaller doses of leptin for 12 weeks found that compared with a placebo treatment, the injection of leptin did not result in reductions in daily food intake or body mass or changes in body composition (Westerterp-Platenga, Saris, Hukshorn, & Campfield, 2001). Although there was evidence of a decrease in hunger and appetite in the group treated with leptin, this effect occurred only before breakfast and not during the rest of the day.

These findings raise an interesting question: If the leptin secretion from fat cells of individuals with obesity functions normally and if their serum level of leptin is increased above that of individuals of normal weight, why is there no reduction of food intake or increase in energy expenditure? There are two possible answers to this question: Either leptin does not function as a satiety signal in humans, or it does so in individuals of normal weight, but because of some deficiency the receptors in the brains of individuals with obesity are insensitive to these signals.

There is evidence that establishes parallels in the function of leptin between humans and animals. First, rare mutations of the leptin gene in humans have been discovered, and symptoms of this deficiency are similar to those shown by *ob/ob* mice. Second, chronic daily leptin treatment in the first human identified with a mutation in her leptin gene resulted in weight loss and reduction in hunger (Farooqi et al., 1999). Third, studies of humans who are obese and those who are lean have repeatedly demonstrated that weight gain significantly increases circulating leptin and weight loss results in a decrease. Most researchers in this area therefore accepted the second explanation, suspecting that something was wrong with the leptin receptors in individuals with obesity that resulted in decreased responsiveness to leptin. However, a recent study of participants with obesity indicated that pathogenic mutations in the leptin-receptor gene are much too rare to account for the high level of obesity prevalence (Farooqi et al., 2007). Thus, unless there are other and as yet unidentified receptors that mediate the actions of leptin, the receptor insensitivity hypothesis must be abandoned.

High Set Point for Body Weight

The notion of regulation according to a set point is likely a familiar one, thanks to the thermostats used in central heating and air conditioning systems. If one adjusts the thermostat of one's central heating system to a given temperature, the system will switch on whenever the sensors register that the temperature has dropped considerably below this set point. Although it is plausible that body temperature is regulated according to a set point, the wide variation in body weight seems to rule out such regulation. However, it has been argued that even though there is wide interpersonal variability, the body weight of most adults remains remarkably stable over time (Keesey, 1986). Keesey (1986) suggested that different people may have different set points and that for some the biological weight is set far above culture's ideal. Thus, having a set point for body weight far above culture's ideal would constitute a risk factor for the development of obesity. It would also explain why individuals who are obese find it so difficult to lose weight or to maintain weight loss.

The most important derivation of set-point theory is that the organism will defend its body weight against pressure to change. Thus, weight reduction and maintenance of a lowered body weight (i.e., weight suppression) is assumed to result in a compensatory decrease in metabolic rate. The intense physiological pressures produced by attempts to maintain weight loss below one's set point is also assumed to be accompanied by significant psychological and behavioral changes (e.g., Keys, Brozek, Henschel, Mickelson, & Taylor, 1950). Thus, weight suppression is expected to be associated with increased irritability and depression, increased hunger, and a preoccupation with food. Finally, it is thought likely that organisms will increase calorie intake to reestablish their original weight (Keys et al., 1950).

Hardly any of these predictions have been supported by empirical evidence (Pinel, Assanand, & Lehman, 2000). First, convincing evidence challenges the assumption that weight is tightly controlled. For example, in the Nurses' Health Study, a substantial proportion of women gained 5 kilograms (11 pounds) or more over the 14-year follow-up period, which suggested that weight gain is normal (i.e., the middle-age spread; Willett et al., 1995). In the Framingham Study, only 30% of participants had weight changes of less than 8 kilograms (18 pounds), even though the mean weight in the population remained relatively stable (Gordon & Kannel, 1973). Although these changes could be attributed to the human organisms defending their set weight against attempts at weight loss, the dramatic increase in body weight that most industrialized countries have experienced during the past 2 decades would be difficult to reconcile with set-point theory. Finally, if body weight were tightly controlled around some set point, it would also be difficult to understand why covert manipulation of the fat content of an individual's diet would result in overconsumption (e.g., Lissner, Levitsky, Strupp, Kalkwarf, & Roe, 1987; Stubbs et al., 1995) or why individuals seem to be unable to compensate for the additional calories they consume in the form of alcoholic beverages or soft drinks (Mattes, 1996). In fact, a recent review by Levitsky (2005) on the nonregulation of food intake suggests that lack of compensation is the rule rather than the exception.

The outcomes of studies that assessed whether weight suppression reduces metabolic rate have been mixed. There is no doubt that ongoing fasting can reduce RMR beyond what one would expect on the basis of loss of body mass and the decrease in TEF (e.g., Ravussin et al., 1985). It has been estimated that this adaptive thermogenesis compensates at most for 25% of a given energy deficit while a person is on a restrictive diet (Flatt, 2007).[6] However, this is a short-term effect. If the body were defending its body weight against pressure to change, one would expect such defensive processes to continue even after weight reduction has stopped as long as the weight loss is maintained. The cross-sectional studies reviewed earlier that compared the RMR of individuals who were formerly obese with that of individuals who were never obese are relevant in this context, because the formerly obese group consisted of individuals who had lost substantial amounts of weight and would therefore be expected to have a lower RMR. The fact that if there is a difference at all it is a very weak one is not supportive of set-point theory. Furthermore, a review of studies of changes in energy metabolism in individuals who repeatedly lost and gained substantial amounts of weight (i.e., *weight cycling*) concluded that the majority of studies that assessed humans after weight cycling demonstrated no evidence of enhanced metabolic efficiency (Atkinson & Stern, 1998).

Finally, there is little evidence for the assumption of set-point theory that dieting or long-term weight suppression is associated with psychological distress. That individuals might be preoccupied with thoughts about food while actively trying to reduce their calorie intake to lose weight is beyond dispute, even though these effects are likely to be much less severe during normal dieting than during extreme dieting such as that practiced by the men in the Minnesota Starvation Study (Keys et al., 1950). However, there is no support for the assumption that dieting is associated with increased levels of distress (French & Jeffery, 1994). Furthermore, there is no support for the prediction of set-point theory that individuals who have lost weight and try to maintain their weight loss experience high levels of distress. Klem, Wing, McGuire, Seagle, and Hill (1998) compared the psychological well-being of a sample of

---

[6]Major, Doucet, Trayhurn, Astrup, and Tremblay (2007) recently claimed evidence for a decline in energy expenditure during weight reduction of a magnitude "that could in some cases be sufficiently important to overcome the prescribed energy restriction, probably leading to incapacity to further lose weight" (p. 206). It is difficult to evaluate this claim because it was based on the "highest male and female responder from the study." (For a critical review of this article, see Flatt, 2007.)

women and men who had lost at least 13.6 kilograms (30.0 pounds) and maintained the weight for at least 1 year with that of community samples of individuals. They found no evidence that these successful weight suppressors experienced levels of distress and depression that were higher than those of comparable community samples.

If there is no set point and no defense of the organism against weight loss, why do people find it so difficult to lose weight and to maintain a lower body weight after weight loss? I discuss the psychological reasons for these problems extensively in chapters 5, 6, and 7 (this volume). In the context of the current chapter, two processes discussed earlier are relevant. First, the body does seems to go into an energy-saving mode during a reducing diet, but this adaptive thermogenesis is assumed to be temporary and to compensate at most for 25% of the energy deficit (Flatt, 2007). A second and more permanent effect is that the lower body weight resulting from weight loss is associated with lower RMR and activity-related thermogenesis. Thus, a reduced-calorie diet that might have led to substantial weight loss initially is likely to become less effective as individuals lose weight (Tataranni & Ravussin, 2002).

A third reason people find it so difficult to lose weight is that body weight is determined by lifestyle. People are creatures of habit. Most people have routines that determine when they eat and how much they eat, when they exercise and how much they exercise. Thus, if one's lifestyle supports a stable weight, one's weight is unlikely to change unless a person dramatically changes his or her lifestyle. Going on a weight-reducing diet typically involves dramatic changes in lifestyle—dieters cut out meals and take up jogging—but once they have reached their target weight or given up their diet they usually revert to their old habits. Because their old lifestyle was associated with a higher weight, reverting to their old routines is likely to result in weight regain.

CONCLUSIONS

Because overweight and obesity are the result of an imbalance between energy intake and energy output, in the first two sections of the chapter I introduced the basic physiological assumptions about energy expenditure and energy intake. All the energy people consume has to be either used or stored. If a person consumes more energy than he or she uses, the excess energy will be stored long-term as fat deposits. Physical activity is the most variable component of daily energy expenditure. It accounts for 20% to 30% of total energy expenditure in sedentary individuals but 50% or more in very active individuals. To balance the energy equation in the case of excess energy, individuals must either reduce food intake or increase physical activity.

Body weight is strongly influenced by genetic factors. Bouchard and Rankinen (2008) speculated that there are four levels of genetic contribution to obesity. True genetic obesity is due to a single gene mutation, as in the rare cases of individuals who are unable to produce leptin or have a pathogenic leptin receptor mutation. They estimated that these cases of genetic obesity account for approximately 5% of obesity and for a larger percentage of severe obesity. With these individuals, obesity is caused by defective biology, and the environment plays only a permissive role. The more common forms of obesity have either a slight or a strong genetic predisposition. People with these forms of obesity are not characterized by a clearly defective biology, but they are slightly or strongly predisposed toward weight gain. They become obese if they live in an environment that favors weight gain. Research into these genetic risk factors for obesity is flourishing, and there is a continuous stream of new discoveries (for reviews, see Aisbitt, 2007; Farooqi & O'Rahilli, 2007). As Aisbitt (2007) observed, many of these genetic polymorphisms or variations are for genes involved in the regulation of appetite. For example, a meta-analysis of 14 case-control studies of a polymorphism in the melanocortin-4 receptor gene found that this variation, which was present in approximately 3% of the population studied, decreased the risk of obesity by about 30% (Heid et al., 2007). The melanocortin-4 receptor is involved in the control of energy intake and expenditure. As a fourth type of genetic disposition, Bouchard and Rankinen suggested that there are individuals who are genetically resistant to obesity and who manage to remain at normal or nearly normal weight even if they live in a land of plenty (for an elaboration of this argument, see Bulik & Allison, 2001).

It is important to realize that even small chronic imbalances in the energy input–output equation can result in considerable weight gain, at least in the long term. Hill et al. (2003) estimated that an intervention that reduced energy gain by 50 kilocalories per day would offset weight gain in approximately 90% of that population.[7] It is therefore likely that the additive effects of potential differences in RMR, TEF, and fat oxidization rate might contribute substantially to the development of obesity. However, the fact that there are genetically determined differences in the regulation of food intake and in levels of physical activity establishes these behavioral factors as major contributors to the risk of weight gain and obesity. In the next chapter's assessment of the environmental changes that are responsible for the secular increase in obesity, I look not only at factors that encourage increased calorie intake but also at factors that encourage a sedentary lifestyle.

---

[7]At 50% efficiency, one would have to consume 100 kilocalories per day for a weight gain of 50 kilocalories per day. If one considers that a boiled egg for breakfast has 78 kilocalories and that an adult weighing 70 kilograms (154 pounds) uses 150 kilocalories by walking at a moderate pace for 37 minutes, small changes in lifestyle could eliminate this weight gain. However, Wyatt et al. (1999) based their estimate on the average weight gain of 0.8 to 0.9 kilograms (1.8 to 2.0 pounds) per year in the study population. Because at that rate it would take most people more than 30 years to move from normal weight to obesity, the chronic energy imbalance experienced by individuals who ultimately become obese is likely to be greater.

4

ENVIRONMENTAL CAUSES OF THE INCREASE IN OVERWEIGHT AND OBESITY

In chapter 3, I reviewed evidence in support of the assumption that individuals differ in their susceptibility to weight gain and that these individual differences are strongly influenced by genetic factors. However, the gene pool in countries such as the United States or Great Britain is unlikely to have changed dramatically within a few decades. There is therefore widespread agreement among researchers that changes in the environment that facilitate overeating and inhibit physical activity have contributed to the steep increase in obesity observed in industrialized countries during the past few decades (e.g., Brownell, 2002; French, Story, & Jeffery, 2001; Hill, Wyatt, Reed, & Peters, 2003; Horgen & Brownell, 2002). As Brownell (2002) stated succinctly,

> the epidemic of obesity seen in the United States, and increasingly so in other countries, is caused by the environment. Genetic and psychosocial factors may determine who in a given population is susceptible to a damaging environment, but the number of people affected, and hence the public health burden, is dictated by the environment. (p. 433)

Support for the assumption that the kind of food-rich environment that is prevalent in the United States and in most Western industrialized countries encourages obesity is found in studies of ethnic groups who left their homeland to move to the United States. For example, the body mass index (BMI) of people from Japan (Curb & Marcus, 1991) or Pima Indians (Ravussin, Valencia, Esparza, Bennett, & Schulz, 1994) who moved to the United States is substantially higher than that of people who stayed in their homelands. But the question of concern here is not whether the environment in the United States or in other industrialized countries encourages overconsumption but why obesity rates have risen so dramatically since the 1980s. After all, most Americans were living quite well even before the start of the "obesity epidemic," but they were not exactly thin, either. Although obesity rates in the United States remained stable at 15% for several decades before suddenly taking off in the mid-1980s, 15% was (and still is) a comparably high rate. Even today the prevalence of obesity is below 15% in many European and Asian countries (see Figure 2.1). Thus, the United States had an obesity problem even before the start of the so-called epidemic, just a much less dramatic one. However, the question remains as to why obesity rates that had remained stable for many decades suddenly increased so dramatically.

In this chapter, I examine the environmental changes that have contributed to the sudden increase in obesity rates. These changes can be categorized into two groups of environmental factors, namely the increase in the availability, marketing, and consumption of high-calorie food and soft drinks and a decrease in physical activity. I begin the discussion by exploring the increased consumption and current culture of fast food, larger portion sizes, soft drinks, and snacking. Then I look more closely at the marketing of high-calorie products and current environmental inhibitors of physical activity.

ENVIRONMENTAL FACILITATORS OF ENERGY INTAKE

The factors that contributed to this increase in obesity prevalence have to be environmental changes that (a) have theoretical plausibility as contributors to weight gain and (b) have accelerated sharply since the 1980s when obesity rates began their steep incline. Research attention has focused on behavioral factors that either increase calorie intake or decrease the need or opportunity for physical exertion and has disregarded less obvious factors such as the decline in smoking rates or the increased use of psychotropic medicine that could also have had an impact (for an exception, see Keith et al., 2006). The most likely suspects with regard to the rise in calorie intake are fast food, snacking, and soft drinks combined with increased portion and container sizes (e.g., French, Story, & Jeffery, 2001; Nestle, 2002). It is easily demonstrated that fast food chains are expanding, that fast food and eating out have become increasingly popular, that portion sizes of commercial foods and drinks in the United States are becoming bigger and bigger, and that soft drink consumption is rapidly increasing (French et al., 2001). What is more difficult to demonstrate is whether there is a causal link between these developments and the long-term increase in obesity.

The fact that consumption of fast food or soft drinks increased substantially during the past few decades at a rate that appeared to parallel the increase in overweight and obesity is suggestive of a causal relationship but in no way conclusive. It demonstrates that these factors could potentially have contributed to the increase in overweight and obesity, but it does not really prove it (for a discussion of criteria to establish mediation, see Baron & Kenny, 1986; Kenny, Kashy, & Bolger, 1998). Let me use the increased popularity of fast food as an example. To demonstrate that the increased popularity of fast food is indeed one of the factors contributing to the obesity epidemic, one has to show (a) that there was indeed a sharp increase in the popularity of fast food, (b) that this increase is correlated with the historical or long-term increase in rates of obesity, (c) that the frequency of eating in fast food restaurants is correlated with increases in calorie intake, (d) that increases in calorie intake are related to the long-term increase in overweight and obesity, and (e) that statistically controlling for changes in calorie intake reduces or eliminates the impact of the increased popularity of fast food restaurants on weight gain.[1] Finally, however, one would need randomized controlled intervention studies that demonstrate that interventions aimed at reducing fast food consumption were successful in reducing consumption with resulting weight loss. Because the increase in calorie intake appears to be the common pathway linking all of the suspected determinants to increases in overweight and obesity, I begin my discussion with a review of the evidence for this association.

Long-Term Trends in Calorie Intake and Obesity

The picture that emerges from surveys based on dietary self-reports about long-term trends in energy intake in the United States has been equivocal. Two recent analyses of large nationally representative samples found total energy intake to have increased from 1971 to 2000 (Briefel & Johnson, 2004) or from 1977 to 1991 (Nielsen, Siega-Riz, & Popkin, 2002), whereas a third review based on different U.S. survey data reported a slight decline in total energy intake between 1987 and 1992 (Norris et al., 1997). In Great Britain the National Food Survey (renamed "Expenditure & Food Survey" since 2002) also found total energy intake to have declined by nearly 500 kilocalories per day from 1974 to 2005 (Department for Environment, Food and Rural Affairs

---

[1]Because the various factors (e.g., frequency of visits to fast food restaurants and soft drink consumption) are likely to be highly correlated, one would have to test the set of suspected determinants simultaneously in a multivariate design.

[DEFRA], 2006). These British data are particularly puzzling, given that this marked decrease occurred when Britain was experiencing a steep increase in rates of overweight and obesity.

Two issues need to be considered in evaluating this discrepancy. First, average energy intake of a country should be related to average BMI rather than obesity rates (i.e., an extreme group). As I discussed in the previous chapter, average weight in the United States has increased much less than obesity rates have. However, even though the discrepancy is less marked, the 10% increase in average BMI would still be inconsistent with the apparent decrease in average energy intake reported by Norris et al. (1997). This inconsistency raises a second issue, namely the extent to which data based on self-reported calorie intake can be trusted. As discussed earlier, self-reported dietary information is seriously biased, and such biases increase with increasing BMI (e.g., Braam, Ocké, Bueno-de-Mesquita, & Seidell, 1998). People underreport their dietary intake, partly out of genuine forgetfulness but also to conceal dietary habits that they may perceive as unhealthy or overindulgent (Prentice & Jebb, 1999). Underreporting is therefore particularly marked for fat intake. It is also substantial. A recent study found that elimination of 42% of the respondents in a sample because of calorie intake reports deemed as biologically implausible (mostly underreports) strengthened the relationship between dietary factors and BMI (Huang, Roberts, Howarth, & McCrory, 2005). Thus, although the total eating frequency per day, meal energy density, and snack frequency per day were unrelated to BMI for the total sample, significant positive relationships emerged once the responses of 42% of respondents had been removed.[2]

In defense of dietary self-reports, one could argue that the bias resulting from underreporting of food intake should remain the same at all points of measurement and that time trends might still give a valid picture, even though absolute numbers cannot be trusted. However, although people might not have become more forgetful during the past few decades, the social pressures toward healthier eating certainly increased considerably during this time period. Thus, unhealthy eaters are likely to have become much more concerned about their eating habits, and the tendency to underreport total calorie intake as well as fat intake is likely to have increased. Consistent with this assumption, a study conducted in Denmark found a substantial increase

---

[2]The criterion of biological plausibility to eliminate survey respondents has to be handled with great care, lest researchers support their biological theories by eliminating all respondents who do not fit them. Huang et al. (2005) used data from the Institute of Medicine (2002) on the relationship between BMI and energy expenditure measured objectively (using the doubly labeled water method) as a benchmark for the validity of their own method. They found that the regression slope of reported energy intake and BMI for their total sample differed significantly from the regression between objectively measured total energy expenditure and BMI calculated by the Institute of Medicine. This difference disappeared when only the reported energy intake of the reduced sample was entered into the regression.

in underreporting bias in 1993 and 1994 compared with 1987 and 1988 (Heitmann, Lissner, & Osler, 2000).

It is therefore informative to compare these self-report data with ecological data reflecting the quantities and types of foods and nutrients available in the United States over the past few decades. Per capita availability of food supply represents the amount of food available for possible consumption rather than the amount of food people actually eat. Because some of the food is wasted or spoiled during the marketing process or in the home, food supply figures overestimate actual consumption (Harnack, Jeffery, & Boutelle, 2000; U.S. Department of Agriculture, 2000). However, if one assumes that food spoilage or wastage remains the same over time, these food supply data should be useful indicators of long-term trends in consumption. On the basis of per capita energy availability estimates from the U.S. Department of Agriculture's U.S. Food Supply Series, Harnack et al. (2000) estimated that total energy availability increased by 15% between 1970 and 1994. According to the U.S. Department of Agriculture (2000), calories from food supply, adjusted for spoilage and waste, increased from 2,220 per person per day in 1970 to 2,680 in 1997, an increase of 460 kilocalories per day. Food supply data for Great Britain suggest that average daily calorie intake between 1982 and 1997 increased by 164 kilocalories.[3]

The findings reported by Harnack et al. (2000) and the U.S. Department of Agriculture (2000) show a substantial increase in U.S. food supply for the period during which obesity rates also increased. Although their results suggest that the increase in energy intake parallels the increase in the prevalence of overweight or obesity, their findings give no indication of the extent of that association. A recent cross-national study by Silventoinen et al. (2004) estimated the association between increases in energy intake and obesity. These authors related data about trends in obesity in 21 European and non-European countries (including the United States, China, and Australia) to estimates of the per capita energy supply from all caloric sweeteners and total fat for these countries. The time trends in obesity were derived from three surveys conducted as part of the World Health Organization MONICA project (the acronym stands for Multinational MONItoring of Trends and Determinants in CArdiovascular Disease) on independent cross-sectional samples in each of these countries.[4] The estimates of changes in energy supply were based on information from the Food Balance Sheets of the Food and Agriculture Orga-

---

[3]These food supply data were obtained by Silventoinen et al. (2004) from the Food Balance Sheets of the Food and Agriculture Organization of the United Nations for the study described later. I am grateful to K. Silventoinen for making these data available to me.

[4]As the authors acknowledge, the MONICA data are based on samples that are limited with regard to both region and age range (35–64 years). Because the data are not representative for the various countries, they are not completely comparable to the food supply data, which refer to whole countries and the entire age spectrum.

nization of the United Nations. Changes in energy supply in these countries were correlated with changes in BMI (correlation of .61 for all sweeteners and .68 for total fat). The long-term trends in total energy supply per capita explained 41% of the differences between populations in the changes observed in BMI. Taking the prevalence of smoking into account resulted in a further 10% increase in explained variance.

This is persuasive support for the assumption that the long-term increase in obesity is partly due to an increase in energy intake. The findings further indicate that success in fighting the war against smoking aggravated the weight problem. However, such ecological comparisons are based on methodologically weak designs and are susceptible to confounding. Psychologists would have preferred evidence from individual data relating dietary intake to weight changes over time. However, the inconsistency in findings of U.S. surveys of dietary intake as well as the evidence that a substantial proportion of respondents who participate in such surveys give responses that are biologically implausible raises serious doubts about the validity of dietary self-reports. Because the use of objective measures is too intrusive and too expensive to use on large samples, we will have to be satisfied with food supply data as the most valid indicator of energy intake.

Fast Food

In his bestselling book *Fast Food Nation*, Schlosser (2002) gave a graphic description of the pervasiveness of our exposure to fast food:

> Over the last three decades, fast food has infiltrated every nook and cranny of American society. An industry that began with a handful of modest hot dog and hamburger stands in southern California has spread to every corner of the nation, selling a broad range of foods wherever paying customers may be found. Fast food is now served at restaurants and drive-throughs, at stadiums, airports, zoos, high schools, elementary schools, and universities, on cruise ships, trains, and airplanes, at K-Marts, Wal-Marts, gas stations, and even at hospital cafeterias. (p. 3)

Fast food did not remain an exclusively American experience. In fact, some of the biggest U.S. chains such as McDonald's and KFC are now earning the majority of their profits outside the United States. McDonald's opened its first European restaurants in 1971 in the Netherlands. The company now has 31,000 restaurants in more than 100 countries (McDonald's, 2007). In Great Britain, McDonald's opened its first restaurant in 1974. Today more than 1,250 restaurants serve more than 2.5 million meals every day in that country.

In the United States, fast food is now offered increasingly as school meals (Nestle, 2002). Although British schools do not seem to have franchised their school meals yet, they sell French fries, hamburgers, and other fried food items prepared by outside caterers. As the young television chef Jamie Oliver disclosed on his TV show *Jamie's School Dinners*, many British children do not even recognize the tastes of vegetables and fruit. On the basis of the program's success, Oliver launched a campaign that was successful in pressuring the British government into introducing higher nutritional standards to British schools.

Most studies of changes in food habits in the United States distinguish between home-prepared food and food prepared away from home, regardless of whether the food prepared away is consumed in a restaurant or eaten at home. Americans now eat food prepared away from home slightly more than 200 times a year, and three fourths of these meals are supplied by fast food restaurants (Tillotson, 2004). Nearly half of the nation's food dollars in 1999 were spent on food prepared away from home (Guthrie, Biing-Hwan, & Frazao, 2002). In Great Britain, the market for food prepared away has grown by a staggering £10 billion ($15 billion) in 10 years (Wintour, 2003). Furthermore, between 1995 and 2004, the expenditure on food eaten out in Great Britain increased from 21% of total expenditure on food to 27% (DEFRA, 2006). It is likely that there was an even greater increase in consumption of take-out food and ready-made meals bought from supermarkets, but unfortunately this information is not available because in the United Kingdom, statistics on food prepared away but eaten at home is subsumed under household consumption (DEFRA, 2006). Yet, from 1990 to 2000 alone, the purchase of convenience food rose by 24% (Select Committee on Health, 2004). Thus, the change in food habits occurred mostly during the period in which the dramatic increase in obesity rates was observed. Because most of the food prepared away from home is fast food, I use the latter term in my review of the literature.

Several factors contributed to the increased popularity of eating out at restaurants and eating food prepared away from home. One important reason is that the percentage of women who joined the workforce and therefore had less time for the preparation of meals doubled between 1950 and 1999 (French et al., 2001). A second factor is technological innovation such as vacuum packing, improved preservatives, deep freezing, and microwaves that have made it possible for food manufacturers to prepare food centrally and ship it to consumers for rapid consumption (Cutler, Glaeser, & Shapiro, 2003). A third factor is the relatively low price of fast food or ready-made meals made possible by the industrialization of food production and the low wages paid to employees at fast food restaurants (Schlosser, 2002).[5] A fourth factor is that the major fast food chains spend enormous amounts on advertising.

---

[5]In fact, all food prices, whether at the store or at the restaurant, have been declining relative to prices of all other items. According to the U.S. Department of Agriculture Economic Research Service (2005), the ratio of food prices to the price of other goods has fallen by 22%.

Food prepared away from home has a higher fat content than does food prepared at home (38% vs. 31%; Guthrie et al., 2002). It has been estimated that if food prepared away had the same fat content in 1995 as food prepared at home, Americans would have consumed nearly 200 calories per day less (French et al., 2001). To be fair to the food industry it should be pointed out that they would not offer what they do if there were no demand. Thus, when many fast food chains, in response to public pressure, began to add lower calorie, healthier options to their menus, they soon discovered that these options did not sell well. (They were not all that low in fat content and calories, either.) Even the Jamie Oliver revolution that led to the replacement of burgers and French fries by healthier meals, including fresh fruits and vegetables, resulted in a decrease of the number of children having school meals by between 9% and 12%, according to a survey conducted by the BBC (Farrington, 2006) among catering contract managers in 2005. In an article with the headline "Jamie May Have Spelled End of School Meals," Liz Lightfood (2007), the education editor of the British national newspaper *Daily Telegraph*, warned that the school meal service in England may be facing a collapse because children are shunning healthy menus. In some places this passive resistance appeared to have even turned into open revolt. As the South Yorkshire newspaper *The Star* reported under the headline "Mums in Burger Backlash Over Healthy Eating" (2006), two angry mothers in the Yorkshire village of Rawmarsh delivered fish and chips, pies, and burgers to hungry children at the local school because pupils were turning up their noses at the "low fat rubbish" served at their school.

Evidence from cross-sectional as well as longitudinal research links consumption of fast food to increased body weight. Thus, in a survey of a small sample of men and women, McCrory et al. (1999) found that the frequency of consuming fast food was positively associated with body fatness. After physical activity was controlled for, this association increased from $r = .36$ to $r = .42$. Similar results were reported by Bowman and Vinyard (2004), who used data from a large national survey. They found that individuals who reported consumption of fast food on the day they were interviewed had a 27% higher chance of being overweight than did individuals who had not eaten fast food on that day. Finally, a small study of children and adolescents conducted in Canada found that in comparison with the group of individuals who were not obese, the respondents who were obese consumed more fast food and sugar-sweetened drinks and overall had a higher energy intake (2,720 kilocalories compared with 2,143 kilocalories; Gillis & Bar-Or, 2003).

These findings have been replicated in several longitudinal studies. O. M. Thompson et al. (2004) found that a small sample of adolescent girls who ate fast food twice a week at baseline had a greater mean increase in BMI z-score 6 years later than did the girls who ate fast food once a week or not at all. There was also a marginally significant difference in total energy intake at baseline between the two groups. Similar results were reported by Taveras et al. (2005), who conducted a 3-year longitudinal study of a sample of more than 16,000 boys and girls aged 9 to 14 years at baseline. Participants were interviewed each year and asked how often they consumed fast food. Boys and girls who had increased their consumption of fast food from "never or once a week" the previous year to "4 to 7 times a week" had gained significantly more weight a year later than did children whose consumption of fast food remained stable at less than once a week. Participants who frequently ate fast food also showed a higher intake of total energy and a greater consumption of sugar-sweetened beverages than did those who consumed fast food infrequently or not at all. Finally, the relationship between increasing consumption of fast food and weight gain was partially mediated by total energy intake.

It is not surprising that frequenting fast food establishments is also related to weight gain in adults. French, Harnack, and Jeffery (2000) assessed frequency of fast food restaurant use and body weight in 891 women of normal weight who participated in a 3-year intervention study aimed at weight maintenance. Women who reported an increase in fast food restaurant use during the 3-year period showed an increase in body weight. On average, an increase of one fast food meal per week was associated with an increase of 56 kilocalories per day and a weight gain of 0.72 kilograms (1.6 pounds) over the 3-year period, above the average weight gain of 1.68 kilograms (3.7 pounds) that was observed for the whole group. On a larger scale, the CARDIA (the acronym stands for "Coronary Artery Risk Development in Young Adults") Study, in which approximately 3,000 young adults were followed for a period of 15 years, found that individuals who ate at fast food restaurants more than twice a week gained 4.5 kilograms (9.9 pounds) more than did individuals who ate there less than once a week (Pereira et al., 2005). Finally, a large 2-year longitudinal study conducted in Spain also found a positive relationship between fast food consumption and weight gain (Bes-Rastrollo et al., 2006).

What can be concluded from these findings? Do they really show that the consumption of fast food leads to weight gain and that increased fast food consumption is a major cause of the obesity epidemic? Because people who eat fast food are likely to engage in other poor eating habits, fast food consumption may only be a marker for a generally unhealthy lifestyle, and these findings might overestimate the role of fast food. However, it could also be argued that the average weight gains reported by French et al. (2000) and Pereira et al. (2005) underestimate the problem. Because individuals are expected to vary in their disposition to gain weight, one would expect even greater weight gain among individuals with a disposition to overweight and obesity. Such individuals are more likely to consume larger portions than are individuals of normal weight on each visit to a fast food restaurant and less likely to compensate for this indulgence by reducing their calorie intake at their next meal.

Support for the latter assumption comes from a random controlled intervention study by Ebbeling et al. (2004), who fed participants who were overweight and those who were of normal weight an extra-large fast food meal in naturalistic settings. Participants were instructed to eat as much as they liked during the 1-hour meal. All participants ate more than 60% of their estimated daily energy needs, but individuals who were overweight consumed even more (1,860 kilocalories) than did the participants who were lean (1,458 kilocalories). Furthermore, dietary interviews taken on a day with the fast food meal and on a day without a fast food meal revealed that unlike participants who were lean, participants who were overweight did not compensate: Their total calorie intake was 409 kilocalories higher on fast food days compared with normal days. In contrast, there was no significant difference between the 2 days in the calorie intake of individuals who were lean. Ebbeling et al. (2004) concluded that "these findings suggest that . . . fast food consumption serves to maintain or exacerbate obesity in susceptible individuals" (p. 2832).

Increase in Portion Size

In combination with an increase in fast food consumption, portion sizes in commercial foods and drinks have dramatically increased in the United States as well. According to one survey, they increased between 1977 and 1998 for all key foods except pizza (Nielsen & Popkin, 2003). During this period, the average energy intake and portion size of salty snacks increased for the total U.S. population from 132 to 225 kilocalories, the average soft drink from 144 to 193 kilocalories, and the average cheeseburger from 397 to 533 kilocalories (Nielsen & Popkin, 2003). These estimates based on self-report data are consistent with information collected by Young and Nestle (2002) from manufacturers. According to Young and Nestle, portion sizes began to grow in the 1970s and have continued to grow in parallel with the increase in obesity rates (see Figure 4.1).

There is ample evidence that the portion size of food has a direct impact on the amount that is consumed. For example, Rolls, Morris, and Roe (2002) served their participants on 4 separate days in a laboratory setting portions of macaroni and cheese that ranged from 500 grams (17.5 ounces) to 1,000 grams (35.0 ounces). Participants consumed 30% more energy (161 kilocalories) when offered the largest compared with the smallest portion. This finding was replicated in a cafeteria on a university campus (Diliberti, Bordi, Conklin, Roe, & Rolls, 2004). Researchers covertly recorded the food intake of customers who purchased a baked pasta dish at lunch. On 5 days, the standard portion size was increased by 50%. Consistent with the findings of the laboratory studies, Diliberti et al. (2004) found that participants who purchased the larger portion increased their energy intake from the pasta dish by 43% (172 kilocalories).

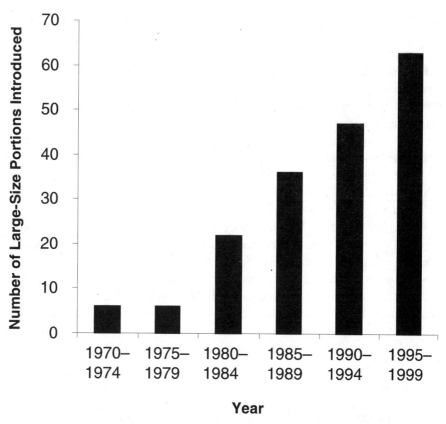

Figure 4.1. Introduction of new, larger portions between 1977 and 1999. From "The Contribution of Expanding Portion Sizes to the US Obesity Epidemic," by L. R. Young and M. Nestle, 2002, *American Journal of Public Health, 92,* p. 248. Copyright 2002 by the American Public Health Association. Reprinted with permission.

To see whether the package size of snacks would have the same effect as portion size at mealtime, Rolls, Roe, Kral, Meengs, and Wall (2004) conducted a laboratory study in which participants came to the laboratory at 3 p.m. for a snack session. They were given a pack of potato chips ranging from 28 to 170 grams (1.0 to 6.0 ounces) with the instruction to eat as many of the chips as they liked. Three hours later, participants returned to the laboratory to eat a meal. Calorie intake from snacks increased significantly with increasing package size. When served the largest compared with the smallest snack, participants consumed on average 143 kilocalories more. Furthermore, they did not compensate by eating less at dinnertime.

It is interesting to speculate about the reasons for the impact of portion size on consumption. One reason could be socialization. Most people have been socialized to clean their plates and might be reluctant to waste food. However, this cannot be the only reason, because portion size affected amount eaten, even when participants who totally cleaned their plates were removed from the analysis. Another possibility could be that with tasty food, it might be difficult to stop before the plate is nearly clean or the bag is empty (in the case of potato chips). However, this possibility could not explain the findings of a study that showed that portion size affected amount eaten even with disliked food (Wansink & Kim, 2005). Moviegoers who were given either medium- or large-sized containers of popcorn, which was either fresh or 2 weeks old and stale, ate considerably more popcorn from the large container. However, taste did affect amount consumed. There was a main effect for taste, with people on average eating less of the stale popcorn. There was also a Taste × Container Size interaction. Container size induced less overeating with the stale (33.6% increase) than with the fresh (45.3% increase) popcorn.

Wansink and van Ittersum (2007) saw two processes as responsible for the portion size effect. First, portion size influences consumption norms. People are flexible in the amount they can eat, and portion size is likely to help them define the size of a reasonable meal. A supersized portion is likely to result in an upward shift of the consumption norm, particularly for people who do not pay much attention to how much they are eating. Second, there is evidence that people systematically underestimate the calorie content of large portions compared with that of smaller portions (Wansink & Chandon, 2006).

Snacking

For exposure to snack food to qualify as an environmental contributor to the overweight and obesity epidemic, people's exposure during the 1980s and 1990s would have had to substantially increase. Evidence suggests that this may have been the case, at least in the United States, and probably also in Europe (Gallo, 1997; McCrory et al., 1999). There was a dramatic increase in the number of candy and snack products (see Figure 4.2) and of high-calorie bakery products introduced into the U.S. market during the 1980s (Gallo, 1997).

Surveys of eating behavior indicate a substantial increase in snacking for the same time period. On the basis of a series of representative cross-sectional surveys of eating behavior of American children and adolescents (2 to 18 years old), Adair and Popkin (2005) found that calorie intake from snacks had increased from 204.2 kilocalories per day in 1977 to 409.6 kilocalories per day in 1996. Findings of cross-sectional representative surveys of young adults (19 to 29 years old) essentially confirm this picture (Zizza, Siega-Riz, & Popkin, 2001). The overall prevalence of snacking had increased between 1977 and 1996 and so had the contribution of snacks to total daily energy intake of snackers (from 20% to 23%). Similar trends can be observed in Great Britain, where within a period of 5 years (1993–1998) the sales of snacks to adults more than tripled (Select Committee on Health, 2004, ¶82).

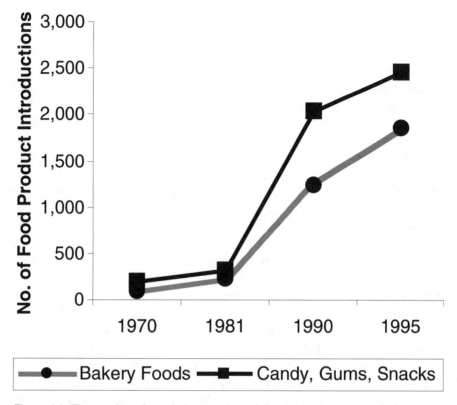

Figure 4.2. The number of new bakery and snack foods introduced in the U.S. market. Data from Gallo (1997).

Yet, the evidence pointing at snacking as a major culprit for the obesity epidemic is not conclusive. One problem that hampers research efforts on this topic is the confusion surrounding the definition of what constitutes a snack: Some scientific definitions of snacks include beverages (e.g., Zizza et al., 2001), and others do not (e.g., Cross, Babicz, & Cushman, 1994). Even dictionaries do not agree on this issue. Whereas the *Oxford American Dictionary* (2005) defined *snack* as "a small amount of food eaten between meals," *Webster's Encyclopedic Unabridged Dictionary of the English Language* (1989) defined *snack* as "a small portion of food or drink." (Both dictionaries added a second meaning of snack: "a light meal that is eaten in a hurry or a casual manner" [*Oxford*] and "between regular meals" [*Webster's*].) These differences are not trivial. If drinks are included in the category of "snacks," they account for a substantial proportion of total amount of snacks consumed. For example, in Zizza et al.'s (2001) survey, regular soft drinks constituted 12.1% of the snacks consumed in 1995, and alcoholic drinks accounted for another 12.4%. In light of the high calorie content of these beverages, including them in the category of snacks will considerably boost the percentage of energy from snacks that is being consumed compared with surveys that exclude beverages from the category of snacks.

Leaving it up to the respondents to define what they consider a snack would seem to offer a convenient way out of this dilemma. The problem with this strategy is that its validity depends on the extent to which respondents agree in their definitions. If respondents differ widely in their interpretation of the concept of "having a snack," their answers will be difficult to interpret. And the possibility of a great deal of variation in people's understanding of the meaning of the concept has been demonstrated in a study by Chamontin, Pretzer, and Booth (2003), who asked three samples of staff and students of a major British university to describe the last occasion when they (a) "had a snack," (b) were "snacking," or (c) "were eating snack food." The answers confirmed the authors' suspicion that "a 'snack' is a term that refers to different eating habits from 'snacking' and that neither pattern of behavior necessarily involves 'snack food' " (p. 21). As Mela and Rogers (1998) pointed out, "many foods such as fruits, yoghurts, and sandwiches are commonly eaten as 'snacks,' yet are not usually perceived or implied by the term 'snack food' " (p. 117).[6]

In light of this variety of interpretations of the meaning of the concept, it is not surprising that epidemiological studies, which mostly related respondent-defined snack-eating frequency to weight gain or obesity, resulted in conflicting findings. Although some studies found a positive link between frequency of snacking and BMI or obesity (e.g., Basdevant, Craplet, & Guy-Grand, 1993; Bertéus Forslund, Torgerson, Sjöström, & Lindroos, 2005; Elgar, Roberts, Moore, & Tudor-Smith, 2005; Howarth, Huang, Roberts, Lin, & McCrory, 2007; Levitsky, Halbmeyer, & Mrdjenovic, 2004), others did not (e.g., Dreon et al., 1988; Field et al., 2004; French, Jeffery, & Murray, 1999; Gatenby, Anderson, Walker, Southon, & Mela, 1994; Hampl, Heaton, & Taylor, 2003; Hawkins, 1979; K. J. Morgan, Johnson, & Stampley, 1983; Phillips et al., 2004; Ruxton, Kirk, & Belton, 1996).

A cross-sectional study that compared a large sample of men and women with obesity to a sample of individuals of normal weight in Sweden reported that the group of obese individuals consumed (self-defined) snacks more frequently than did the comparison group and that energy intake increased with increasing snacking frequency (Bertéus et al., 2005). Similarly, a study conducted in France among 173 women with obesity found that both daily energy intake and mealtime intake among "snackers" were higher than among "non-snackers" (Basdevant et al., 1993). Individuals were classified as "snackers" when they ate between their usual times for meals and when snacking was

---

[6]If one finds differences in the understanding of these terms even within one culture, one wonders about the validity of the cross-cultural comparisons among Chinese, Russian, and Philippine Islander participants reported by Adair and Popkin (2005).

responsible for at least 15% of their daily intake. Finally, two longitudinal studies reported an association between snacking and BMI or weight gain. Elgar et al. (2005), who followed a cohort of 355 adolescents for a period of 4 years, found the number of snacks consumed per day at intake predictive of BMI 4 years later. Similarly, in a longitudinal study of predictors of weight gain among 68 1st-year university students during the first 12 weeks, Levitsky et al. (2004) found that evening snacks (self-defined) accounted for approximately 12% of the variance in weight gain (average weight gain: 2.4 kilograms [5.3 pounds]).

In contrast, Hampl et al. (2003), who used dietary recall data (2 nonconsecutive days) from 1,756 men and 1,511 women in a cross-sectional study, found no association between people who snacked (self-defined) and those who did not, even though multiple snackers had a significantly higher energy intake (2,535 kilocalories) than did individuals who never snacked (2,043 kilocalories). Similarly, Hawkins (1979), who investigated the self-defined "meal" and "snack" frequencies of 240 students who were either of normal weight or overweight, found no association between overweight and snack frequency. Negative results were also reported by Dreon et al. (1988), who took 7-day dietary records from 155 sedentary men with obesity. In this study, snacks were defined by designated time periods (postbreakfast, postlunch, postdinner). Their findings did not indicate any relation between body fatness and number of meals or snacks. A study of 75 adults also failed to find an association between measures of fatness and the total frequency of self-defined "meals" or "snacks" (Gatenby et al., 1994). Two longitudinal studies of adolescents also reported negative results (Field et al., 2004; Phillips et al., 2004). A 3-year longitudinal study of 8,203 girls and 6,774 boys (aged 9 to 14 at intake) found that "snack food was not a meaningful predictor of change in BMI z-score among children from lean or overweight mothers" (Field et al., 2004, p. 1214). Eating of snacks was measured with a 22-item list of snack foods, and participants consumed between 300 and 400 kilocalories per day from snacks. Similar negative findings were reported in a longitudinal study of 132 girls who were 8 to 12 years old at intake and were followed up until 4 years after menarche. Eating of snacks was measured with a snack list, and the girls consumed approximately 14% of their daily calorie intake from snack food (Phillips et al., 2004).

Since the confusion surrounding the definition of what constitutes a snack is likely to be exacerbated by a tendency of overweight and obese individuals to underreport eating energy-dense snacks, it is not surprising that the evidence on snacking and weight gain is equivocal. However, the failure of many studies to observe a relationship between snacking and weight gain could be the result of compensatory adjustment of energy intake. People might intentionally or automatically compensate in their main meals for the energy they consume as snacks. The evidence of such compensatory adjustment of energy intake following a snack is mixed, with some studies demonstrating compensatory adjustment (Johnstone, Shannon, Whybrow, Reid, & Stubbs, 2000) but others failing to do so (e.g., Marmonier, Chapelot, Fantino, & Louis-Sylvestre, 2001; Porrini et al., 1997). A potential reason for this inconsistency could be that even automatic adjustment processes need to be learned; they occur only after participants have repeatedly experienced the snack food offered. Thus, in a study in which young boys were offered the same high- or low-calorie version of an afternoon snack before dinner for several days, Louis-Sylvestre, Tournier, Verger, Chabert, and Delorme (1989) found that their respondents did not compensate during the first few days but that after several days, precise caloric adjustment occurred. Similarly, an experimental study in which participants had to supplement their diet with commercial snack products for a period of 2 weeks found that individuals who habitually consumed these type of snack products compensated better than those who were not used to eating such snacks (Whybrow, Mayer, Kirk, Mazlan, & Stubbs, 2007).

Soft Drink Consumption

In less than a quarter of a century (1977 to 2001), Americans more than doubled the proportion of total energy obtained from soft drinks (Nielsen & Popkin, 2003). Although soft drinks already accounted for 3.9% of total energy in 1977, this percentage had increased to 9.2% by 2001 (Nielsen & Popkin, 2003). During this period, the daily calorie intake from soft drinks increased from 70 to 166 kilocalories. There is evidence to suggest, however, that the recent increase may be only the continuation of a long-term trend. Between 1947 and 1995, the per capita consumption of carbonated soft drinks increased in the United States from just over 10 to more than 50 gallons per year. At the same time, milk consumption dropped nearly by half (U.S. Department of Agriculture, 2000).

Several environmental changes could have contributed to the most recent increase in calories from soft drink consumption. First, the mid-1980s witnessed an explosion in introductions of new beverages just as it did with new snack foods (Gallo, 1997). Second, and probably more important, the container sizes in which soft drinks were being sold were increased. For example, in 1916 Coca-Cola was sold in 6.5-ounce (0.19-liter) bottles. Then the 12-ounce (0.36-liter) bottle was introduced, which has now been replaced by the 20-ounce (0.59-liter) bottle as the standard size sold from vending machines and convenience stores (French et al., 2001). Even a 12-ounce can contains about 40 grams of sugar and 154 kilocalories, but the other ingredients have so little nutritional value that it has been referred to as "liquid candy" (Nestle, 2002).

In a recent review of 15 cross-sectional and 10 prospective cohort studies of the association between soft drinks and weight gain, mostly conducted in the United States and focusing on children and adolescents, Malik, Schulze, and Hu (2006) concluded that there was a positive association between intake of sugar-sweetened soft drinks and obesity in both children and adults. Consistent with these epidemiological findings, several experimental studies showed that participants who were randomly assigned to consume drinks with caloric (rather than artificial) sweeteners showed a significant increase in body weight (Raben, Vassilareas, Moller, & Astrup, 2002; Tordoff & Alleva, 1990). Finally, a British school-based randomized controlled educational intervention resulted in a decrease in soft drink consumption in the intervention group (James, Thomas, Cavan, & Kerr, 2004). Whereas obesity rates increased in the control group (7.5%), there was a slight decrease in the prevalence of obesity in the intervention group (−0.2%). According to the review of Malik et al. (2006), in epidemiological studies, regular soft drink consumption appears to be associated with a 50% to 100% increase in the risk of becoming overweight or obese.

The major mechanism linking soft drink consumption to weight gain and obesity risk is lack of compensation (e.g., Mattes, 1996). People do not eat less because they have had a Coke with their meal. In fact, compensation for calories ingested in liquid form is much poorer than that for calories ingested in solid form (DiMeglio & Mattes, 2000). This lack of compensation has been demonstrated experimentally by Mattes (1996), who induced his research participants to drink just over a liter of cola on several test days with their midday meal. Dietary records indicated that participants ate as much food on test days as on nontest days.

In summary, then, the consumption of sugar-sweetened soft drinks in the United States has increased substantially during the past 2 decades, adding nearly 100 kilocalories to the daily energy intake of the average American. If people had compensated for the added calories by decreasing their calorie intake from other nutrients, this change would have been weight neutral. However, because of a pervasive failure to compensate for the added calorie intake, soft drink consumption is likely to be a major contributor to the long-term increase in body weight.

The Marketing of Fast Food, Snacks, and Soft Drinks

The increase in the sales of fast food, snack products, and soft drinks has been facilitated by the gigantic advertising budgets of the food industry, and television has been the mass medium of choice (Brownell & Horgen, 2004). The reasons for this are simple. TV has great reach. Television sets are present in virtually every household in the United States (French et al., 2001). Furthermore, between 1965 and 1985, television viewing time increased by 44% in the United States. In Britain, it doubled from 1963 to 1993 (Fox, 1999). By the mid-1990s, both the average American and the average Briton spent 3 to 4 hours per day watching television, and American children spent more time watching television than doing anything else apart from sleeping (Brownell & Horgen, 2004). It is therefore not surprising that the food industry invests a sizable part of its advertising budgets in television advertisements—and these budgets are gigantic. For every $1 spent by the World Health Organization to improve the nutrition of the world's population, $500 is spent by the food industry on advertising processed food (International Association of Consumer Food Organizations [IACFO], 2003).

Content analyses of advertisements shown during prime-time television reflect the effects of these investments. An analysis of 101.5 hours of prime-time television in the United States revealed that of the 3,062 advertisements that appeared during these programs, 553 (18%) were food advertisements (Henderson & Kelly, 2005). The largest proportion of these food advertisements featured fast food restaurants. Henderson and Kelly (2005) estimated that with 9.4 food advertisements appearing every hour, an individual watching 2 hours of prime-time television per day, 5 days a week, all year long could be exposed to 40 hours of food marketing over the course of the year. This estimate is very conservative given that Americans spend 3 to 4 hours every day watching television (Brownell & Horgen, 2004). However, not only are viewers of prime-time television in the United States persuaded to eat junk food through food advertisements, but their favorite prime-time actors also model this behavior in their shows. On the basis of a content analysis of occasions of eating in popular TV shows, Story and Faulkner (1990) concluded that 72% of the foods consumed in those shows were snacks eaten between meals and less than 10% of these snacks were fruits and vegetables.

There is some indication that children are exposed to an even larger percentage of food advertisements on television than are adults. An analysis conducted by Taras and Gage (1995) found that children viewed on average 21.3 commercials per hour and that food advertisements accounted for 47.8% of these commercials. Ninety-one percent of the advertised food was high in fat, sugar, or salt and thus not very healthy. Numerous studies conducted in the United States between 1970 and 2000 arrived at similar estimates (for a review, see L. M. Powell, Szczypka, & Chaloupka, 2007), but an analysis conducted in 2003–2004 found a slightly reduced but still high proportion (36%) of food advertisements (L. M. Powell et al., 2007).

Similar patterns were reported in Australia (Neville, Thomas, & Bauman, 2005) and Britain (Hastings et al., 2003). An exhaustive review of research on the effects of food promotion to children prepared for the UK Food Standards Agency in 2003 concluded that televised children's food promotions were dominated by breakfast cereals, confectionary, savory snacks, soft drinks, and fast food (Hastings et al., 2003). McDonald's, KFC, Burger King, and Pizza Hut were among the top five brands advertised in 2002, with McDonald's in first position, spending more than twice as much as the number two brand (Coca-Cola; Hastings et al., 2003).

The fact that fast food, snacks, and soft drinks are being heavily advertised on television does not necessarily imply that these advertisements are also effective in influencing behavior. However, two lines of evidence support such an association. First, there is evidence from cross-sectional and longitudinal studies that self-reported television viewing is linked to increased risk of obesity. Second, there is also evidence to show that food promotion has an effect on food preferences and purchasing behavior particularly in children. I discuss both types of evidence next.

In a large cross-sectional study conducted in the United States, Crespo et al. (2001) used data on 4,069 boys and girls from the National Health and Nutrition Examination Surveys III (NHANES III) collected between 1988 and 1994 to assess the association between self-reported hours of television watching and obesity (see Figure 4.3). Obesity was lowest among children watching TV 1 hour or less a day and increased with each additional hour of television viewing. There was also a positive relationship between total energy intake and hours of television watched, more so among girls than among boys. Girls who watched television for 5 or more hours consumed on

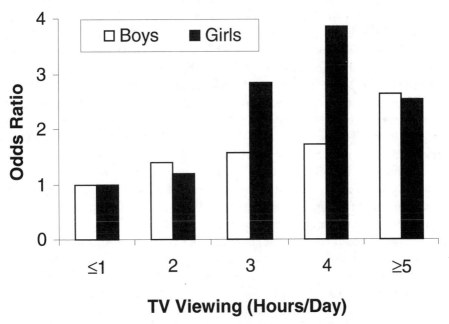

Figure 4.3. Association between television watching and obesity for U.S. boys and girls aged 8 to 16 years. From "Television Watching, Energy Intake, and Obesity in US Children," by C. J. Crespo, E. Smit, R. P. Troiano, S. J. Bartlett, C. A. Macera, and R. E. Andersen, 2001, *Archives of Pediatric and Adolescent Medicine, 155,* p. 363. Copyright © 2001 by the American Medical Association. All rights reserved. Reprinted with permission.

average 175 kilocalories more than did girls who watched television for 1 hour or less. A cross-sectional study of 1,318 Canadian schoolchildren aged 11 to 16 replicated the association between frequency of television viewing and obesity (Janssen, Katzmarzyk, Boyce, King, & Pickett, 2004). Both girls and boys with the highest viewing frequency were more than twice as likely to be obese than were children who watched very little television. The association between television viewing and BMI was replicated for adults in a large study of 14,189 men and women conducted in England in 1997 (Jakes et al., 2002). Men who watched more than 4 hours of television had a BMI that was 1.0 kg/m^2 greater than that of men who watched television for less than 2 hours. The difference between these two groups for women was 1.6 kg/m^2. Other cross-sectional studies reported similar findings (e.g., Giammattei, Blix, Marshak, Wollitzer, & Pettitt, 2006).

The association between self-reported hours of television watching and obesity risk has been replicated in several longitudinal studies (e.g., Dietz & Gortmaker, 1985; Hancox, Milne, & Poulton, 2004; Hancox & Poulton, 2004; Kaur, Choi, Mayo, & Harris, 2003; Proctor et al., 2003). In one of the larger studies, Kaur et al. (2003) used data for 3,376 adolescents to relate hours of television watching at baseline (1,993) to self-reported height and weight at follow-up (1,996). Controlling for weight at baseline, the researchers found that watching more than 2 hours of television at baseline resulted in twice the odds of being overweight at follow-up. Similar results were reported by other longitudinal studies conducted in the United States (e.g., Dietz & Gortmaker, 1985; Hu et al., 2003; Jeffery & French, 1998; Proctor et al., 2003) and Australia (Hancox et al., 2004; Hancox & Poulton, 2004).[7] The time individuals devote to TV watching or computer games in childhood and adolescence has even been found to predict obesity in adult life (e.g., Hancox et al., 2004; Viner & Cole, 2006). Thus, even though there are also some negative findings (e.g., Katzmarzyk, Malina, Song, & Bouchard, 1998; T. N. Robinson et al., 2001), the overwhelming majority of studies on this topic found self-reported television viewing to be associated with an increased risk of obesity. Furthermore, an experimental study by T. N. Robinson (1999), who reduced television viewing among children, found this reduction to be associated with weight loss. T. N. Robinson exposed 106 third- and fourth-grade students from one school to lessons to reduce television, videotape, and videogame use, with 100 students from a second school serving as an assessment-only control group. The intervention was successful in reducing television viewing, videotape, and videogame use. It also had a small but significant effect on BMI.

Yet, these findings provide only weak evidence for the effect of TV advertising on body weight, because there are at least two plausible alternative expla-

---

[7]The association between television watching and BMI tends to be stronger for girls and women than for boys and men (e.g., Hancox & Poulton, 2004; Jakes et al., 2002; Jeffery & French, 1998).

nations. First, children who spend a great deal of time watching television (or playing video games) are likely to be less physically active in general. Though the association seems obvious, the evidence on the association between television watching and physical activity is mixed. Whereas some studies have reported a small negative correlation (e.g., Crespo et al., 2001; T. N. Robinson et al., 2001), others have found no correlation (e.g., Jeffery & French, 1998; Katzmarzyk et al., 1998). Furthermore, several studies have reported an effect of television viewing on weight gain even after physical activity levels were controlled for (Janssen et al., 2004; Koh-Banerjee et al., 2003; Proctor et al., 2003).

A second alternative mechanism could be that individuals who watch a great deal of television eat more unhealthy food because they snack or even eat meals while watching TV. To demonstrate that increased food consumption during TV watching is responsible for the association between television viewing and overweight or obesity, one has to demonstrate (a) that television viewing while eating is associated with increased calorie intake and (b) that this increased calorie intake is responsible for the relationship between TV watching and BMI. Whereas there is ample support for the first assumption, there is little evidence for the second.

In an experimental test of the first assumption, Blass et al. (2006) had 20 students eat a high-calorie meal while either watching a popular TV show or listening to Rachmaninoff's Second Symphony. Watching TV had a significant impact on calorie intake. Students consumed on average 255.5 kilocalories more when watching TV than when listening to the concert. The reasons for these differences are not clear. It would seem plausible students were more distracted by TV and thus less able to cognitively control their food intake. If this had been the case, one would have expected that restrained eaters, who tend to control their consumption cognitively would have been more strongly affected by the experimental manipulation than individuals who score low on a measure of restrained eating (Boon, Stroebe, Schut, & Ijtema, 2002; Boon, Stroebe, Schut, & Jansen, 1997; see chap. 6, this volume). Although Blass et al. (2006) measured eating restraint with the Three Factor Eating Questionnaire (TFEQ; Stunkard & Messick, 1985), they did not report whether their experimental manipulation interacted with restraint. Finally, a short-term observational study among 76 undergraduate students found total energy intake to be higher on days when at least one meal was consumed while watching television compared with days without eating while viewing television (Stroebele & de Castro, 2004).

Most long-term observational studies confirm the association between television watching and increased consumption of snacks and other less healthy food but fail to demonstrate that this overconsumption contributes to obesity (e.g., Coon, Goldberg, Rogers, & Tucker, 2001; Matheson, Killen, Wang, Varady, & Robinson, 2004). For example, a study that examined the relationships between the presence of television during meals and children's food consumption found that children from families with high television use derived more of their daily energy intake from meats, pizzas, snack foods, and carbonated soft drinks and less from fruits and vegetables than did families with low television use (Coon et al., 2001). Controlling for socioeconomic status did not eliminate this association. However, the relationship between TV food consumption and BMI was not reported, and there were no significant differences in either fat intake or total calorie intake. Such differences would have been expected if the impact of television viewing on food consumption were a contributor to the obesity risk. Similar findings were reported by Matheson et al. (2004), who also failed to find significant differences between the fat content and energy density of foods consumed while viewing television compared with food consumed while not watching television. Finally, a 4-year longitudinal study of 173 White girls who were 5 years old at baseline found a positive association between snacking in front of the TV and television watching (Francis, Lee, & Birch, 2003). However, television watching predicted overweight only for girls from families in which neither parent was overweight, and snack consumption did not mediate this relationship. For girls from overweight families, daily TV viewing was unrelated to changes in BMI during the period of the study. Thus, although there can be little doubt that frequent television viewing is associated with increased calorie intake, there is little evidence that this overconsumption constitutes a risk factor for weight gain.

The fact that there is only weak support for the alternative explanations for the association between television watching and obesity tends to strengthen the case for a direct effect of advertising. Fortunately, in addition to this negative evidence, some studies directly link television advertisements to food choice and consumption. For example, Stoneman and Brody (1982) assessed the effects of children's food advertisements on influence attempts by these children when food shopping with their mothers. In two apparently unrelated studies, children and parents were first shown either a film containing food commercials (for confectionary, salty snacks, and soft drinks) or a film that contained no commercials. Afterward, the mother–child pairs were observed while shopping in a grocery store. Children exposed to the advertising tape engaged in more attempts to influence their mothers' food-buying behavior in general and particularly in attempts to influence their mothers' selection of the specific products advertised on the tape. These findings are consistent with the findings of Galst and White (1976), who reported a positive and significant association between the attentiveness of children to advertisements shown on tape during the experimental session and their subsequent behavior in the supermarket. The more attention the children had paid to the food advertisements while watching the tape, the more they tried to influence their mothers' shopping purchases in the supermarket.

Even more impressive are the findings of a recent experimental study by Halford, Gillespie, Brown, Pontin, and Dovey (2004), who exposed

42 schoolchildren ages 9 to 11 years—including both those who were obese and those who were normal weight—to cartoon films containing a collection of food and nonfood advertisements. When recognition of advertisements was tested afterward, children who were obese recognized significantly more food (but not nonfood) advertisements than did children who were of normal weight. In an ad libitum food consumption test after the video, not only did the children eat more after having been exposed to food rather than nonfood advertisements, but also, the number of food ads recognized correlated significantly with the amount of food eaten ($r = .49$).

In summary, there can be little doubt that at least for children and adolescents, food advertising on television contributes to the positive association between television viewing and overweight and obesity. Children are exposed to a great number of food advertisements on TV, and these ads influence their desire to purchase and consume the advertised food items. These food advertisements motivate children to either buy the advertised food themselves or influence their parents to buy the food or to take them to a fast food restaurant. At least in the United States, children have a great deal of money to spend themselves, and by pestering their parents, they can influence the spending of even more money. According to one estimate, U.S. children aged 4 to 12 years had a combined discretionary income of more than $27 billion per year and influenced parental spending worth $188 billion (Nestle, 2002). The situation is likely similar in Western European countries. Children in Britain enjoyed a 45% increase in pocket money between 1997 and 2001. Thus, 5- to 16-year-olds were able to spend an average of £6.53 (about $10 US) of pocket money per week in 2001 (Select Committee on Health, 2004). All of these factors may have contributed to the fact reported in chapter 2 (this volume) that, at least in the United States, the well-to-do have recently experienced the fastest increase in obesity rates.

Although they are the most important, advertisements on regular television are only one of many marketing channels by which the food industry reaches it consumers. Advertisers increasingly use schools to target children with their marketing messages (IACFO, 2003). For example, in the United States, a private TV channel (Channel One) is beamed into 12,000 participating schools, which, in exchange for allowing this, receive television sets and installation hardware (Nestle, 2002). In 80% of the classrooms, students are required to watch the program on most school days. Two minutes of every program are devoted to commercials, and food companies are particularly prominent among these advertisers (Nestle, 2002).

Another pervasive and persuasive example of marketing to children in U.S. schools are so-called "pouring rights." Pouring rights are exclusive contracts between soft drink companies and school districts that ensure that only drinks produced by that company are available to children. In return for these contracts, school districts receive large payments from these companies (IACFO, 2003; Nestle, 2002). These payments are sometimes linked to sales to encourage school administrators to influence students to increase their soft drink consumption during school hours.

Food advertisements have also increasingly made it into textbooks used in schools. For example, Brownell and Horgen (2004) found a mathematics textbook for elementary school students that used breakfast cereals, soft drinks, and chocolate snacks in their exercise examples. In the United Kingdom, many primary and secondary schools accept commercially sponsored exercise books. The books are paid for by advertisements from food companies and can therefore be given free to children (IACFO, 2003). In addition to these traditional promotion techniques, new technologies, including the Internet, e-mail, and text messages on mobile phones, allow advertisers direct access to children that is usually not monitored by parents. Even in Scandinavian countries where advertising to children is restricted, no specific rules have yet been introduced to govern this kind of marketing (IACFO, 2003).

Some Final Comments on Environmental Facilitators

The research reviewed in this section points to fast food and soft drinks as the major environmental contributors to the long-term increase in obesity. The evidence is most persuasive with regard to fast food, demonstrating clearly that in the United States, exposure to fast food increased dramatically at the same time the rate of obesity steeply increased. Concurrently, soft drink consumption also substantially increased. Both of these effects have been magnified by two marketing strategies, namely the increase in portion size and the increase in advertising, particularly advertising aimed at children. These trends have added sufficient calories to the average American diet to explain the increase in obesity even without assuming a decrease in physical activity.

However, there is evidence to suggest that the U.S. version of an environment that facilitates overconsumption is not the only road toward obesity. If this were the case, the fall of the wall in Germany in 1992 should have led to a dramatic increase in obesity among the former East Germans, who found themselves suddenly exposed to Western capitalist living, including a dramatic increase in television exposure to food advertisements and the spread of fast food chains all over the region. Instead, between 1991 and 1998, the obesity prevalence increased less for East German than for West German men and even decreased for East German women (see chap. 2, this volume; see also Benecke & Vogel, 2005). The explanation must lie in the environmental conditions that led to the high obesity rates in the German Democratic Republic (GDR) before the fall of the wall. One factor could have been the extraordinary high percentage of fat (40%) in the GDR diet (Benecke & Vogel, 2005). Furthermore, like in the West in the immediate postwar period, huge portions were taken as a sign of quality, and vegetables were not considered an essential part of a meal by the newly liberated East Germans. However, because obesity rates in the "old" federal states (i.e., states of the Federal Republic before reunification) were also already high in the late 1980s and increased much less than they did in Britain or the United States, my guess would be that the traditional German diet was already facilitating obesity before the advent of the fast food revolution. Germans merely exchanged sausage and beer for hamburgers and soft drinks.

ENVIRONMENTAL INHIBITORS OF PHYSICAL ACTIVITY

As mentioned before, weight gain is the result of an imbalance between energy intake and energy expenditure. Now that I have reviewed evidence for the environmental factors that might have contributed to increased energy intake, in this last section of the chapter I focus on environmental inhibitors of physical activity. I address three questions: (a) whether physical activity has really decreased since the 1980s, (b) how changes in the built environment may have affected physical activity levels, and (c) whether low levels of physical activity really are a strong determinant of weight gain.

Long-Term Trends in Physical Activity

The major surveys conducted in the United States are fairly similar in their approach to assessing physical activity. They typically ask about the extent to which respondents have recently (e.g., in the past 2 weeks, in the past month) engaged in physical activities such as walking for exercise, jogging or running, hiking, gardening or yard work, aerobics, or aerobic dancing. For example, the 1994 version of the Behavioral Risk Factor Surveillance System (BRFSS) initiated by the U.S. Centers for Disease Control (CDC) and based on monthly, year-round telephone interviews of adults aged 18 years and older opened inquiry into physical activities with the following question: "During the past month, did you participate in any physical activities or exercises, such as running, calisthenics, golf, gardening, or walking for exercise?" If respondents answer yes, they are then asked detailed questions about their two most frequent activities (CDC, 1994). Most reports on physical activity distinguish between three patterns of leisure-time activity, namely *physical inactivity* (no activity reported during the period asked), *regular sustained physical activity* (at least five times per week and at least 30 minutes per occasion of any physical activity of any type and any intensity), and *regular vigorous activity* (at least three times per week and at least 20 minutes per occasion of vigorous exercise performed at 50% or more of one's age-specific cardiorespiratory capacity; U.S. Department of Health and Human Services [USDHHS], 1996). Thus, the category *regular sustained physical activity* reflects the sum of all the activities engaged in, including regular vigorous activities.

It is easiest to measure "physical inactivity during leisure." People are categorized as physically inactive if they report no leisure-time physical activities during the past 2 to 4 weeks. Because the BRFSS changed the way it asked about the various types of activities, the category *physical inactivity* is the only one for which comparable data can be obtained for the period from 1990 to 2002 (CDC, 2007; see Figure 4.4). As can be seen, nearly one third of American men and women reported having been inactive, and women appear to have higher levels of inactivity than do men. Most important, however, the prevalence of physical inactivity has been declining slightly during the past decade; Americans reported having become slightly more active in their leisure time. At the same time, there is some indication that the level of physical activity undertaken as part of daily routines has decreased (French et al., 2001).

The scarce longitudinal data available for American adolescents and young adults also suggest an increase in the prevalence of physical activity. Thus, according to a national survey of 12- through 21-year-olds, the prevalence of inactivity decreased from 13.7% in 1992 to 10.4% in 1995 (USDHHS, 1996). The prevalence of vigorous physical activity increased during the same period from 53.7% to 63.7% even though the percentage of students who participated in daily physical education at high school was at an all-time low (USDHHS, 1996).

The limited information available for Great Britain also suggests a slight increase in leisure-time activity during the past few decades (Allender, Peto, Scarborough, Boxer, & Rayner, 2006; Fox, 1999). However, this positive

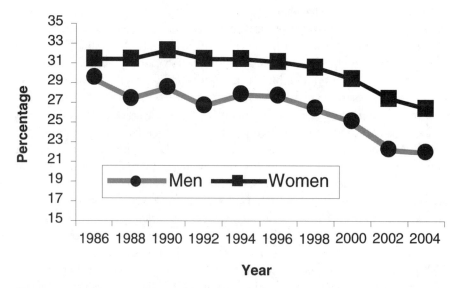

Figure 4.4. Prevalence of leisure-time physical inactivity among American men and women from 1990 to 2002. Based on the Behavioral Risk Factor Surveillance System. Data from U.S. Department of Health and Human Services (2007).

effect might have been more than compensated for by a decrease in the level of physical activity undertaken as part of daily routine. According to the National Travel Survey, during the past few decades, the number of miles per year traveled by foot and by cycle fell by 25% to 30% (Allender et al., 2006).

Data on levels of physical inactivity across Europe are even more scarce. Only two multinational surveys have looked at levels of physical activity across 15 European countries, and the more recent one of these was conducted in 2002 (Allender et al., 2006; see Figure 4.5). Although these data are difficult to compare with the U.S. figures, the fact that more than 40% of adults in these European countries reported no moderate level of physical activity in the past week suggests that physical activity levels in Europe are, on average, not strikingly different from those in the United States.

In summary, then, the evidence available on trends in leisure-time physical activity suggests that both Americans and Britons increased rather than decreased their level of leisure-time physical activity during the period for which data are available. However, these estimates are based on self-reports and thus open to the same problems discussed earlier for self-reports of food consumption, with the difference being that with physical activity, social norms encourage overreporting rather than underreporting. Furthermore, physical activity surveys focus exclusively on leisure-time activities, disregarding occupational or domestic activities (USDHHS, 1996). This

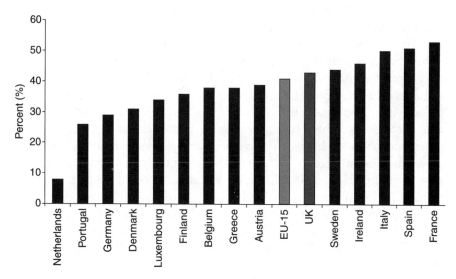

Figure 4.5. Percentage of adults who do no moderate-intensity physical activity in a typical week, 2002, in European Union-15 (EU-15) countries. From *Diet, Physical Activity and Obesity Statistics* (p. 131), by S. Allender, V. Peto, P. Scarborough, A. Boxer, and M. Rayner, 2006, BHF Coronary Heart Disease Statistics at http://www.heartstats. org. Copyright 2006 by the British Heart Foundation. Reprinted with permission.

serious limitation can result in an underestimate of physical activity, not only for people with physically demanding jobs but also for women, who still do most of the housework. Therefore, it cannot be ruled out that activity levels required in the domestic and occupational domains decreased during this time period and that this decrease more than compensated for the increase in leisure-time physical activity.

The Environmental Facilitators of Physical Inactivity

Next to the elevator and the escalator, the car is probably the most widely used labor-saving device ever invented. Car use has increased in the United States during the past few decades, and people have become less likely to walk or bike for transportation (French et al., 2001). Similar trends have been observed in Great Britain and Australia. For example, in Great Britain, the average number of miles per year traveled by car increased by just under 70% over the past 25 years (Allender et al., 2006). However, unlike in the United States, where car ownership has remained stable (French et al., 2001), the increase in automobile use has been accompanied by an increase in car ownership in Britain as in Australia (Wen, Orr, Millett, & Rissel, 2005). That car ownership is indeed associated with an increased risk of weight gain was demonstrated in a study conducted in China (Bell, Ge, & Popkin, 2001). With adjustments for socioeconomic status, men and women in households who owned a motorized vehicle (car or motorcycle) were found to have an 80% greater chance of being obese than those living in households without motorized transport.

Having spent my adult life in small or midsize university towns in the United States, Great Britain, Germany, and the Netherlands, I have been most dependent on cars when living in the United States. If I placed these countries on a continuum from encouraging least to encouraging most physical activity, I would have the United States at one extreme and the Netherlands at the other. Whenever I moved to the United States, I had to buy a car immediately because life would have been impossible without one. Regardless of whether I wanted to get to work, play tennis, swim, or go shopping, all these places could be reached only by car. Because one could always find a parking place at the university or at the shopping center, using the car was easy.

Evidence from research on the impact of urban sprawl on physical activity supports these observations (Ewing, 2005; Ewing, Schmid, Killingsworth, Zlot, & Raudenbush, 2003; Saelens, Sallis, & Frank, 2003). According to Ewing (2005), *urban sprawl* refers to an environment characterized by

> 1) a population widely dispersed in low-density residential development; 2) a rigid separation of homes, shops, and workplaces; 3) a lack of distinct, thriving activity centers; and 4) a network of roads marked by very large block size and poor access from one place to another. (p. 70)

Residents of neighborhoods that are not characterized by urban sprawl have been found to report twice as many "walking trips" per week than those who live in neighborhoods that suffer from urban sprawl (Saelens et al., 2003). Furthermore, when Ewing et al. (2003) linked their sprawl index to BMI data from the BRFSS, they found that with relevant risk factors controlled for, residents of sprawling counties had a higher BMI and were more likely to be obese than were their counterparts living in compact counties.

Urban sprawl and the trend toward constructing schools away from the center of communities have also resulted in a decline in children walking or biking to school. Whereas 48% of students walked or biked to school in 1969, by 2001 fewer than 15% of students aged 5 to 15 walked to school, and just 1% biked (Story, Kaphingst, & French, 2006). Long distance and traffic danger were the most frequently reported reasons parents did not want their children to walk or bike to school. It has been estimated that walking to school uses up 30 to 40 kilocalories per day.

The Netherlands has insufficient space to allow urban sprawl, and urban areas are compact, with thriving city centers.[8] It also has an excellent public transport system. Thus, living in the Netherlands, one would not even need a car. People walk everywhere in town or go by bicycle. Dutch mothers usually transport their children to kindergarten by bicycle, and Dutch adolescents carry their girl- or boyfriends on the back of their bicycle. This behavior is encouraged by the presence of bicycle paths everywhere and the scarcity and extremely high costs of parking places in Dutch cities. Because public transport is good, people mostly take the bus if they want to go to the airport or the train station. There are also convenient train connections to most places in the Netherlands, which encourages people to use trains rather than their cars. Finally, most of the older Dutch houses have several floors and very steep staircases, forcing people to move a great deal even at home. It is therefore not surprising that the percentage of Dutch who do not engage in moderate-intensity physical exercise is not only the lowest in Europe but is also 3 times lower than that of Portugal, which has the next lowest rate (see Figure 4.5).

That supermarkets in the Netherlands are typically within walking distance of housing areas and often have no parking facilities also has consequences for shopping frequency and shopping habits. The fact that people walk or bike to a supermarket prevents them from doing large amounts of shopping. As a result, they have to shop more frequently and cannot stock up on as much food as they could if they were able to drive there by car. Fur-

---

[8]Unfortunately, children who grow up in city centers often have no gardens or public green areas to play in. A study conducted by researchers at the University of Wageningen (the Netherlands) demonstrated that with socioeconomic status and ethnicity controlled for, children who grow up in city centers without green areas are fatter than children who grow up in suburbs or villages that have gardens and public parks (Vreke, Donder, Langers, Salverda, & Veeneklaas, 2006). The percentage of children who were overweight was 15.6% in areas with green and 19.3% in areas without green.

thermore, because large containers are difficult to carry in shopping bags, most food is sold in small containers. Because stockpiling food and large containers increase consumption (Wansink, 2004), having neighborhood shops to walk to not only encourages exercise but also discourages overconsumption. Yet, as I mentioned in chapter 2 (this volume), rates of overweight and obesity are increasing even in the Netherlands.

The Association Between Physical Inactivity and Weight Gain

It is a truism that a sedentary lifestyle is a risk factor for overweight and obesity, and the findings of numerous cross-sectional studies are consistent with this assumption (e.g., Hemmingsson & Ekelund, 2007; Janssen et al., 2004; L. O. Schulz & Schoeller, 1994; M. S. Tremblay & Willms, 2002; Wen et al., 2005; Willamson et al., 1993). For example, a study based on a nationally representative sample of 7,216 Canadian children aged 7 to 11 years who were assessed in 1994 compared physical activity and sports participation with BMI measured by parental report (M. S. Tremblay & Willms, 2002). Both organized and unorganized sports and physical activity were found to be associated with lower levels of overweight and obesity. Active participation in sports and physical activity was associated with a reduced risk of overweight of 10% to 24% and of obesity of 23% to 43%. Another cross-sectional study, of a nationally representative sample of 11- to 16-year-old Canadian male and female adolescents conducted in 2001, reported similar findings (Janssen et al., 2004). Finally, Williamson et al. (1993), who used data from the NHANES I Epidemiological Follow-Up Study (1971–1975 to 1982–1984), found in their cross-sectional analyses an inverse association between BMI and physical activity at both baseline and follow-up.

A survey conducted in 2003 in New South Wales (Australia) among 6,810 adults is particularly interesting because it not only reported a significant association between physical activity and obesity but also linked car use to obesity (Wen et al., 2005). Individuals whose physical activity level was judged inadequate (less than 150 minutes per week of physical activity over five separate occasions) had a 10% higher chance of being overweight or obese than did individuals with adequate activity levels (53.1% vs. 43.7%). Car use was also associated with an increased risk of weight problems. Of respondents driving more than 10 times a week, 47% were overweight or obese, compared with 41% of those driving 6 to 10 times and 30% of those driving fewer than 6 times. Because frequent car users had lower activity levels than did non–car users, the association between car use and weight problems is likely to have been at least partly mediated by differences in physical activity. However, even with physical activity levels controlled for, car users still ran an increased risk of overweight and obesity.

Though all of these studies used self-report data, cross-sectional studies employing objective measures of physical activity reported similar results. L. O. Schulz and Schoeller (1994), who used the doubly labeled water method to measure energy expenditure, found a correlation between percentage of body fat and nonbasal energy expenditure of $r = -.55$ for men and $r = -.83$ for women. Similarly, Hemmingsson and Ekelund (2007), who used accelometry to measure physical activity in adults with obesity and adults of normal weight for a period of 7 days also found an inverse association between BMI and physical activity.

As pointed out repeatedly, cross-sectional studies cannot disentangle cause–effect relationships. Although it would seem plausible that this association is due to the fact that physical activity induces weight loss, it is equally plausible that the discomfort of their weight prevents individuals who are overweight from engaging in physical activity. However, these explanations are not mutually exclusive, and there is evidence to support both assumptions. A study by Voorrips, Meijers, Sol, Seidell, and van Staveren (1992) suggested that overweight and obesity can precede physical inactivity. On the basis of a retrospective study of the weight of a group of physically active and sedentary 71-year-old women, they reported that the sedentary group was significantly heavier than was the physically active group from age 25 onward, although no differences were found in physical activity scores between these groups at ages 12, 25, 40, and 55. Thus, in this retrospective study, overweight appeared to precede the differences in physical activity, leading the authors to suggest that the current physical activity was probably a result rather than a cause of higher body weight in older age. However, the retrospective estimate of body weight based on old photographs may have been more reliable and valid than the retrospective assessment of physical activity based on a structured interview.

Use of well-controlled longitudinal studies can usually help at least to establish the long-term sequence. Unfortunately, in the case of the impact of physical activity on body weight, the evidence from longitudinal studies is equivocal. Although numerous longitudinal studies were successful in linking physical inactivity to risk of weight gain, overweight, and obesity (e.g., Elgar et al., 2005; French et al., 1994; Guo, Zeller, Chumlea, & Siervogel, 1999; Haapanen, Miilunpalo, Pasanen, Oja, & Vuori, 1997; Kimm et al., 2005; Koh-Banerjee et al., 2003; Schmitz, Jacobs, Leon, Schreiner, & Sternfeld, 2000), other studies have failed to do so (e.g., Bak, Petersen, & Sorensen, 2004; French et al., 1999; Heitmann et al., 1997; Petersen, Schnohr, & Sorensen, 2004; Williamson et al., 1993).

One of the positive findings of longitudinal studies is illustrated by a work site study conducted in the United States that assessed behavioral predictors of body weight in 1,629 men and 1,913 women and found over the 2-year period that an increase in one walking session per week was associated with a decrease in body weight of 0.8 kilograms (1.76 pounds) for women and

0.4 kilograms (0.88 pounds) for men. The addition of one high-intensity activity session per week predicted 0.6 kilograms (1.32 pounds) weight loss for women and 1.6 kilograms (3.52 pounds) weight loss for men (French et al., 1994). Similarly, a study based on 16,587 healthy men (a subsample of the Health Professionals Follow-up Study) conducted between 1986 and 1996 in the United States found an increase in total vigorous activity significantly related to a reduction in waist circumference after 9 years (Koh-Banerjee et al., 2003). Finally, a 10-year longitudinal study of a cohort of 2,564 men and 2,695 women conducted in Finland found physical activity at baseline signif- icantly and inversely related to BMI at follow-up for women but not for men (Haapanen et al., 1997).

Longitudinal studies of children and adolescents reported similar find- ings. Thus, a 9-year longitudinal study of 1,213 Black and 1,166 White girls, who were followed up annually from ages 9 and 10 to 18 and 19 years, assessed extracurricular sports and physical activities during the past year at each point of measurement (Kimm et al., 2005). On the basis of their over- all level of physical activity over the 9-year period, these girls were defined as active, moderately active, or inactive. There was a significant decrease in activity levels with increasing age. Girls who stayed more active over the period of the study showed significantly less increase in BMI than did girls who stayed less active, with activity levels having a greater effect on the BMI of Black than of White girls. Finally, a 4-year longitudinal study that assessed physical activity and body weight of a cohort of 355 Welsh adolescents twice in 1994 and 1998 found physical activity at baseline to predict change in BMI at Time 2, with the physically more active children gaining less weight during the course of the study (Elgar et al., 2005).

In view of the support from longitudinal studies for the assumption that physical activity helps to prevent weight gain and facilitates weight loss, it would be tempting to explain the failure of other longitudinal studies (e.g., Bak et al., 2004; French, Jeffery, & Murray, 1999; Heitmann et al., 1997; Petersen et al., 2004; Williamson et al., 1993) to support this association with use of unreliable measures of physical activity. This interpretation is ren- dered implausible by the fact that several of the studies that failed to find an association in their longitudinal analyses did find strong inverse associ- ations when analyzing their data cross-sectionally (e.g., Bak et al., 2004; Petersen et al., 2004; Williamson et al., 1993). So how can this puzzling inconsistency be resolved?

In chapter 8 (this volume), which covers the treatment and prevention of overweight and obesity, I discuss several randomized controlled intervention studies that demonstrate that exercising results in weight loss (R. Ross et al., 2000; Sopko et al., 1985). These studies also show that comparatively high lev- els of physical activity are necessary to induce sizable weight loss. For exam- ple, to induce a deficit of 500 kilocalories/day by exercise alone, individuals have to walk nearly 2 hours per day, every day (see Table 3.1, this volume, p. 38). If one assumes that the reliable and substantial association between BMI and physical activity so regularly observed with cross-sectional studies reflects the joint effects of (a) increased activity reducing overweight and (b) increased overweight reducing activity, and if one further assumes that the second effect is much stronger than the first, it becomes plausible that cross-sectional and longitudinal analyses conducted on the same data set often result in discrepant outcomes.

CONCLUSIONS

The evidence about environmental contributors to the long-term increase in overweight and obesity in the United States that I have reviewed points to calorie intake as the major culprit. The food supply data suggest that between 1970 and 1997, Americans increased their calorie intake by 460 kilocalories per day, an increase sufficient to account for the increase in overweight and obesity observed since the mid-1980s. The evidence is less clear for Great Britain, partly because there is less information but also because the information is conflicting. The survey data for Britain suggest that food consumption has decreased during the critical period. Because this decrease in calorie intake was paralleled by a steep rise in rates of overweight and obesity, these data are difficult to accept. Furthermore, the food supply data paint a somewhat different picture and suggest a modest increase in calorie intake. These data are also more in line with other information that suggests substantial changes in British eating habits.

The research reviewed in this chapter also has identified the environmental factors that are likely to have been responsible for the increase in calorie intake. Studies have demonstrated that the increased consumption of fast food and soft drinks as well as increased portion and container sizes contribute substantially to calorie intake and weight gain. Marketing strategies such as television advertising aimed at children and food and drink marketing in American schools have contributed to the increase in popularity of fast food and soft drinks.

The evidence on long-term trends in physical activity is less clear. Information on trends in leisure-time physical activity suggests that activity levels have increased in the United States as well as in Britain. At the same time, there is some indication that levels of physical activity undertaken as part of daily routines have decreased in both countries. In light of a long-term decrease in occupational activity, it is likely that overall there has also been a decrease in physical activity. Such a trend would be consistent with the findings of longitudinal studies that identify physical inactivity as a risk factor for weight gain and obesity.

That biological and environmental factors contribute to the obesity epidemic should not distract from the fact that obesity is ultimately the result of an imbalance between energy consumption and energy expenditure. People gain weight if they eat too much and exercise too little. Environmental factors, particularly those that favor increased calorie intake, facilitate the development of overweight and obesity, and their impact is greatest for individuals with a biological disposition toward weight gain. However, unless they suffer from genetic obesity that is due to a single gene mutation (Bouchard & Rankinen, 2008), people can counteract these influences by controlling their food intake. In the next three chapters, I discuss the self-regulation of body weight and the factors that increase the risk of self-regulatory failure.

5

DETERMINANTS OF WEIGHT REGULATION IN INDIVIDUALS WITH OBESITY

Why do some people become overweight or even obese, whereas others appear to be able to keep their weight within the normal range? This question has interested social and clinical psychologists for many decades. In chapter 3 (this volume), I discussed genetically influenced risk factors, and chapter 4 (this volume) focused on environmental changes likely to have facilitated the development of overweight and obesity. However, as emphasized before, weight gain is due to an imbalance between calorie intake and energy expenditure, too much food and too little physical activity. This chapter and the next two chapters present psychological theories developed to explain why people overeat.

Psychological theories of overweight and obesity (psychosomatic theory; externality theory) share the assumption that there is a major difference in the regulation of eating between individuals with obesity and individuals of normal weight. These theories assume that (a) individuals with obesity are less responsive than are individuals of normal weight to internal hunger and satiation cues (the differential sensitivity hypothesis) and that (b) their eating is activated by cues unrelated to hunger or satiation, such as anxiety and stress (Bruch, 1961; H. I. Kaplan & Kaplan, 1957), or by eating-related external stimuli (H. I. Kaplan & Kaplan, 1957; Schachter, 1971). These theories and some of the experimental studies conducted to test them are discussed in this chapter. Many of these empirical findings are highly relevant for the more recent theories that are reviewed in chapters 6 and 7 (this volume).

PSYCHOSOMATIC THEORY

In 1957, H. I. Kaplan and Kaplan published an influential article on the psychosomatic concept of obesity, in which they expressed the then-novel view that obesity was not caused by an organic disorder in metabolism but was the result of overeating. To explain why some people have a tendency to overeat, H. I. Kaplan and Kaplan (1957) suggested a number of hypotheses (differential sensitivity hypothesis; comfort hypothesis) that were based mainly on learning theory concepts. According to these researchers, obesity can be due to two types of abnormal overeating. The first, and the one relevant to the differential sensitivity hypothesis, results from a "disturbance in hunger or appetite" (H. I. Kaplan & Kaplan, 1957, p. 197) as a consequence of appetite having become (classically) conditioned to nonnutritional factors. For example, hunger and appetite may come to be elicited by previously neutral stimuli (e.g., one's regular lunchtime or dinnertime), because these stimuli have been regularly associated with hunger and eating. Similarly, if in the case of a neglected infant, hunger has repeatedly been associated with fear or loneliness, then fear or loneliness is likely to evoke appetite or a desire to eat later in life.

A second type of overeating that is not mediated by disturbances in hunger or appetite can result from instrumental conditioning. According to H. I. Kaplan and Kaplan (1957), eating was found to reduce fear or anxiety. Because fear and anxiety are assumed to be negative drive states, behavior that reduces fear or anxiety results in drive reduction and is thus reinforced. Individuals who have learned that eating reduces fear or anxiety will therefore be motivated to eat whenever they experience fear or anxiety without feeling any "conscious increase in hunger or appetite" (p. 198). Because fearful or anxious individuals are assumed to eat because they have experienced eating as anxiety reducing or comforting, this hypothesis has also been referred to as the comfort hypothesis (e.g., Polivy, Herman, & McFarlane, 1994).

With these learning principles, H. I. Kaplan and Kaplan (1957) offered a cogent analysis of the learning processes through which nonnutritional factors could induce eating. It is less clear, however, why the appetite of some individuals (i.e., those who are obese) and not of others becomes associated with stimuli such as lunchtime or dinnertime, and why only individuals with obesity, and not others, are expected to experience eating as fear-reducing. Even though H. I. Kaplan and Kaplan described a number of processes that might cause overeating, they believed that knowledge was insufficient at that time to offer any explanation of why only individuals with obesity and not individuals of normal weight are affected.

In another pioneering article, Bruch (1961), a psychiatrist with a psychoanalytic background, was less reluctant to offer hypotheses about familial factors that might have contributed to the loss of sensitivity for hunger cues and the development of obesity. She concluded from clinical observations of patients with obesity that these individuals were unable to differentiate sensations of hunger from other states of bodily arousal. She attributed this inability to differentiate between these states to experiences in childhood, with the ultimate cause being the failure of parents to teach their children to recognize hunger signals. When mothers use food as an expression of love, or to pacify or reward the child rather than offering food to their child in response to nutritional needs, the child does not learn to recognize internal hunger signals or to distinguish hunger from other states of bodily arousal.

Thus, there are two mechanisms through which anxiety could result in overeating. According to the differential sensitivity hypothesis, anxiety (or any other strong emotion) can stimulate eating in individuals who failed to learn to distinguish hunger cues from cues that signal emotional states (Bruch, 1961, 1974) or for whom appetite has been regularly associated with fear, loneliness, or some other nonnutritional cue (H. I. Kaplan & Kaplan, 1957). In the second mechanism, according to H. I. Kaplan and Kaplan (1957), overeating may have become a learned response to anxiety that serves to reduce anxiety. The major difference between these two theoretical accounts of the relationship between anxiety and eating is that the first, but not the second, assumes it to be mediated by differential sensitivity to internal cues, and that the second, but not the first, assumes that eating will reduce anxiety.

Early empirical support for the differential sensitivity hypothesis was provided by a study of Stunkard and Koch (1964) that showed that gastric motility was related to self-report of hunger in individuals of normal weight but not individuals with obesity. The problem with this study is that gastric motility plays at best a minor role as a hunger signal (Blundell & Stubbs, 1998).

A more direct test of the mechanisms through which anxiety is expected to stimulate eating in individuals with obesity was conducted by Schachter, Goldman, and Gordon (1968), who examined the effects of manipulated anxiety and satiation on the number of crackers eaten in an alleged taste test. Anxiety was manipulated by leading respondents to expect to receive either a weak or a strong electric shock. Satiation was manipulated by having research participants either eat or not eat roast beef sandwiches (i.e., preload) before the taste test. Whereas individuals of normal weight ate significantly fewer crackers after a preload than without a preload, the amount of crackers consumed by participants with obesity[1] was not affected significantly (see Figure 5.1,

---

[1]In most studies reported in this chapter, obesity was defined in terms of norms published by the Metropolitan Life Insurance Company (1959). Participants were categorized as obese if they were 15% or more above their expected normal weight. This is a rather low cut-off point that suggests that some of the participants categorized as obese would have been considered overweight according to the definition of obesity used in this volume.

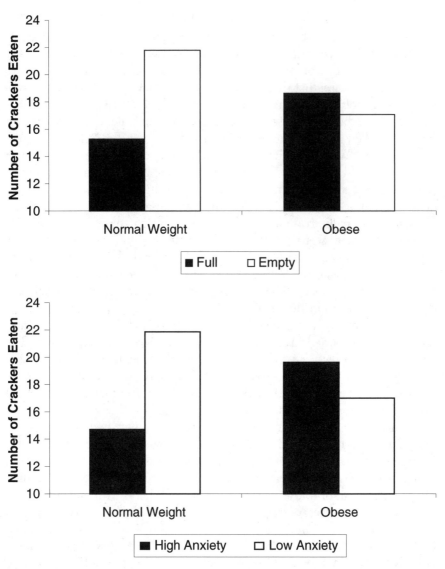

Figure 5.1. The impact of a preload (top panel) and anxiety (bottom panel) on food consumption of individuals who are obese and individuals who are of normal weight. Data are from Schachter et al. (1968, p. 95, Table 2).

top panel). These findings support the differential sensitivity hypothesis that eating behavior of respondents with obesity is not regulated by internal cues of hunger or satiation (i.e., nonregulation).

There was no support, however, for the second and more central assumption of psychosomatic theory that eating behavior of individuals with obesity is triggered by emotional arousal or, more specifically, by fear or anxiety. The anxiety manipulation failed to have a significant impact on food consumption of individuals with obesity but reduced consumption of individuals of normal weight (see Figure 5.1, bottom panel). Individuals with obesity also did not show indication of greater anxiety reduction following eating.

Neither the preload effects nor the pattern of effects of anxiety on amount eaten reported by Schachter et al. (1968) have ever been replicated in comparisons of individuals with obesity and individuals of normal weight. Four studies have assessed the impact of preloads on eating with individuals with obesity and individuals with normal weight (Hibscher & Herman, 1977; Nisbett, 1968; Ruderman & Christensen, 1983; Spencer & Fremouw, 1979), and, with the exception of Ruderman and Christensen (1983), none of these studies found a significant Weight × Preload interaction. With Ruderman and Christensen (1983), simple effect analyses indicated that the interaction was due to preloaded individuals with obesity eating less rather than more.

The impact of anxiety on food intake of individuals with obesity and individuals of normal weight has been examined in eight experimental studies (Abramson & Wunderlich, 1972; McKenna, 1975; Pine, 1985; Reznick & Balch, 1977; Ruderman, 1985; Slochower, 1983, Experiments 1, 2, and 4) and two quasi-experimental studies (Slochower, 1983, Experiments 3 and 5). Only one of these studies replicated the Schachter et al. (1968) finding that anxiety reduced the amount eaten by individuals of normal weight, but only for palatable and not for bland food (McKenna, 1975). None of the other studies found an effect of anxiety on amount eaten by individuals of normal weight.

With regard to individuals who are overweight, findings have been similarly unsupportive. Only 2 of the 10 studies found anxiety to have no significant effect on amount eaten by individuals who are overweight (Abramson & Wunderlich, 1972; Reznick & Balch, 1977), and one study found that those who were obese ate less ice cream under low than under high anxiety (Ruderman, 1985).[2] The majority of studies (McKenna, 1975; Pine, 1985; Slochower, 1983, Studies 1 to 5) found anxiety to facilitate eating among individuals with obesity, at least under some conditions. McKenna (1975) had individuals with obesity and individuals of normal weight, who were either threatened with physiological measurements (e.g., large blood sample) or not threatened, taste either very bland or very tasty cookies. All participants were extensively preloaded (e.g., roast beef sandwiches, a cup of hot bouillon) before the taste test. There was a Weight × Anxiety interaction, with participants with obesity eating more under high- than low-anxiety

---

[2]It is extremely likely that this latter effect can be attributed to the way anxiety was manipulated in this study. In the high-anxiety condition, the female participants had to speak to a male stranger "with the goal of impressing him" (Ruderman, 1985, p. 237). It seems plausible that if a young woman with obesity had to impress a male stranger, weight concerns might have been made highly salient. These weight concerns could then have reduced these individuals' eating in the subsequent ice cream tasting session.

conditions, and this effect was more marked in the condition with the tasty rather than the bland cookies. Thus, the pattern of findings in the condition with tasty cookies was in line with predictions from psychosomatic theory. There was no evidence, however, that overeating reduced anxiety in those with obesity.

A similar pattern of results was reported by Pine (1985). Participants with obesity and participants of normal weight were exposed to an anxiety manipulation similar to the one used by Schachter et al. (1968), before having to taste two brands of peanuts. There was a main effect of weight, with individuals with obesity eating more peanuts than did individuals of normal weight (see Figure 5.2). However, this main effect was moderated by an Anxiety × Weight interaction. Tests of simple effects indicated that individuals with high anxiety and obesity ate significantly more than did participants in any of the other three conditions. None of the other differences were significant.

Slochower (1983) reasoned from a psychoanalytic perspective that anxiety manipulations that exposed individuals to clear-cut external threats may

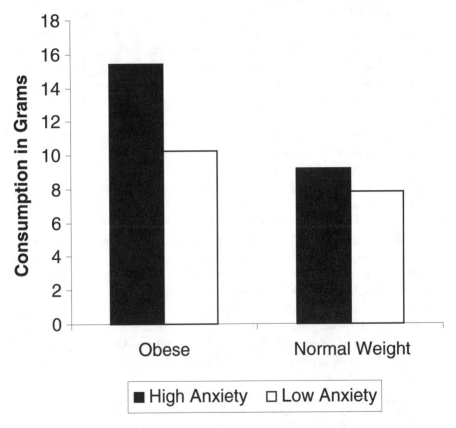

Figure 5.2. Effects of anxiety on food consumption. Data are from Pine (1985, p. 777).

not constitute optimal tests of psychosomatic theory. She speculated that overeating typically occurs in response to internal emotional conflicts. Because such conflicts are often unconscious, individuals might not even be aware of the source of their anxiety. Slochower suggested that this diffuseness of the affective response is the precise trigger for overeating and makes overeating such an effective means of anxiety reduction. In Experiment 1 of her impressive research program, Slochower manipulated arousal and the explanation or label participants were given for their arousal in a factorial design. Male participants who were overweight or of normal weight were led to believe that their heart rate would be measured as part of a study of the "physiological and psychological correlates of thinking" (p. 22) and that they could hear their own heartbeats during this measurement period. At an alleged baseline measurement period, participants in the high-arousal condition were exposed to a sound recording of fast heartbeats (84 to 92 per minute) compared with slow heartbeats (66 to 74) in the low-arousal condition. To provide a neutral (i.e., nonanxiety) explanation or label for their apparent arousal, half the participants were then given the misleading information that wearing earphones in the laboratory would tend to increase heart-rate levels. The other participants were offered no explanation for their arousal. It was assumed that participants who experienced unexplained high arousal would feel anxious, an assumption that was supported by manipulation checks. Participants were then asked to think "for the next few minutes" about a set of objects placed in front of them. One of those objects was a bowl of nuts. Participants were encouraged "to touch the objects . . . or to eat the nuts" (p. 33). The amount of nuts eaten constituted the dependent measure.

Participants with obesity ate significantly more nuts when they were aroused, and this effect was mainly due to the condition in which they had no explanation for their arousal (i.e., high anxiety). In contrast, the eating by participants of normal weight was not affected by any of the manipulations. Difference scores of anxiety before and after eating also indicated that the more the anxious individuals with obesity ate, the less anxious they felt subsequently. No such relationship was observed for individuals of normal weight. Thus, in line with the instrumental conditioning assumption of psychosomatic theory, eating appeared to have reduced anxiety among individuals with obesity but not among individuals of normal weight. This finding was replicated in a second experiment in which perceived control over the arousal state was added as a variable, although having control somewhat reduced eating under high arousal.

Given the artificial nature of the anxiety manipulation used in the first two experiments, Slochower (1983) thought it wise to replicate her findings conceptually using exam stress as a more real-life source of uncontrollable stress and anxiety. In this and the following studies, female undergraduates served as participants. Using the eating situation of Experiments 1 and 2 as a measure of eating, participants were assessed twice, once during and once after the exam period. It is not surprising that students felt more anxious and less in control of their feelings during rather than after the exam period, and this effect was the same for individuals who were overweight and those of normal weight. However, individuals who were overweight ate significantly more nuts than did individuals of normal weight during the exam period, whereas there was no difference afterward. Whether eating reduced anxiety among those with obesity was not assessed in this study.

In her last two studies, Slochower (1983) pitted psychosomatic theory against a hypothesis derived from Schachter's (1971) externality theory by manipulating both anxiety or stress and the cue salience of the food. Whereas salience of food items as an external cue rather than anxiety should affect the amount eaten by individuals with obesity (but not individuals of normal weight) according to externality theory, which assumes that individuals with obesity are overly sensitive to external food-relevant cues, psychosomatic theory makes the opposite prediction (i.e., that anxiety but not cue salience should increase food intake). In Experiment 4, Slochower induced anxiety by leading her female participants to expect either a highly threatening or a benign personality test. The threatening test was described as uncovering hidden "neurotic emotional problems, and severe pathological tendencies" (p. 69). In her fifth study, she again used the exam period as a time of high anxiety. Eating was assessed during a 10-minute "waiting period," when the experimenter placed a box of M&Ms candy in front of the participants, telling them "to feel free to help yourself to the candy while you are waiting" (p. 70). In both studies, salience was manipulated by presenting the 600 grams (21.16 ounces) of M&Ms either in a box made of clear plastic or in a box lined with brown paper so that the M&Ms were not visible once the box was put down. In addition, the box was placed farther away from participants in the low-salience condition of Study 5. In both studies, participants with obesity, but not participants of normal weight, ate significantly more candy under high anxiety and high salience. Although the Weight × Anxiety × Salience interactions did not reach significance in either study, the data patterns suggest that salience influenced eating mainly under conditions of high anxiety (see, e.g., Figures 5.3 and 5.4). In Experiment 4 eating reduced anxiety among those with obesity, a relationship that was not assessed in the exam situation used in Study 5.

Two factors seem to distinguish studies that found anxiety or stress to induce overeating by those who are obese from those that did not: namely, the type of food offered and cue salience. Tasty snack food that is liked by most people, such as peanuts (Pine, 1985), candy, or chocolate cookies (McKenna, 1975; Slochower, 1983), appears to work better than crackers (Abramson & Wunderlich, 1972; Schachter et al., 1968) or "bland, practically tasteless, dry . . . greenish-gray Scotch shortbread" (McKenna, 1975).

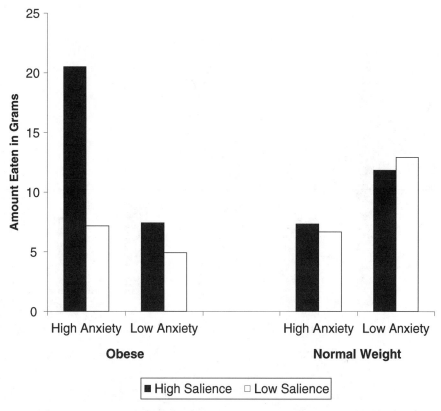

Figure 5.3. Amount eaten by individuals with obesity and those of normal weight. From *Excessive Eating: The Role of Emotions and the Environment* (p. 71), by J. A. Slochower, 1983, New York: Human Sciences Press. Copyright 1983 by Springer Science + Business Media. Adapted with kind permission of Springer Science + Business Media.

Cue salience seems to be a second factor necessary to induce overeating in individuals with obesity who have been made anxious. With the usual food-tasting paradigm, food salience is automatically high. After all, participants who are requested to rate the taste of various food items obviously must attend to, and think about, the taste of the food offered. However, with the type of incidental eating task used by Slochower (1983) in her first three experiments, food salience would normally be low. If snack food is put in front of participants with the remark that they could eat some, these individuals, who are busy with some other task, might not really attend to the food. However, Slochower increased food salience with her cover story. She used the pretense of a thinking task and asked her participants to think about the various objects placed in front of them. It would seem rather plausible that participants with obesity thought mainly about the bowl of peanuts, which thus would have become a highly salient object.

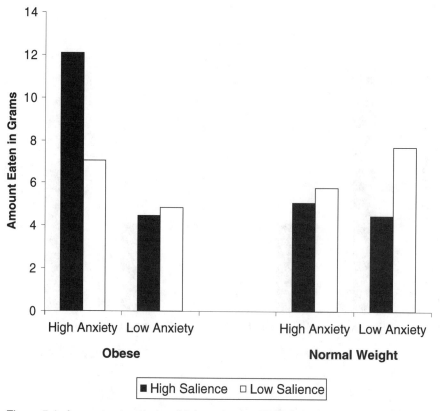

Figure 5.4. Amount eaten during (high anxiety) and after (low anxiety) final exams. From *Excessive Eating: The Role of Emotions and the Environment* (p. 82), by J. A. Slochower, 1983, New York: Human Sciences Press. Copyright 1983 by Springer Science + Business Media. Adapted with kind permission of Springer Science + Business Media.

In contrast, Slochower's (1983) hypothesis that anxiety induces overeating in individuals with obesity only if it is diffuse and cannot be attributed to an external cause such as an electric shock does not help to explain the pattern of findings. Pine (1985) induced overeating with electric shocks, and McKenna induced it (1975) with threatening physiological assays. In contrast, Abramson and Wunderlich (1972) failed to induce overeating with a threatening personality test, which, according to Slochower (1983), should have been a cause of diffuse anxiety.

In conclusion, consistent with psychosomatic theory, inducing anxiety or stress in individuals with obesity stimulates overeating, at least in situations where food stimuli are salient. Although I am not reviewing the clinical literature here, it is worth noting that studies of persons with obesity seeking treatment have consistently reported a positive association between anxiety and other states of emotional arousal and food intake (Slochower,

1983). Furthermore, on the basis of self-report descriptions of relapse situations of individuals who were overweight and dieting, Grilo, Shiffman, and Wing (1989) concluded that nearly half of the relapse crises occurred in the presence of negative affect, with anxiety being the affect most frequently cited.

Evidence is more equivocal with regard to the two processes suggested by psychosomatic theory as potential mediators of the impact of anxiety on overeating by individuals with obesity (i.e., differential sensitivity; instrumental conditioning). The fact that eating was found to reduce anxiety in two of the three studies in which anxiety reduction was assessed (Slochower, 1983, Experiments 1 and 4) is more consistent with the instrumental conditioning or comfort hypothesis than with the differential sensitivity assumption. If individuals with obesity had responded to anxiety by eating because anxiety had become classically conditioned to appetite (H. I. Kaplan & Kaplan, 1957) or because they had never learned to distinguish hunger from other states of bodily arousal (Bruch, 1961, 1974), then eating would not have been expected to reduce anxiety. However, there is simply insufficient evidence to draw confident conclusions.

EXTERNALITY THEORY

The diffusion of knowledge of the theoretical work of H. I. Kaplan and Kaplan (1957) and Bruch (1961) was limited to a specialist group interested in eating and eating disorders. Social psychologist Stanley Schachter (see, e.g., Schachter, 1971; Schachter & Rodin, 1974) made a much wider audience of psychologists aware that overweight and obesity were exciting research topics that could be studied experimentally. It was more the daring and innovative nature of his experimental work than the sophistication of externality theory that aroused enthusiasm. For a little more than a decade, his externality theory became the dominant theory in this area.

The Original Theory

As mentioned earlier, the development of externality theory was strongly influenced by the findings of two studies, namely the study of Stunkard and Koch (1964) and the experiment of Schachter et al. (1968). Both studies suggested that eating by those who are obese is not guided by internal stimuli. What then activated eating by individuals with obesity? Bruch's hypothesis seemed to have been ruled out by the findings of the Schachter et al. study. Thus, there appeared to be no support for the assumption that individuals with obesity ate because they misinterpreted the experience of strong emotions as hunger signals. This lack of support led Schachter et al. to conclude "that internal state is irrelevant to eating by obese, and that external, food-relevant cues trigger eating for such people" (p. 97). Such food-relevant cues could be any noncaloric properties of food (e.g., palatability) or any aspect of the environment that had been regularly associated with eating (e.g., dinnertime) and signaled palatable food (e.g., sight or smell of food; salience of food cues). The assumption that the food intake of individuals with obesity is triggered by external, food-relevant cues rather than by bodily feedback of sensations of hunger and satiation would explain why these individuals often overeat in food-rich environments.

This assumption was tested in a series of innovative and by now classic studies that assessed the impact of external eating-relevant cues on eating behavior of individuals with obesity (e.g., Goldman, Jaffa, & Schachter, 1968; McArthur & Burstein, 1975; Nisbett, 1968; L. Ross, 1974; Schachter, 1971; Schachter et al., 1968; Schachter & Friedman, 1974; Schachter & Gross, 1968; Tom & Rucker, 1975). In one of the early experiments, Schachter and Gross (1968) manipulated the external, food-relevant cue "dinnertime." Student participants of normal weight and student participants who were overweight, both of whom had a regular dinnertime of 6 p.m., were scheduled for the experiment at 5 p.m. They were asked to hand in their watches, supposedly because the electrode jelly applied for (fake) physiological measurements would corrode metal. Thus, they had to rely on a wall clock for their time, and this clock was doctored to run slow for half of the participants and fast for the other half. After a period of fake physiological measurements, participants were asked to fill in a questionnaire and were encouraged to eat some crackers from a box left on the table by the experimenter. The true period during which they could eat crackers lasted from 5:40 to 5:50 p.m. However, participants in the slow condition were led to believe that it was 5:25 to 5:35 p.m. (i.e., before dinnertime), whereas participants in the fast condition thought it was 6:10 to 6:20 p.m. (i.e., after dinnertime). The amount of crackers eaten was the dependent measure. Schachter and Gross predicted that because their eating was guided by external cues, participants with obesity would eat more crackers if they thought it was past their dinnertime than if they thought it was early. Individuals of normal weight, on the other hand, whose eating behavior is supposed to be regulated by internal hunger and satiety cues, should have been much less affected in their eating by the doctored clock.

The results for individuals with obesity were consistent with these predictions. They ate substantially more when they thought that dinnertime had passed than when they thought that it was still ahead of them (see Figure 5.5). However, the eating behavior of individuals of normal weight was unexpectedly also affected by the doctored clock. They ate considerably less if they thought it was past their usual dinnertime. To explain this unexpected finding, Schachter and Gross (1968) argued that individuals of normal weight ate less in the slow condition because they did not want to spoil their dinner. It is interesting to note that according to this interpretation, the external cue

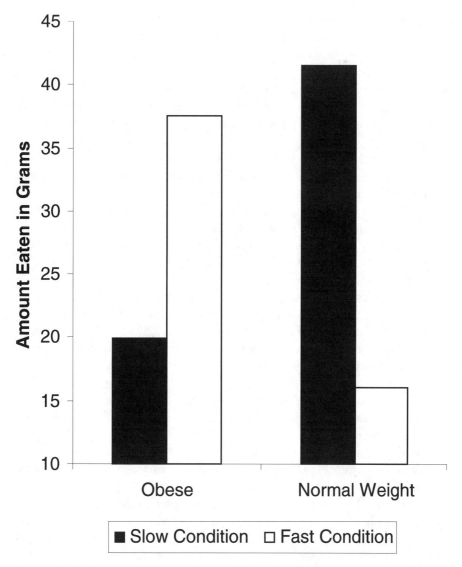

Figure 5.5. Amount eaten by participants with obesity and those of normal weight. Data are from Schachter and Gross (1968, p. 101, Table 2).

"dinnertime" has as much impact on eating by individuals of normal weight as on eating by individuals with obesity. The only difference is that the cue has different meanings for the two groups.

Nisbett (1968) manipulated the external cue "taste" or "palatability" in an experiment in which individuals who were underweight, normal weight, or overweight had to rate the taste of vanilla ice cream. For half of the participants, quinine sulphate was added to give the ice cream a slightly bitter and unpleasant taste. Nisbett assumed that ice cream consumption by individuals who were underweight would be least affected and that by individuals who were overweight most affected by this external eating-relevant cue. A significant Weight × Palatability interaction supported this hypothesis: The impact of the palatability manipulation was strongly influenced by the body-weight category of the individual, and this pattern was consistent with theoretical predictions because individuals who were overweight ate considerably more of the good ice cream than did participants who were underweight or normal weight. However, the data for the bad-tasting ice cream were not quite as expected: There were no significant differences in the amount eaten by the three weight groups.

The reason for this unexpected finding was probably that Nisbett (1968) had been too enthusiastic in trying to make his ice cream taste bad. Therefore, many participants ate only the token amount requested by the experimenter. As Woody, Costanzo, Liefer, and Conger (1981), who tried to replicate Nisbett's taste conditions, remarked, "a pilot study indicated that subjects would refuse ice cream so strongly adulterated" (p. 384). An unpublished study by Dekke tends to support this assumption (Schachter, 1971, pp. 103ff). When the bad-tasting food (milkshakes in this case) is only slightly unappealing instead of being truly awful, those who are obese do indeed eat less than do participants who are normal weight.

Findings from a field study provided further support for the assumption that individuals who are overweight are more responsive than are individuals who are normal weight to variations in palatability (Goldman et al., 1968). At Columbia University, undergraduates can sign up for a prepaid food plan at the beginning of the school year that allows them to eat in the dining hall of their dormitory. Three months into the academic year, students are offered the possibility to cancel the food contract and to get a refund, albeit at a small financial penalty. As in practically all university dining halls, the food offered at Columbia is not all that great. Because individuals with obesity are more responsive to the taste of food than are individuals of normal weight, one would predict that more 1st-year students with obesity would use the opportunity to cancel their food contract than would individuals of normal weight. In line with these assumptions, a significantly larger proportion of 1st-year students with obesity (86.5%) than 1st-year students of normal weight (67.1%) dropped out of their meal plan.

If individuals with obesity find it difficult to resist the temptation of palatable food (Nisbett, 1968) that is highly salient (Slochower, 1983), it would explain why they have difficulties dieting in a food-rich environment. They should find fasting much easier in an environment that has few external food cues. Goldman et al. (1968) hypothesized that the more time religious Jews who were overweight would spend on Yom Kippur (a religious day of fasting) in synagogue and thus away from tempting food stimuli, the less unpleasant they would experience the fasting. Consistent with this assumption, the correlation between the hours spent in synagogue during Yom Kippur and how unpleasant people experienced fasting to be was significantly higher for religious Jews with obesity (−.50) than for those of normal weight (−.18).

Experiments that manipulated food salience more directly were conducted by Schachter and Friedman (1974) and McArthur and Burstein (1975). They reasoned that the responsiveness of individuals with obesity to food-relevant cues should be strengthened if one increased the salience of these cues. Both studies manipulated food cue salience by offering participants with obesity and participants of normal weight a bag of either shelled (high salience) or unshelled (low salience) almonds while they had to fill out a lengthy personality test. Whereas cue salience did not affect the eating behavior of the participants of normal weight, it had a strong effect on individuals with obesity: 19 out of 20 ate shelled nuts, and only 1 out of 20 ate unshelled nuts. McArthur and Burstein (1975) found that all participants ate fewer nuts when the nuts were presented in shells rather than unshelled, but that the difference was much greater for individuals who were overweight than for those who were normal weight.

The problem with these findings is that salience is confounded with effort: Nuts that are still in shells are not only less salient but also more cumbersome to eat. Thus, the finding might merely indicate that individuals with obesity eat less when eating requires greater effort. An interpretation in terms of effort rather than salience would also reconcile these results with those of Studies 4 and 5 of Slochower (1983), who found salience to affect food intake of individuals with obesity mainly under conditions of high anxiety (see Figures 5.3 and 5.4). Because participants in the studies of McArthur and Burstein (1975) and Schachter and Friedman (1974) were unlikely to have been anxious, salience should not have affected the amount of nuts eaten by individuals with obesity.

A more conclusive test of whether salience influences eating behavior of individuals with obesity was reported by L. Ross (1974). He conducted an experiment in which he manipulated salience in a way that was not confounded with effort. The procedure he used was similar to that of Slochower (1983). The experiment was introduced as a study of the physiological correlates of thinking, and participants were told that they had to think about one of the sets of objects displayed on the table in front of them. One of these objects was a bowl containing 800 grams (28.22 ounces) of salted cashew nuts. The instructions regarding which object they should think about were given by a tape recorder. Participants were told that they could touch the objects and eat the nuts.

Cue salience was manipulated by having the table lit either very brightly or very dimly. In addition, L. Ross (1974) manipulated "cognitive salience" with a procedure that would now be considered priming.[3] In the high cognitive salience conditions, participants were instructed to think about the taste of cashew nuts. In the low salience condition, they were instructed to think about the marbles in front of them. Figure 5.6 presents the results for individuals with obesity (top panel) and for individuals of normal weight (bottom panel). It is obvious that the salience manipulation had a much greater impact on individuals with obesity than on individuals of normal weight: For individuals with obesity, both salience manipulations resulted in main effects, whereas these effects were not significant for individuals of normal weight. Participants with obesity ate more nuts when the nuts were brightly lit and when instructed to think about their taste than when the nuts were dimly lit or when participants had to think about the marbles instead of the nuts. More interesting, however, was an apparent interaction between cue salience and cognitive salience for those with obesity. The priming procedure used to manipulate cognitive salience seemed to have had a greater impact under low rather than high cue salience. Thus, when the nuts were brightly lit, individuals with obesity did not need to be primed to eat them. However, when the nuts were not displayed saliently, then having to think about their taste and texture substantially increased eating. Unfortunately, L. Ross analyzed the effect of each of the salience manipulations separately, so there is no information as to whether this interaction is significant.

That priming individuals who are obese with food stimuli increases the amount they eat has also been demonstrated by Tom and Rucker (1975), who exposed their participants with obesity and those of normal weight either to slides "of pictures of meat dishes, vegetable dishes, and desserts" or to slides showing "scenic areas of the United States." After participants had rated the extent to which they found these slides appealing, they had to evaluate the tastes of different kinds of crackers and indicate their willingness to buy each kind of cracker. In line with externality theory, exposure to food slides but not nonfood slides significantly increased the cracker consumption and buying intention of individuals with obesity. No difference was observed for individuals of normal weight.

Taken together, the findings of L. Ross (1974) and Tom and Rucker (1975) show that food salience affects the food intake of individuals with obesity even under conditions of low anxiety. Anxiety may enhance the impact of salience on food intake, as has been suggested by Studies 4 and 5 by Slochower (1983), but it does not appear to be a necessary condition for the occurrence of salience effect. It is at this point unclear why the studies reported by Slochower did not find an effect of salience under conditions of low anxiety.

---

[3]As explained in chapter 7 (this volume), *priming* refers to procedures that increase the cognitive accessibility of stimuli.

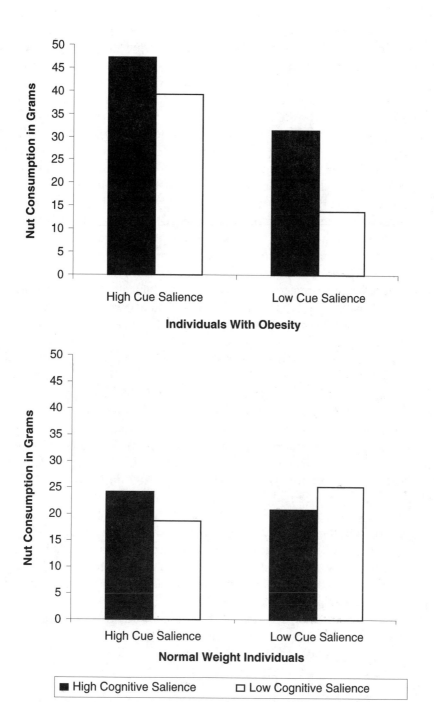

Figure 5.6. Grams of cashew nuts consumed by individuals with obesity (top panel) and those of normal weight (bottom panel) under high- or low-salience conditions. From *Obese Humans and Rats* (p. 49), by S. Schachter and J. Rodin (Eds.), 1974, Potomac, MD: Erlbaum. Copyright 1974 by Erlbaum. Adapted with permission.

What about effort? Did the fact that nuts in their shell are not only less salient as food items but also harder to eat have no effect on the eating behavior of individuals with obesity in the studies of Schachter and Friedman (1974) and McArthur and Burstein (1975)? A study reported by Johnson (1974) goes some way toward disentangling the effects of salience and effort on eating behavior of individuals with obesity. Johnson argued that individuals with obesity work harder to obtain palatable food than do individuals of normal weight, but only if the palatable food is made salient. In this study, participants had to lift a 3-kilogram (6.6-pound) weight with their index finger to obtain food portions, and the dependent measure was the number of times individuals flexed their index finger. Food salience was manipulated in two ways: (a) by displaying an attractive-looking sample sandwich either in a transparent wrap or wrapped in white nontransparent shelf paper and (b) by having participants taste a slice of a tasty sandwich. A significant Food Visibility × Weight interaction indicated that individuals with obesity worked harder for palatable food than did individuals of normal weight, but only when this food was highly visible. The Weight × Prior Taste interaction was not significant (nor was the third-order interaction), even though descriptively it appears as if prior taste did have an effect on the effort expended by individuals of normal weight when food was not visible (see Figure 5.7).

In a more recent study, Saelens and Epstein (1996) replicated the finding that individuals with obesity work harder for palatable food items (chocolate bars, ice cream, chocolate chip cookies) than do individuals who are not obese. Although they did not manipulate salience, participants had to rate their liking for the snack food and to taste samples before their effort was measured. Thus, even though the food was not visible during the task, it can be assumed that it was highly salient to participants.

In summary, then, these findings offer impressive support for the assumption that the food intake of individuals who are overweight and those with obesity is strongly influenced by external cues such as palatability, visibility, salience, and time of day. Findings from preload studies are less supportive of the second assumption of externality theory, namely that individuals with obesity are relatively insensitive to internal cues. However, this lack of support does not really pose a problem for externality theory. Responsiveness to internal versus external cues should probably not be considered one-dimensional but as two independent dimensions. It is less clear at this point, however, how these two dimensions should be assumed to interact. Slochower (1983) reasoned that anxiety "might act to enhance the overweight person's reactivity to external cues" (p. 99), but except for her own studies, little evidence supports this assumption. I explore alternative assumptions in my discussion of the role of cognitive processes in eating regulation in chapters 6 and 7 (this volume). Suffice it to say here that the core assumption of externality theory, that external cues have a greater impact on food

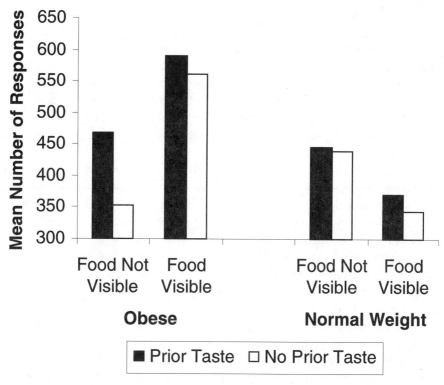

Figure 5.7. Mean effort expended on food as a function of weight and cue prominence. Data are from Johnson (1974, p. 846, Table 2).

intake of individuals who are overweight and those with obesity than they do on individuals of normal weight, has been supported by a wealth of empirical evidence.

The Revised and Extended Externality Theory

In revising and extending externality theory, Schachter and Rodin (1974) tried to remedy a shortcoming of the original version of the theory, namely that it did not offer an explanation for the origin of the difference in external responsiveness assumed to exist between individuals with obesity and those of normal weight. As early as 1971, Schachter had speculated that the evidence of greater responsiveness of individuals with obesity to food-relevant external cues "may be a manifestation of a generalized sensitivity to external cues" (Schachter, 1971, p. 136). Schachter (1971) originally tried to link obesity to more general personality dimensions such as field dependence and independence (Witkin et al., 1954). The idea that field-dependent individuals orient more on the basis of external visual cues than they do on gravitational cues from their own bodies could easily be extended to other internal and external food cues. This connection had been suggested by Karp and Pardes (1965), who found that women who were obese scored higher than did women of normal weight on three widely used measures of field dependence such as the rod-and-frame test, the body-adjustment test, and the embedded-figures test. However, after two failures to replicate the Karp and Pardes findings, Schachter abandoned the idea of conceiving of the externality of individuals with obesity as a specific instance of their more general field dependence.

Schachter did not give up the idea that the greater sensitivity to food cues could be a manifestation of a more generalized sensitivity to external cues of individuals with obesity. In a landmark publication with the provocative (and also somewhat derogatory) title *Obese Humans and Rats*, Schachter and Rodin (1974) examined the behavioral similarities of humans with obesity and animals whose satiety center (the ventromedial hypothalamus) had been lesioned. Similar to individuals with obesity, animals whose satiety center has been destroyed are insensitive to internal satiety and hunger cues and hypersensitive to external cues.

In a series of studies, Schachter, Rodin, and their associates explored further similarities. Individuals who were obese were found to be more reactive than individuals of normal weight to salient external cues that affected their pain perception, ideation, emotionality, and distractibility in contexts that had nothing to do with eating (Schachter & Rodin, 1974). For example, those who were obese differed from those who were not obese in terms of immediate recall of objects and words that were briefly presented on a slide (Rodin, Herman, & Schachter, 1974), in the extremity of affective ratings given to positive versus neutral stimuli (Rodin, Elman, & Schachter, 1974), and in the influence of external cues on judgments of time (Rodin, Slochower, & Fleming, 1977).

These findings were exciting because they suggested the integration of obesity into a much broader neurophysiologic framework. Unfortunately, however, the association between obesity and generalized external responsiveness could not always be replicated. For example, Rodin et al. (1977) found no correlation between degree of overweight and degree of external responsiveness as well as low intercorrelations between different measures of external responsiveness. Acknowledging these problems, Rodin (1981) denounced externality theory in an article entitled "Current Status of the Internal–External Hypothesis for Obesity: What Went Wrong?" Even though her refutation was directed mainly at the revised externality theory, this article delivered the death blow to externality theory in general because most readers did not realize that Rodin was referring to generalized external responsiveness rather than the specific responsiveness to food-relevant cues implied by the original version of the theory. The article also gave the wrong answer to the rhetorical question about what went wrong with externality theory. What really went wrong was that the sound insight that individuals with obesity are overly responsive to external food-relevant cues was over-extended to a sensitivity to all external cues, food-relevant or not. It is this latter assumption that has not stood up to empirical tests.

CONCLUSIONS

The research reported in this chapter supports predictions from both psychosomatic theory and the original version of externality theory. Consistent with psychosomatic theory, anxiety or stress induced overeating in participants who were overweight and those who were obese. Individuals with obesity were also willing to exert greater effort than were individuals of normal weight to gain access to food, particularly when the food was made salient. Predictions from externality theory about factors that should trigger eating in individuals with obesity were also supported: Palatability and salience of food as well as dinnertime were all shown to stimulate eating in participants with obesity but not those of normal weight. It would have been easy to integrate the two theories. Most external stimuli examined in research on externality theory (e.g., dinnertime, sight or smell of food) derive their quality as cues from their past association with eating. This fact suggests a process based on classical conditioning or expectancy learning, which would be consistent with the learning theory principles suggested by H. I. Kaplan and Kaplan (1957).

Yet, as it stands, the original externality theory can be criticized for being limited because it is mute about the causes of externality. The concept of eating restraint (Herman & Mack, 1975), which I discuss in chapter 6, was originally developed as a theoretical rationale for why eating behavior of individuals with obesity is often triggered by external stimuli. Drawing on the set-point theory of Nisbett (1972), Herman and Mack (1975) argued that many individuals with obesity were chronically dieting in their hopeless battle against a set point that pegged their weight above a culturally unacceptable level. Thus, it was not their obesity per se but their chronic state of food deprivation that was responsible for their overresponsiveness to external food cues.

6

RESTRAINED EATING AND THE BREAKDOWN OF SELF-REGULATION

Restraint theory was originally conceived as an extension of externality theory (Herman & Polivy, 1980). By linking externality to food deprivation, it provided a theoretical explanation for the overresponsiveness of individuals with obesity to external food-relevant cues. Because food deprivation rather than obesity was assumed to determine an individual's overresponsiveness to external food-relevant cues, dietary restraint was seen as a better predictor than was obesity. As a result, differences in eating restraint replaced differences in body mass index (BMI) as the predictor of overeating. Enthusiasm for the concept of eating restraint and for the theoretical elaboration of this idea into the boundary model of eating was further fueled by the promise that this model held for the explanation of the development of eating disorders, particularly bulimia nervosa (Herman & Polivy, 1984).[1] This enthusiasm was hardly dampened when, faced with the fact that restrained eaters typically have BMIs in

---

[1]*Bulimia nervosa* is characterized by recurrent episodes of binge eating (eating large amounts of food in short periods of time), a sense of lack of control over eating, and inappropriate compensatory behavior to prevent weight gain (e.g., self-induced vomiting; misuse of laxatives). These behaviors occur at least twice a week (*Diagnostic and Statistical Manual of Mental Disorders*, 4th ed.; American Psychiatric Association, 1994).

the high normal range, Herman, Polivy, and their colleagues abandoned the claim that restrained eaters were food-deprived (see, e.g., Heatherton, Herman, Polivy, King, & McGree, 1988, p. 20).

This chapter presents the boundary model of eating and reviews research stimulated by this model. I first evaluate the different scales that have been developed to measure restrained eating. Then, after describing the boundary model of eating, I review the innovative research that has been conducted to test this model. The boundary model proposes that restrained eaters regulate their eating according to their *diet boundary*—a self-imposed limit on their daily calorie intake. This effortful cognitive control of food intake is easily disrupted, such as when restrained eaters are distracted by emotional experiences or lose their motivation after a breach of their diet. Research findings have supported these predictions, but there have also been inconsistent findings, particularly from studies testing the cognitive processes assumed to regulate food intake. These inconsistencies motivated my colleagues and me to develop a new theory, the goal conflict theory of eating, which I describe in chapter 7 (this volume).

EATING RESTRAINT AND ITS MEASUREMENT

Eating restraint refers to the intentional effort to restrict one's food intake to control one's body weight. Herman and Mack (1975) developed the Restraint Scale (RS) to assess the degree of self-imposed restriction of food intake and weight fluctuation. The revised version of this scale (see Table 6.1) consists

TABLE 6.1
The Revised Restraint Scale

Question	Factor
1. How often are you dieting?	CD
2. What is the maximum amount of weight (in pounds) you have lost in a month?	WF
3. What is your maximum weight gain within a week?	WF
4. In a typical week, how much does your weight fluctuate?	WF
5. Would a weight fluctuation of 5 lbs affect the way you live your life?	CD
6. Do you eat sensibly in front of others and splurge alone?	CD
7. Do you give too much time and thought to food?	CD
8. Do you have feelings of guilt after overeating?	CD
9. How conscious are you of what you're eating?	CD
10. How many pounds over your desired weight were you at your maximum weight?	WF

Note. CD = concern for dieting; WF = weight fluctuations. From "The (Mis)measurement of Restraint: An Analysis of Conceptual and Psychometric Issues," by T. F. Heatherton, C. P. Herman, J. Polivy, G. A. King, and S. T. McGree, 1988, *Journal of Abnormal Psychology, 97*, p. 20. Copyright 1988 by the American Psychological Association.

of a 10-item questionnaire (Heatherton et al., 1988). Several studies have been conducted primarily on individuals of normal weight to identify the factor structure of the RS (Gorman & Allison, 1995; Heatherton et al., 1988). Most of these studies resulted in two factors, namely Weight Fluctuations (RS-WF) and Concern for Dieting (RS-CD).

Eating restraint as measured with the RS has been consistently found to be related to percentage overweight (Lowe, 1984: $r = .38$; Ruderman, 1983: $r = .37$; Ruderman, 1985: $r = .38$) and to BMI (Mensink, Stroebe, Schut, & Aarts, 2003: $r = .42$). Whether these positive correlations reflect a greater concern for dieting among individuals with obesity or are the result of greater weight fluctuations has been a matter of debate. This problem could easily be avoided if researchers in this area would also report scores on the subscales of the RS and if they would use the RS as a continuous measure rather than dichotomizing their samples into restrained and unrestrained eaters.

The ambiguities surrounding the RS motivated researchers to develop measures of dietary restraint that were truly one-dimensional. However, instead of focusing on a single factor of restrained eating, researchers typically decided to develop instruments that contained several subscales to tap other theoretically interesting facets of eating behavior. Thus, the Three Factor Eating Questionnaire (TFEQ) developed by Stunkard and Messick (1985) measures three dimensions, namely Cognitive Control of Eating, Disinhibition, and Susceptibility to Hunger. Although the Cognitive Restraint Scale of the TFEQ contains some of the restraint items of the RS, it appears to reflect a somewhat different type of restraint. Many of the items contained in that scale seem to assess a tendency to be aware of or focused on one's food intake (e.g., "I have a pretty good idea of the number of calories in common food"; "I often stop eating when I am not really full as a conscious means of limiting the amount I eat"; "I consciously hold back at meals in order not to gain weight"). Heatherton et al. (1988) suggested therefore that the TFEQ measured successful food restriction, whereas the RS assessed unsuccessful dieting. The correlation between the RS and the Restraint scale of the TFEQ (TFEQ-R) is substantial (e.g., $r = .68$; Stice, Fisher, & Lowe, 2004).

The Dutch Eating Behavior Questionnaire (DEBQ) was developed by van Strien, Frijters, Bergers, and Defares (1986) to provide one-dimensional scales to test the three primary theories of overeating and obesity: namely, psychosomatic theory, externality theory, and restrained eating. The DEBQ measures three dimensions, namely Restraint, External Eating, and Emotional Eating. Like the TFEQ-R, the Restraint scale of the DEBQ (DEBQ-R) tries to identify restrained eaters who are consciously restricting their food intake (e.g., "Do you try to eat less at mealtimes than you would like to eat?"; "Do you watch exactly what you eat?"; "Do you deliberately eat foods that are slimming?"). Thus, again, in contrast to the RS, which seems to identify unsuccessful dieters who oscillate between dieting and splurging, the DEBQ-R appears to measure successful dieting. Stice et al. (2004) reported a correlation of .76 between the RS and the DEBQ-R.

A study of Laessle et al. (1989), who administered the three scales and some additional measures to a small sample of women, provides support for the interpretation that Heatherton et al. (1988) offered for the differences between the RS on the one hand and the TFEQ-R and DEBQ-R on the other hand. A principal components factor analysis conducted by Laessle et al. on the RS, the TFEQ-R, the DEBQ-R, and measures of caloric intake, disordered eating, and body shape consciousness resulted in a three-factor solution, with the RS-CD loading on the first factor, the RS-WF on the second, and the TFEQ-R and the DEBQ-R on the third. This pattern is consistent with the assumption that these measures assess different dimensions.

If one analyzes the other measures that load on each of the three factors, an interesting picture emerges. The Eating Disorders Inventory (EDI) Body Dissatisfaction subscale, EDI Drive for Thinness subscale (Garner, Olmsted, & Polivy, 1983), and Body Shape Questionnaire (P. J. Cooper, Taylor, Cooper, & Fairburn, 1987) load highly on the first factor (which includes the RS) and also on the third factor (which includes the TFEQ-R and the DEBQ-R). These findings suggest that eating restraint (as assessed by all three scales) is motivated by concerns about shape and weight and results, in women, from a drive to be thin to comply with current standards for female beauty. However, the restrained eaters identified with the RS appeared to be less successful in reaching this goal. The other measures that also loaded only on the first factor were the TFEQ Disinhibition subscale and the EDI Bulimia subscale. Thus, consistent with the interpretation offered by Heatherton et al. (1988), the RS appears to reflect a tendency toward disinhibited eating.

In contrast, the measure that loaded only on the third factor, the factor on which the TFEQ-R and the DEBQ-R are located, was daily caloric intake. This dimension appears to reflect actual restriction of food intake. Indeed, daily calorie intake assessed with a food diary correlated $-.46$ with the TFEQ-R and $-.49$ with the DEBQ-R. Thus, higher levels of restraint on those measures were associated with lower daily calorie intake. In contrast, scores on the RS were unrelated to calorie intake ($r = -.04$).

The association between the TFEQ-R and DEBQ-R on the one hand and daily calorie intake on the other reported by Laessle, Tuschl, Kotthaus, and Pirke (1989) appears to be inconsistent with results of four studies of food intake of restrained eaters conducted by Stice et al. (2004). These authors unobtrusively observed food intake of restrained and unrestrained eaters in two laboratory studies and two studies conducted in a restaurant setting. In none of the studies did the correlations between calorie intake and eating restraint reach acceptable levels of significance. Stice et al. attributed the inconsistency between their findings and those of Laessle et al. to the inaccuracy of self-report measures. Although this possibility cannot be ruled out, the discrepancy could also be due to problems with the observational studies. In their classic analysis of studies of the association between attitude and behavior, Ajzen and Fishbein (1977) identified the noncorrespondence between the measures of attitude and behavior as one of the main reasons for the failure of attitudes to predict behavior. Noncorrespondence is caused by differences in the globality of the two measures, most commonly the fact that global attitude measures are used to predict behavior in specific situations. Stice et al. committed this sin by trying to predict eating behavior in specific situations (i.e., during one specific meal) from a global measure of an individual's intention to diet, namely the TFEQ-R and the DEBQ-R. To construct a measure of eating behavior that corresponds with global measures of dieting intentions such as these Restraint Scales, one would have to aggregate observations of eating behavior across a great number of meals and eating situations. This is precisely the strategy Laessle et al. chose when they estimated food intake with a 7-day food diary. It is thus quite likely that Laessle et al.'s findings provide a more valid picture of the relationship between eating restraint and eating behavior than do the observations about behavior made by Stice et al.

Finally, the measures that loaded on the second factor, the dimension with which the RS-WF scale was mainly associated, were BMI, maximum BMI, and the difference between maximum and minimum. This dimension appears to reflect weight fluctuation. The fact that the RS-CD and RS-WF were located on separate factors, but that the RS-CD and not the RS-WF subscale was most closely linked to measures of Bulimia and Disinhibition, suggests that this scale reflects both attempts at restraint and problems with disinhibition. In contrast, the RS-WF subscale appears to be a pure measure of weight fluctuations. This finding reinforces the point made earlier that studies that use the RS should report their results for the separate subscales.

The pattern that emerges from this factor analysis is consistent with the assumption that the RS identifies individuals who alternate between restraint and splurging, whereas the TFEQ-R and the DEBQ-R identify individuals who are more successful in their restraint. As Ouwens (2005) concluded from her thorough review of research in this area, this impression is validated by the fact that studies that use the TFEQ or the DEBQ rarely find disinhibition effects in restrained eaters. Individuals with high scores on the TFEQ-R or the DEBQ-R seem to be better able than individuals who score high on the RS to resist the temptation to splurge and binge while they are actually dieting. They might thus be more successful in losing weight, at least in the short run.

THE BOUNDARY MODEL OF EATING BEHAVIOR

Herman and Polivy (1984) incorporated their hypotheses regarding eating restraint into a boundary model of the regulation of eating that has dictated the research agenda of eating researchers for decades and has stimulated an immense amount of research (see Figure 6.1). They proposed that biological pressures work to maintain food intake within a certain range. The aversive qualities of hunger keep consumption above a minimum level and the aversive qualities of satiety keep it below some maximum. Between these two zones is a zone of biological indifference, where eating is regulated by nonphysiological social and environmental influences.

Restrained eaters or chronic dieters are assumed to differ from nonrestrained eaters (or nondieters) in two respects: First, restrained eaters impose a diet boundary within their zone of biological indifference. This boundary consists of a set of dieting rules that specify more or less precisely the amounts and types of food individuals allow themselves. In many instances, these dieting rules reflect the dietary prescriptions of the currently fashionable diet. These dieting rules are used to limit food intake to maintain or achieve desirable weight. Restrained eaters are assumed to regulate their food intake cognitively through the application of these dieting rules. In contrast, unrestrained eaters

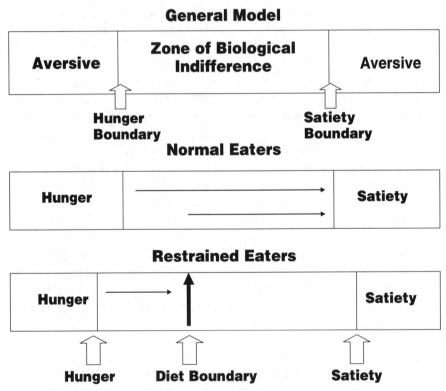

Figure 6.1. The boundary model of eating. From *Eating and Its Disorders* (p. 153), by A. J. Stunkard and E. Stellar (Eds.), 1984, New York: Raven Press. Copyright 1984 by Raven Press. Adapted with kind permission of Springer Science + Business Media.

are assumed to regulate their eating through bodily feedback: They eat when they are hungry and stop eating when they are full. Second, restrained eaters are assumed to have a larger zone of biological indifference. Because of their frequent dieting and overeating, restrained eaters are assumed to have become less sensitive to bodily hunger and satiation signals. According to Herman and Polivy (1984), dieters "may be seen as in some sense under reduced physiological control, compared to nondieters" (p. 145). In comparison, the nondieters can be seen as "animals" (p. 146) whose eating is unaffected by cognitive controls and guided by internal cues.

As long as restrained eaters are motivated to concentrate on the regulation of their eating, they are capable of keeping to their diet boundary. However, if their motivation to restrict their food intake is impaired, physiological regulation takes over and they eat until they are satiated. Two sets of factors are assumed to impair the ability and motivation of restrained eaters to control their eating: (a) emotional distress and (b) actual or perceived dietary violations (Herman & Polivy, 1984). The following sections review the role of these factors in impairing the eating regulation of restrained eaters. Because Herman and Polivy gave up the claim that restrained eaters were actually food deprived, they no longer emphasized overresponsiveness to external cues as a factor triggering overeating.

The Impact of Emotional Distress on Eating: The Emotion Hypothesis

In view of the substantial correlation between BMI and eating restraint (e.g., Mensink et al., 2003; Ruderman, 1983, 1985), the hypothesis that distressing emotions result in overeating in restrained eaters is consistent with the instrumental conditioning or comfort hypothesis of psychosomatic theory (H. I. Kaplan & Kaplan, 1957). According to this hypothesis, restrained eaters overeat because eating reduces their distress. Thus, they break their diet because the need to reduce their distress motivates them to eat.

A somewhat different perspective has been suggested by Herman and Polivy (1984), who argued that distressful experiences undermine the restrained individuals' motivation to diet because of the "the imposition of a more urgent concern" (p. 152). Thus, when one has just experienced the loss of a loved one or is worried about an impending exam, concern for dieting might temporarily appear to be of diminished importance. According to this theory, distressed restrained eaters overeat not because eating reduces their distress but because concerns for diet appear unimportant compared with the event that caused the emotional upheaval.

A third and rather more complicated motivational explanation has been suggested by Heatherton and Baumeister (1991). According to their "escape from self-awareness" model, dieters hold a negative view of self, particularly of their appearance. Therefore, they generally experience self-focused attention (i.e., self-awareness) as unpleasant (Heatherton, Striepe, & Wittenberg, 1998). Unfortunately, to control their food intake, restrained eaters need to be aware of their personal standards for consumption (i.e., their diet boundary) as well as of their actual food intake (Heatherton et al., 1998). Thus, a state of self-awareness is essential for the self-monitoring of food intake that is necessary for the restrained eaters' cognitive regulation of eating. Therefore, they have to tolerate the negative feelings about the self that are activated during states of self-awareness. However, self-awareness may become too painful when individuals encounter negative information about themselves that threatens their self-image. Failure experiences and other threats to their ego are likely to motivate them to escape from self-awareness "by constricting their cognitive attention to the immediate situation" (Heatherton et al., 1998, p. 302). Not all types of distress threaten the self-image, however. Physical threats have little implication for one's self-worth and should not motivate restrained eaters to escape from aversive self-awareness (Heatherton, Herman, & Polivy, 1992). Therefore, overeating should be induced in restrained eaters only by threats that have some implications for the individual's self-esteem and not by physical threats, such as the threat of electric shocks.

Despite considerable differences, these explanations share the assumption that the distressing nature of the emotional experiences is what undermines an individual's motivation to monitor food intake. In contrast, my colleagues and I have argued that the disinhibitory effect of distress on the eating behavior of restrained eaters has little to do with the emotional quality of the experience; rather, coping with distress requires cognitive resources (cognitive investment hypothesis; Boon, Stroebe, Schut, & Ijtema, 2002; Boon, Stroebe, Schut, & Jansen, 1997; see also Lowe & Kral, 2006). For restrained eaters, regulating their food intake is a controlled process and, as with any controlled process, it is effortful and requires attentional resources (Bargh, 1996). Restrained eaters must monitor their current food intake, calculate calorie content, keep track of their daily consumption, and evaluate all of this information against their dietary standards (i.e., their diet boundary). Thus, restrained eaters are assumed to invest more cognitive resources in regulating their eating than do unrestrained eaters. As a consequence, cognitive capacity restrictions (e.g., cognitive load) should affect the eating behavior of restrained eaters more than that of unrestrained eaters. Factors that interfere with cognitive control are therefore assumed to impair the regulation of eating in restrained eaters because these factors decrease their ability to monitor their food intake. Because all strong emotions, whether they are distressful or pleasant, are likely to be distractive, one would expect that strong positive emotions should also result in overeating among restrained eaters. In a more general way, our theory would predict that any experience that distracts individuals while they are eating palatable food is likely to lead to overeating among restrained eaters.

It would seem easy to devise experiments to test theories that make such divergent predictions. The most specific predictions are made by the escape from self-awareness theory (Heatherton & Baumeister, 1991). According to this theory, only threats to the self-image should induce overeating in restrained eaters. Physical or any other type of threats should have no impact on their eating. Predictions from psychosomatic theory and the hypothesis suggested by Herman and Polivy (1984) are somewhat broader. According to these theories, any experience that results in emotional distress should induce overeating in restrained eaters. According to our own theory, not only distressing experiences but also extreme pleasure, even nonemotional experiences that are distractive, are likely to induce overeating in restrained eaters (Boon et al., 1997, 2002).

Yet, empirical evidence is somewhat equivocal, even though in my not unbiased view it is most consistent with our own perspective (e.g., Boon et al., 1997, 2002). The emotion hypothesis has typically been tested in experiments that compared the eating behavior of restrained and unrestrained eaters after the induction of negative mood compared with either a neutral or a positive situation. A variety of manipulations have been used to induce negative mood. Participants were stressed with the threat of shock (Heatherton, Herman, & Polivy, 1991; Herman & Polivy, 1975), task failure (Baucom & Aiken, 1981; Eldredge, 1993; Heatherton et al., 1991; Heatherton, Polivy, Herman, & Baumeister, 1993; Polivy & Herman, 1999; Ruderman, 1985; Stephens, Prentice-Dunn, & Spruill, 1994; Tanofsky-Kraff, Wilfley, & Spurrell, 2000), the anticipation of public speaking (Heatherton et al., 1991; Tanofsky-Kraff et al., 2000), interpersonal rejection (Tanofsky-Kraff et al., 2000), expecting blood samples to be taken (Bleau, 1996), watching unpleasant videos (Cools, Schotte, & McNally, 1992; Schotte, Cools, & McNally, 1990; Wardle & Beales, 1988), reading Velten self-referent statements (Frost, Goolkasian, Ely, & Blanchard, 1982; Lowe & Maycock, 1988; Ridgeway & Jeffrey, 1998), remembering negative autobiographical experiences (Tuschen, Florin, & Baucke, 1993), performing Stroop tasks with forbidden food words (Mitchell & Epstein, 1996), and watching a sad film (Sheppard-Sawyer, McNally, & Harnden Fischer, 2000). Most of these studies used amounts eaten in an (alleged) taste test as dependent measures.

In most of these studies, induction of negative emotions increased eating among restrained eaters (e.g., Bleau, 1996 [16-year-old-girls]; Cools et al., 1992; Frost et al., 1982; Heatherton et al., 1991 [task failure, anticipated speech]; Heatherton et al., 1993 [simple failure, failure with distraction]; Heatherton et al., 1998; Herman & Polivy, 1975; Polivy & Herman, 1999; Polivy, Herman, & McFarlane, 1994; Ruderman, 1985; Schotte et al., 1990; Tanofsky-Kraff et al., 2000 [interpersonal manipulation]; Tuschen et al., 1993; Wallis & Hetherington, 2004; Wardle & Beales, 1988, Experiment 2). Whereas most of these studies used questionnaires (mainly the RS) to assess restrained eating, two studies used current dieting status: Baucom and Aiken (1981) induced negative mood with a failure experience, and Wardle and Beales (1988) used a frightening film. Both studies found that negative mood increased consumption of individuals who were currently dieting, but not of those who were not currently on a diet. Rotenberg and Flood (1999) also found an effect for current dieting, after their questionnaire measure proved ineffective (Eating Attitude Test; Garner, Olmsted, Bohr, & Garfinkel, 1982). However, this effect emerged only for a distress manipulation based on memory of lonely but not of sad events. Because experiences of loneliness are likely to be more ego threatening than are experiences of sadness, this pattern would be consistent with the escape from self-awareness model.

Several other experiments (or experimental conditions) failed to observe an increase in eating among restrained eaters following induction of a distressing emotion (e.g., Eldredge, 1993; Heatherton et al., 1991 [physical threat condition]; Lowe & Maycock, 1988; Oliver, Wardle, & Gibson, 2000; Ridgeway & Jeffrey, 1998; Rotenberg & Flood, 1999 [memory of sad events]; Sheppard-Sawyer et al., 2000; Stephens et al., 1994; Tanofsky-Kraff et al., 2000 [failure experience, anticipated speech threat]). It is important to note that only one of these studies found that distress reduced eating among restrained eaters (Eldredge, 1993).[2] All other studies found either no effect, or if they found a difference in the right direction, it did not reach acceptable levels of significance. One could therefore argue that the evidence supports the conclusion that distress induces overeating in restrained eaters. However, in light of the considerable number of inconsistent results, such a global conclusion would prove unsatisfactory.

Two criteria have been suggested that might differentiate experiments that failed from those that succeeded in finding that emotion induced overeating in restrained eaters. According to the escape from self-awareness model, one distinguishing factor should be whether studies used distress manipulations that posed a threat to the individual's self-worth. Only ego-threatening manipulations should be effective. A second factor that has been suggested by Ouwens (2005) is the type of measure used to assess restrained eating. Ouwens argued that practically all the studies that found a disinhibitory effect of distressing emotions on eating by restrained eaters had used the RS of Herman and Polivy (1980). Only rarely have disinhibitory effects been found with other measures of dietary restraint.

In Table 6.2, the various studies or conditions of studies are categorized according to the eight cells that result from the above categorization.

---

[2]Participants in Eldredge's (1993) study had to respond to a body image scale before the taste test. Because restrained eaters have low body satisfaction anyway, inclusion of this measure might have focused them on dietary restraint, a focus that might have been strengthened by the fact that the body image scale was embedded in a self-esteem and a neuroticism scale. As a result of this focus, the failure experience might have increased the motivation of restrained eaters to diet ("I cannot do anything about being stupid, but at least I can try to improve my figure"). Forming this intention might have helped them to cope with the blow to their self-esteem in the failure condition.

TABLE 6.2
Pattern of Findings of Studies on the Impact of Emotional Distress on Eating Among Individuals Who Are Obese and Individuals of Normal Weight

| Type of threat | Measure | |
	RS scale or current dieting	TFEQ, DEBQ, or others
Ego threat	**Effective**	
	Baucom & Aiken, 1981	Bleau, 1996 (16-year-olds)
	Frost et al., 1982	Wallis & Hetherington, 2004
	Heatherton et al., 1991 (task failure, anticipated speech)	
	Heatherton et al., 1993 (simple failure, failure/distraction)	
	Heatherton et al., 1998	
	Polivy et al., 1994	
	Polivy & Herman, 1999	
	Rotenberg & Flood, 1999, (memories of loneliness)	
	Ruderman, 1985	
	Tuschen et al., 1993; Tanofsky-Kraff et al., 2000 (interpersonal manipulation)	
	Wardle & Beales, 1988	
	Ineffective	
	Eldredge, 1993	**Haynes et al., 2003**
	Heatherton et al., 1993 (failure videotaped)	**Lowe & Maycock, 1988**
	Mitchell & Epstein, 1996	**Oliver et al., 2000**
	Ridgeway & Jeffrey, 1998 (failure to find effects with RS); Stephens et al., 1994	**Rotenberg & Flood, 1999 (memory of loneliness; failure to find effects with Eating Attitude Test)**
	Tanofsky-Kraff et al., 2000 (anticipated speech, failure experience)	**Ridgeway & Jeffrey, 1998 (failure to find effects with TFEQ)**
No ego threat	**Effective**	
	Cools et al., 1992	
	Herman & Polivy, 1975	
	Schotte et al., 1990	
	Ineffective	
	Heatherton et al., 1991 (physical shock)	**Rotenberg & Flood, 1999 (memory of sad events; failure to find effects with Eating Attitude Test)**
	Heatherton et al., 1998 (Experiment 3, other condition)	
	Rotenberg & Flood, 1999 (memory of sad events)	

Note. Boldface type indicates studies or conditions that are consistent with predictions based on two criteria. Emotional distress should result in overeating in restrained eaters only (a) if distress is induced with a threat to the individual's self-worth rather than a physical threat and (b) if restrained eating is measured with the RS (or indicated by current dieting) rather than with the TFEQ, DEBQ, or other measures of restraint. RS = Restraint Scale; TFEQ = Three Factor Eating Questionnaire; DEBQ = Dutch Eating Behavior Questionnaire.

Studies or conditions that are consistent with predictions based on these two criteria are printed in bold. As can be seen, type of measure used is a good predictor of the success of a study. Only two studies that did not use either the RS or current dieting were successful in finding an effect of emotional distress on eating among restrained eaters (Bleau, 1996; Wallis & Hetherington, 2004).

The distinction between ego threats and other threats does less well in differentiating successful and unsuccessful studies. In fact, the greatest number of inconsistent findings is in the category of studies that used ego threats to induce emotional distress but failed to find overeating among restrained eaters, despite using the RS. However, as I mentioned earlier, all but one study (Eldredge, 1993) reported no difference or some insignificant differences in the right direction. For example, Mitchell and Epstein (1996) found a significant Restraint × Condition interaction, but the simple effects reached significance only for unrestrained eaters (who ate significantly less). In the Heatherton et al. (1993) study, restrained eaters did not eat more after failure when the failure was videotaped (but did so without the videotape). The videotape probably increased participants' self-awareness. This increase in self-awareness is likely to remind restrained eaters of their diet plans and to stop them from violating them. Stephens et al. (1994) also used videotaping to manipulate self-awareness and found that failure experience did not induce overeating in restrained eaters in the high self-awareness condition. Without the videotape, restrained eaters consumed considerably more ice cream in the failure than in the success condition (213.4 grams [7.53 ounces] vs. 165.6 grams [5.84 ounces]), but the third-order interaction did not reach significance (which could be a power problem).

Studies that succeeded in inducing overeating in restrained eaters despite using a non-ego-threatening stressor (see Table 6.2) are also inconsistent with the escape from self-awareness model. One of these inconsistent studies is the original study by Herman and Polivy (1975), who induced overeating with the threat of electric shocks. Cools et al. (1992) and Schotte et al. (1990) caused overeating with frightening and even comic films, again manipulations that are unlikely to threaten the ego of adult viewers. Yet, the few studies that tested the model directly by manipulating ego threat within the same design tended to support the notion that ego-threatening experiences induce more overeating than do threats that do not affect participants' self-esteem (Heatherton et al., 1991, 1998; Rotenberg & Flood, 1999).

How can this inconsistency be accounted for? These findings suggest that (a) any type of threat can induce overeating in restrained eaters but that (b) the effects of ego-threatening experiences are often (but not always) stronger than those of events that are not ego-threatening. In my opinion, the reason for this powerful effect of ego-threatening experiences is not escape from self-awareness, but that coping with some ego-threatening experiences may often require more cognitive resources than would coping with experiences that are not ego-threatening. For example, coping with the threat of an inescapable electric shock is likely to require few cognitive resources. Because one cannot do much about the threat of an electric shock, one will probably try not to think about it, which should not be very distractive. In contrast, as anybody knows who has done so, anticipating giving a speech is likely to require a great deal of cognitive activity. In fact, studies show that individuals anticipating having to speak usually do not hear (or remember) anything that has been said by the speaker before them (the *next-in-line effect;* Brenner, 1973). However, non-ego-threatening experiences can also be distractive. For example, watching a frightening film in a darkened room is likely to draw most of an individual's attention (Cools et al., 1992; Schotte et al., 1990). Because watching a good comedy should also be involving, one would expect that funny films also induce overeating in restrained eaters. Indeed, Cools et al. (1992) found that restrained eaters also overate while watching a comedy film.[3]

The most direct support for the cognitive investment hypothesis that my colleagues and I proposed comes from studies showing that even distracting events that are unlikely to arouse emotions may still induce overeating in restrained eaters. For example, Boon et al. (2002) had restrained and unrestrained eaters listen to a radio conversation and count the number of animal words used in that conversation while tasting various ice creams. Whereas restrained eaters ate slightly less ice cream than did unrestrained eaters when undistracted, they ate considerably more when distracted. Ward and Mann (2000) also found that putting restrained eaters under cognitive load disinhibited their eating. Similar results were reported by Rutledge and Linden (1998) and Lattimore and Caswell (2004). The study of Lattimore and Caswell is particularly interesting because they used a distracting stressor (reaction task) and a nondistracting stressor (cold pressor task). They found that both stress tasks produced significant increases in self-rated anxiety and that there was no difference in anxiety ratings between tasks. Yet, overeating was induced only by their distracting task. This finding supports our hypothesis that distraction and not emotion induces overeating in restrained eaters.

How do the findings on the impact of emotional distress on the eating behavior of restrained and unrestrained eaters compare with the research that manipulated distress with individuals with obesity and those of normal weight? This comparison is important because, originally, the concept of restrained

---

[3]In response to a critique by Schotte (1992), Heatherton et al. (1992, 1998) modified their escape from self-awareness model in a way that would allow them to account even for these distraction effects. They argued that people can experience escape from self-awareness with any type of movie as long as it is compelling and as long as they can "lose themselves" in the movie (Heatherton et al., 1992). Because experiences that require cognitive resources make it more difficult for individuals to focus their attention on the self, any strong distraction should result in escape from self-awareness. Although this argument is reasonable, it is inconsistent with their earlier prediction that only ego threats would motivate people to escape from self-awareness.

eating had been introduced to account for the problems individuals with obesity have in regulating their eating. Although Herman and Polivy (e.g., 1984) became more interested in the application of their model to eating disorders, the equivalence hypothesis was once one of the core assumptions of the boundary model. It is therefore surprising that it has never been tested properly in research studies on the distress–eating relationship. With one exception, all studies on the impact of emotions on eating on restrained eaters involved individuals of normal weight.

The one exception is the study of Baucom and Aiken (1981), which used a Weight × Dieting status design. A 2 (distress) × 2 (weight) × 2 (dieting status) analysis of variance revealed a significant Distress × Dieting Status interaction: Emotional distress manipulated through failure on a concept formation task increased eating among dieters and decreased it among nondieters. In contrast, the Distress × Obesity interaction did not even approach significance. Although the finding, with dieting status controlled for, that emotional distress did not induce overeating in individuals with obesity is consistent with the equivalence hypothesis, it does not fully answer the question whether eating restraint mediates the impact of emotional distress on eating in those who are obese. To test this assumption, the authors would first have to demonstrate that there is an effect to be mediated (i.e., that without dieting status controlled for, emotional distress does induce overeating in those who are obese).[4] The findings of Wardle and Beales (1988) are similarly inconclusive because their sample consisted exclusively of individuals who were overweight.

The Impact of Dietary Violations on Eating

The diet boundary is the strength of but also the Achilles' heel for the eating regulation of restrained eaters. As long as they are motivated and able to regulate their eating cognitively, they are able to keep to their diet. However, as has been seen in the previous sections, once their motivation or ability to regulate is somehow impaired, they are likely to overeat. According to the boundary model, one of the main factors that destroys the motivation of restrained eaters to keep to their diet is the recognition that they have already violated their diet boundary. Once they have (or think they have) breached this boundary, restrained eaters are assumed to see no further reason for main-

---

[4]According to Kenny, Kashy, and Bolger (1998), four conditions must be met to demonstrate that eating restraint is the mediator of the impact obesity has on eating behavior: One must show that (a) obesity is related to outcome (i.e., that there are obesity-related differences in eating behavior); (b) obesity is correlated with the assumed mediator (i.e., eating restraint); (c) the mediator affects the outcome (i.e., that the differences in eating behavior between restrained and unrestrained eaters parallel those between individuals who are obese and those who are of normal weight); and, finally, (d) controlling for the mediator (i.e., eating restraint) eliminates or significantly reduces the association between obesity and eating.

taining their diet goals. Herman and Polivy (1984) have called this state the "what-the-hell effect," suggesting that once restrained eaters realize that they have broken through their diet boundary, they totally abandon all dietary concerns.

The effects of dietary violations on eating by restrained eaters have been tested with a modified version of the preload paradigm of Schachter, Goldman, and Gordon (1968). In the modification introduced by Herman and Mack (1975), preloads are no longer used to manipulate satiation but instead to induce violation of the diet boundary and disinhibited eating in restrained eaters. Respondents are instructed to preload with a prescribed amount of some rich (and therefore normally forbidden) food. Herman and Mack (1975) preloaded their restrained and unrestrained participants with either one or two milkshakes before an ice cream tasting session that functioned as a dependent measure of eating. Whereas unrestrained eaters ate less ice cream under preload than they did under control conditions (i.e., regulation), restrained respondents ate more after the preload (see Figure 6.2). Thus, restrained eaters were not merely insensitive to preloads (i.e., nonregulation) as in the study of Schachter et al., but increased their ice cream consumption under preload conditions (i.e., counterregulation). However, the amount of ice cream consumed by restrained eaters after two milkshakes was unexpectedly not significantly greater than after one. Herman and Polivy (1984) argued that after two milk-

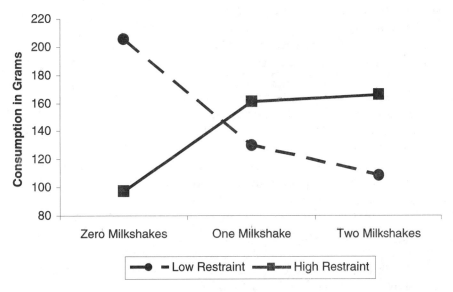

Figure 6.2. Grams of ice cream consumed by restrained and unrestrained eaters under different preload conditions. From "Restrained and Unrestrained Eating," by C. P. Herman and D. Mack, 1975, *Journal of Personality, 43,* p. 656. Copyright 1975 by Blackwell Publishing. Adapted with permission.

shakes, restrained eaters needed to eat less ice cream to reach their satiety boundary than they did after only one milkshake.

Following the Herman and Mack (1975) study, the preload paradigm became popular (Dritschel, Cooper, & Charnock, 1993; Herman, Polivy, & Esses, 1987; Hibscher & Herman, 1977; Jansen, Oosterlaan, Merckelbach, & van den Hout, 1988; Lowe, 1995; Lowe, Whitlow, & Bellwoar, 1991; P. J. Morgan & Jeffrey, 1999; J. Ogden & Wardle, 1991; Polivy, 1976; Polivy, Heatherton, & Herman, 1988; Polivy, Herman, Hackett, & Kuleshnyk, 1986; Rotenberg & Flood, 2000; Ruderman & Christensen, 1983; Spencer & Fremouw, 1979; van Strien, Cleven, & Schippers, 2000; Wardle & Beales, 1987; Westenhoefer, Broeckmann, Münch, & Pudel, 1994; Woody, Costanzo, Liefer, & Conger, 1981). A few of these studies replicated the original experimental paradigm (Dritschel et al., 1993; Herman et al., 1987; Hibscher & Herman, 1977; Jansen, Oosterlaan, Merckelbach, & van den Hout, 1988; Rotenberg & Flood, 2000; van Strien et al., 2000; Westenhoefer et al., 1994); others manipulated the perceived rather than the actual calorie content of the preload (Polivy, 1976; Spencer & Fremouw, 1979; Woody et al., 1981). Some of the studies also controlled for variables in addition to restraint, such as obesity (e.g., Hibscher & Herman, 1977; Ruderman & Christensen, 1983), dieting status (Lowe, 1995; Lowe et al., 1991), or self-esteem (Polivy et al., 1988). These latter studies are particularly interesting because they tested the assumption that eating restraint and not some third variable correlated with restraint is responsible for the observed effects. I limit my review to studies that used the RS (either alone or in addition to other measures). For reasons discussed earlier, none of the studies that used the TFEQ or the DEBQ found a significant interaction between eating restraint assessed with either of these measures and preload (e.g., Lowe & Kleifield, 1988; P. J. Morgan & Jeffrey, 1999; J. Ogden & Wardle, 1991; Wardle & Beales, 1987).

Three of the pure replications of the original preload study reported a significant interaction between preload and restraint (Herman et al., 1987; Hibscher & Herman, 1977; Jansen et al., 1988), but only two of these found evidence of counterregulation (Herman et al., 1987; Hibscher & Herman, 1977, according to reanalysis by Ruderman & Wilson, 1979). In the Jansen et al. (1988) study, the significant interaction was due to restrained eaters eating the same, regardless of whether or not they had consumed a preload (i.e., nonregulation), while unrestrained eaters ate less in the preload condition. In the Rotenberg and Flood (2000) study, the Preload × Restraint interaction failed to reach significance, but, supportive of the boundary model, consumption increased with increasing restraint within the preload condition.

None of the three studies that employed the RS in addition to either the TFEQ or DEBQ reported an interaction between restraint measured with the RS and the preload manipulation (Dritschel et al., 1993; van Strien et al.,

2000; Westenhoefer et al., 1994). However, at least two of these studies used a procedure that was likely to make the restraint questionnaires highly salient. In the study of van Strien et al. (2000), participants were asked to complete a set of eating measures and to bring them along to the experiment (DEBQ, TFEQ, RS, and the Bulimia subscale of the Revised EDI). Similarly, participants in the study of Westenhoefer et al. (1994) were sent the TFEQ and told they would be selected on the basis of their questionnaire results. Thus, participants knew that researchers were somehow concerned about eating restraint, which could have influenced their behavior during the study.

Perceived Versus Actual Calorie Content

Studies that extended the preload paradigm by manipulating the perceived calorie content of the preload provide evidence that the preload effect is mediated by cognitive rather than physiological processes. These studies demonstrated that it is not the actual number of calories in the preload but the (manipulated) beliefs about the calorie content that determine whether restrained eaters overeat (Polivy, 1976; Spencer & Fremouw, 1979; Woody et al., 1981). Counterregulation is inferred in these studies if participants eat more of a preload that is perceived as high in calories than a preload that is perceived as low in calories. The consumption of equal amounts in both conditions would be evidence for nonregulation.

Polivy (1976) was the first to report that restrained eaters ate more when they thought they had consumed a high-calorie preload, whereas unrestrained eaters showed the reverse effect, independent of the actual calorie content of the preload. She reported a marginally significant Restraint × Perceived Calories interaction. Because of the marginal level of significance and the failure of many participants to believe the instructions that the preload was high or low in calories, she conducted a post hoc analysis in which she regrouped her participants according to their reported beliefs.

In an early attempted replication of this study, Ruderman and Wilson (1979) failed to find an effect of perceived calorie content of a milkshake preload that was described as either high or low in calories on the amount of ice cream consumed in a subsequent taste test. However, this study also failed to observe counterregulation in restrained eaters with a preload of perceived high-calorie content or regulation in unrestrained eaters. The findings of Ruderman and Wilson are thus discrepant with the research on preloading effects reported earlier. As the authors concluded themselves, the likely reason for these discrepant results was the fact that the preload factor involved repeated measures on the same participants.

A more convincing demonstration of the importance of perceived calorie content was published by Spencer and Fremouw (1979), who gave participants a milkshake preload of approximately 500 kilocalories but told them that the drink was either very high or very low in calories. A manipulation check attested to the effectiveness of this manipulation. In line with predictions, restrained eaters ate significantly more ice cream in a subsequent ice cream tasting test when they thought the milkshake was of high rather than low calorie content. Perceived calories had no significant impact on the ice cream consumption of unrestrained eaters (i.e., nonregulation).

This study was replicated by Woody et al. (1981), who preloaded with milkshakes of identical composition that were presented as either high or low in calories. However, Woody et al. added two variations to this basic design. Cross-cutting the perceived calorie manipulation, they made the milkshake preload bad tasting (with quinine) for half of the participants. Similarly, the ice cream used in the subsequent tasting test was adulterated with quinine for half of the participants. Thus a 2 (perceived calorie of preload) × 2 (taste of preload) × 2 (taste of ice cream) × 2 (restraint) factorial design was used. Because the taste of the preload had no effect on amount eaten, Woody et al. collapsed across preload taste conditions in their analyses. Subsequent analyses revealed a significant Restraint × Ice Cream Taste × Calorie Information interaction. Restrained eaters ate significantly more ice cream with a preload than without a preload, but only if the preload was perceived as being high in calories and the ice cream in the taste test tasted good. There was no evidence for counterregulation if the preload was perceived as being low in calories or if the ice cream tasted bad. None of these factors affected amount of ice cream eaten by unrestrained eaters.

To test whether the calorie content of the preload or the fact that the preload consisted of normally forbidden food led to the results obtained, Knight and Boland (1989, Experiment 2) preloaded with either forbidden food (milkshake) or nonforbidden food (cottage cheese) of equal calorie content. There was a significant Restraint × Type of Food interaction. Restrained eaters increased their consumption only when preloaded with a milkshake, but not when the preload consisted of cottage cheese.

In summary, then, these studies provide consistent evidence for the assumption that the perceived rather than the actual content of the preload induces restrained eaters to overeat. This pattern of finding is consistent with expectations based on the boundary model. Because the perception of having breached one's diet boundary is assumed to be responsible for abandoning restraint in restrained eaters, it makes sense that this consequence is less likely to occur when restrained eaters are assured that the preload has a very low calorie content.[5]

---

[5]As in the pure preload studies, counterregulation in these extended preload studies can be demonstrated only when the RS is used to identify restrained eaters. Studies that use the DEBQ (e.g., J. Ogden & Wardle, 1991) or TFEQ (e.g., Chapelot, Pasquet, Apfelbaum, & Fricker, 1995; Huon, Wootton, & Brown, 1991) to identify restrained eaters fail to observe counterregulation or nonregulations following preload manipulations.

Anticipation of Future Consumption

Some authors reasoned that the disinhibiting effect of a preload on restrained eaters would be strengthened if, in addition to having consumed a rich preload, they had to anticipate having to eat a highly caloric meal in the near future (Knight & Boland, 1989; Ruderman, Belzer, & Halperin, 1985; Tomarken & Kirschenbaum, 1984). As Tomarken and Kirschenbaum (1984) argued, "the prospect of an additional bout of overeating in the future would further intensify feelings of hopelessness about one's ability to adhere to personal norms of dietary restraint during the present day" (p. 45). The only indication of a disinhibiting effect of the anticipation of future consumption comes from studies that used the meal anticipation manipulation without also exposing participants to a preload (Knight & Boland, 1989, Experiment 3; Ruderman et al., 1985, Experiment 2). Restrained eaters in the Ruderman et al. (1985) study ate more crackers in a taste test if they anticipated having to consume a milkshake in a second taste test than did restrained eaters who did not anticipate a second taste test. Similarly, Knight and Boland (1989) found increased cracker consumption among restrained eaters who anticipated having to consume some forbidden food after the taste test, compared with restrained eaters who did not anticipate further consumption. The findings of Tomarken and Kirschenbaum (1984, Experiment 2), who combined the manipulation of anticipatory consumption with a preload manipulation, are less conclusive. Although they managed to find evidence for counterregulation in their preload-only control group, anticipating a high-calorie meal did not increase consumption any further among restrained eaters.

What can be concluded from these findings? The results of Knight and Boland (1989) and of Ruderman et al. (1985) suggest that anticipatory consumption of a high-calorie meal can have a disinhibitory effect on restrained eaters. The fact that anticipation of a high-calorie meal on top of a high-calorie preload did not result in greater disinhibition among restrained eaters than did eating a preload without anticipation of further consumption (Tomarken & Kirschenbaum, 1984, Experiment 2) suggests that once restrained eaters are disinhibited (i.e., as a result of the consumption of a preload), they do not need further disinhibition to overeat.

Equivalence Hypothesis

The dietary violation studies were stimulated by the findings of Schachter et al. (1968) that individuals with obesity did not reduce their cracker consumption following a preload of roast beef sandwiches. According to the equivalence assumption, the nonregulation demonstrated by individuals with obesity is due to the high prevalence of restrained eaters among those who are obese. Dietary violation studies therefore offer an important testing ground for the equivalence assumption. The first test of this assumption was conducted by Hibscher and Herman (1977) in a preload study that varied dietary restraint as well as body weight in a 2 (unrestrained vs. restrained) × 3 (skinny, normal weight, obese) × 2 (preload vs. no preload) design. To deal with an extremely uneven distribution of participants across conditions, Hibscher and Herman decided to conduct two separate analyses of variance, one collapsing across levels of restraint and one collapsing across weight categories. The only significant effect in these analyses was an interaction of restraint and preload: Unrestrained eaters regulated (i.e., ate less after a preload), whereas restrained eaters counterregulated (i.e., ate more after the preload). Although the response pattern to the preload manipulation of restrained and unrestrained eaters replicated the findings of the pure preload studies reported earlier, the failure to find an interaction between body weight and preload is inconsistent with the findings of Schachter et al. It also violates the first requirement for the demonstration of mediation, namely that there is an effect that could be mediated (Kenny et al., 1998).

A second failure to confirm the equivalence assumption was reported by Spencer and Fremouw (1979) in a study discussed earlier. Relevant to the present context is the fact that they also varied the weight of their participants (underweight, normal weight, and overweight) in addition to perceived calorie content. Again, because of an empty cell problem, they followed the example of Hibscher and Herman (1977) and analyzed their data with two separate analyses of variance. One analysis contained weight and beliefs about the calorie content of the preload; the other used restrained and beliefs as factors. The only significant interaction was a Restraint × Belief interaction, with restrained eaters counterregulating after having consumed a preload they believed to be of high-calorie content. Again, the effect supposed to be mediated according to the equivalence assumption could not be demonstrated.

A third failure to confirm the equivalence hypothesis comes from a study of individuals with obesity recruited into a research study comparing different weight-loss programs (Lowe, Foster, Kerzhnerman, Swain, & Wadden, 2001). Before the start of the weight-loss program, participants were exposed to the usual milkshake preload and ice cream tasting paradigm. There was no evidence of counterregulation. In fact, these individuals with obesity ate significantly less in the preload than they did in the no-preload condition. However, the findings of this study conflict with findings of an earlier study of attendees of a weight loss clinic who were obese. These individuals consumed twice as much ice cream after a milkshake preload than they did without a preload (McCann, Perri, Nezu, & Lowe, 1992). Lowe, Miller-Kovach, and Phelan (2001) attributed this discrepancy to a difference in sample composition. Whereas the study of Lowe et al. (2001) excluded binge eaters from their sample, the McCann et al. (1992) study had a high proportion of participants with binge-eating tendencies. Furthermore, the degree of counterregulatory eating was directly related to participant's binge-eating problems. This finding might indicate that counterregulatory eating is more closely related to binge-eating tendencies than to dietary restraint.

It is important to note, however, that the failure to find counterregulation among individuals with obesity who consumed a preload is not necessarily inconsistent with the equivalence assumption. Because the obese–normal weight differences in eating are supposed to be mediated by eating restraint according to the boundary model, and because eating restraint is only moderately correlated with BMI, one would expect the Preload × Weight interaction to be weaker than the Restraint × Preload interaction. It is thus possible that a Preload × Obesity interaction would have emerged with a bigger sample size.

More problematic for the boundary model is another failure to support the equivalence hypothesis reported by Ruderman and Christensen (1983). They used a 2 (restrained vs. unrestrained eaters) × 2 (obese vs. normal weight) × 2 (preload vs. no preload) design. If differences between the responses to the preload of individuals with obesity and the responses of those of normal weight were indeed due to eating restraint, then this difference should be eliminated in a design that controls for eating restraint. The findings of the Ruderman and Christensen study did not support these predictions. They reported two significant second-order interactions (Restraint × Preload; Obesity × Preload). Simple effect analysis revealed that the preload significantly reduced the consumption of unrestrained eaters (regulation) but did not affect consumption of restrained eaters (nonregulation). This finding is consistent with the boundary model. However, with eating restraint controlled for, there should have been no Obesity × Preload interaction. The fact that there was one suggests that obesity affects eating in ways that are unrelated to restraint. Even more puzzling, simple effect analyses revealed that the preload significantly reduced the consumption of the obese group: With restraint controlled for, individuals with obesity regulated for the preload in their ice cream eating. Furthermore, in reanalyses of the Hibscher and Herman (1977) and the Spencer and Fremouw (1979) data (solving the empty cell problem by combining individuals who were normal weight and those who were skinny), Ruderman and Wilson (1979) demonstrated similar patterns for the individuals with obesity in these studies.

Ruderman and Christensen (1983) concluded from these findings "that restrained eaters as selected by [Herman, Polivy, Pliner, Threlkeld, and Munic's] (1978) scale are not appropriate as analogues of obese. Whereas they demonstrate predictable and interesting eating patterns, these patterns do not correspond to those of obese individuals" (p. 214). Ruderman and Christensen suggested that the finding that individuals with obesity showed a greater reduction in intake following the preload than did individuals of normal weight could reflect problems with the RS rather than greater ability in regulating consumption. Because the RS-WF is more highly correlated with body weight than is the RS-CD, scores on the RS of individuals who are overweight may reflect less restraint in individuals who are overweight than in those who are normal weight. As a result, the individuals with obesity in their study could have been less restrained than were the individuals of normal weight, which might have accounted for the findings. It is a pity that Ruderman and Christensen did not test this hypothesis by separating the effects of RS-WF and RS-CD in their analysis.

CONCLUSIONS

The boundary model of eating behavior has stimulated an impressive amount of empirical research. Despite some inconsistencies, the overall findings of this research tend to be supportive of two of the major predictions derived from the model, namely that emotional distress and violation of one's diet boundary can induce overeating in retrained eaters. Thus, the boundary model has been quite successful in predicting outcomes. However, the model also claims to describe the psychological processes that are responsible for the disinhibition induced by emotional distress or dietary violations. These predictions about the psychological processes by which restrained eaters are assumed to regulate their eating have fared less well in empirical tests. Although it still dominates experimental research on eating control, the boundary model has attracted a great deal of criticism on both empirical and theoretical grounds (e.g., Boon, 1998; Heatherton & Baumeister, 1991; Lowe, 1993; Lowe & Butryn, 2007). Instead of giving a comprehensive review of these criticisms, I focus on three major concerns that motivated my coworkers and me to develop our goal conflict model of eating, which I describe in chapter 7.

Our first concern was metatheoretical rather than substantive. When Herman, Polivy, and their colleagues (see Heatherton et al., 1988) abandoned the original claim (Herman & Mack, 1975) that individuals with high restraint scores were significantly food deprived, the boundary model no longer offered an explanation for the overresponsiveness to food-relevant external stimuli displayed by individuals with obesity. The boundary model takes the existence of eating restraint as given and offers no explanation about its development. As a result, eating restraint is considered dysfunctional and even dangerous because of its association with binge eating and its suspected role in the development of eating disorders. Although there appears to be little empirical support for set-point theory from which Herman and Mack (1975) originally derived their claim (see chap. 3, this volume), there is evidence for genetically determined individual differences in susceptibility to weight gain (e.g., Bouchard, 2007a; Bouchard & Rankinen, 2008). It seems therefore likely that restrained eaters are mostly individuals who (a) are genetically disposed toward gaining weight and (b) developed a concern for dieting to counteract this disposition. They are not starving themselves, but they monitor carefully what they eat and how much they eat. The positive correlation between BMI and restraint indicates that these attempts are not always successful. However, without restricting their food intake, these individuals might have gained even more weight.

Our second concern relates to the motivational assumptions underlying the disinhibition effects. Herman and Polivy (1984) attributed the difficulties of restrained eaters in regulating their calorie intake to their presumed insensitivity to internal cues. Because of this insensitivity, they have to rely on calorie counting in regulating their eating. However, why should lack of sensitivity always result in overeating? It would seem equally likely that individuals who rarely experience feelings of hunger would forget to eat and slowly starve to death. I therefore proposed in an earlier article (Stroebe, 2002) that disinhibition effects are not caused by lack of sensitivity to internal cues of hunger and satiation but by the fact that restrained eaters enjoy the taste of palatable food. This assumption would explain why all successful empirical demonstrations of disinhibition effects among restrained eaters used ice cream or some other highly palatable food rather than the bland food used in the Schachter (1971) studies. Of the 29 preload studies with restrained eaters considered by Ouwens (2005) in her extensive review of this research, 16 used ice cream to assess the impact of their preloads on eating. Most of the remaining studies used cookies, candies, or nuts to measure food intake. Similarly, 8 of the 19 studies of the impact of emotions on food intake of restrained eaters also used ice cream, with many of the others tempting their participants with chocolate cookies or nuts. A study that manipulated the taste of ice cream in a preload study found the preload effect only with the good-tasting ice cream (Woody et al., 1981).

Yet, palatability and eating enjoyment are not considered major determinants of eating by the boundary model. Even though Herman and Polivy (1984), in their classic presentation of the boundary model, listed palatability as one of the factors that influences appetitive control within the range of biological indifference (Herman & Polivy, 1984, Figure 1, p. 142), they failed to discuss it in the remainder of their chapter. In one of their most recent analyses of the regulation of eating, in which they devote a paragraph to desire and the resistance to temptation, their discussion focuses mainly on the role of hunger as a factor that either depletes "the resources necessary for resistance" or "renders forbidden food even sweeter" (Herman & Polivy, 2004, p. 505).

Pinel, Assanand, and Lehman (2000) attributed the focus on hunger and satiety in theories of eating regulation to the lasting impact of set-point theory. According to set-point theory, reduction of the body's energy resources below some energy set point is the main factor motivating organisms to consume food. Pinel et al. (2000) shared our view that "humans and other animals living in food-replete environments rarely, if ever, experience energy deficits" (p. 1109). Pinel et al. contrasted set-point theory with positive incentive theory, according to which the primary stimulus for hunger and eating is the positive incentive value of food: "According to positive-incentive theory, people are not driven to eat by declines of their energy resources below set points. Rather, people are drawn to eat by the anticipated pleasure of eating (i.e., by food's positive-incentive value)" (p. 1109). A similar suggestion has been made by Lowe and Butryn (2007), who proposed a distinction between *homeostatic* and *hedonic* eating. They argued that homeostatic hunger is mainly determined by the prolonged absence of energy intake. The palatability of food to which the individual is exposed to between instances of eating is assumed to have little influence on homeostatic hunger. In contrast, hedonic hunger is strongly influenced by the availability and palatability of foods in the individual's immediate environment. Whether individuals have recently eaten is assumed to be relatively unimportant for their state of hedonic hunger.

Not only human beings overeat when food is very tasty; even rats do so. This was demonstrated by Rogers and Blundell (1980), who increased the positive incentive value of the food fed to laboratory rats by adding bread and chocolate, two items that rats apparently find highly palatable. If consumption were really driven by energy deficits as claimed by set-point theory, this manipulation of palatability should have had little effect on ad libitum consumption. In fact, the caloric intake of rats increased by an average of 84%, and their body weight increased by 49% within 120 days. The rats developed a weight problem.

There is also a great deal of evidence from studies of human participants that palatability is associated with greater food intake (for a review, see Yeomans, Blundell, & Leshem, 2004). Furthermore, the degree to which flavor is rated as palatable at the beginning of a meal typically predicts overall food consumption. As Yeomans et al. (2004) proposed, "the palatability of foods constitutes a behavioral risk fact that promotes over-consumption" (p. 59). Thus, the main problem with dieting may not be (homeostatic) hunger but appetite (i.e., hedonic hunger). Diets are abandoned not because they oblige people to eat "less than what the body demands" (Herman & Polivy, 2004, p. 494) but because they deny them the pleasure of enjoying continuous and unlimited access to their favorite foods.

Our third concern relates to the process assumptions made by the boundary model. No evidence has so far been found for the existence of "what-the-hell cognitions," which are supposedly activated by violations of this boundary, even in studies that specifically searched for these cognitions (e.g., French, 1992, Experiment 2; Jansen et al., 1988). Furthermore, a number of findings have reported disinhibition effects under conditions in which no disinhibition would have been expected according to the boundary model. For example, Jansen and van den Hout (1991) found that restrained eaters who merely smelled a preload counterregulated in a subsequent taste test in which they were asked to taste the various food items (e.g., licorice, biscuits, cake). This finding is problematic for the boundary model, because smelling the food does not transgress any diet boundary. Thus, according to the boundary model, restrained eaters should not have reacted with overeating. Similar effects were reported for restrained eaters by Fedoroff, Polivy, and Herman (1997, 2003), who exposed half of their respondents to the smell of pizza before they had to rate the taste of four freshly baked individual pizzas. Significant Restraint × Prime interactions demonstrated that exposure to the smell of pizza increased pizza consumption of restrained but not of unrestrained eaters, even though smelling pizza does not involve transgression of a diet boundary and should therefore not induce overeating.

To answer these limitations of the boundary model, my colleagues and I developed the goal conflict theory of eating (Papies, Stroebe, & Aarts, 2007a, 2007b, 2007c; Stroebe, 2002; Stroebe, Mensink, Aarts, Schut, & Kruglanski, 2008). Chapter 7 of this volume explains this theory.

7

BEYOND THE BOUNDARY MODEL: A COGNITIVE PROCESS THEORY OF RESTRAINED EATING

The goal conflict theory of eating was developed by my colleagues and me to provide a more realistic model of the cognitive processes by which restrained and unrestrained eaters regulate their food intake (Papies, Stroebe, & Aarts, 2007a, 2007b, 2007c; Stroebe, 2002; Stroebe, Mensink, Aarts, Schut, & Kruglanski, 2008). Our aim was to develop a theory that could not only account for all the findings (i.e., also the inconsistent ones) that emerged from empirical tests of the boundary model but would also help us to explain the findings of the research program stimulated by externality theory.

THE GOAL CONFLICT THEORY OF EATING

The basic assumption of our goal conflict theory of eating is that the eating behavior of restrained eaters is dominated by a conflict between two incompatible goals, namely the goal of enjoying palatable food (i.e., eating enjoyment) and the goal of losing (or at least not gaining) weight (i.e., weight control). We assume that weight control is normally the focal goal for restrained eaters and that they normally attach greater importance to this goal than to the goal of eating enjoyment. But as I show in chapter 6, this volume, restrained eaters are not always successful in the pursuit of this focal goal. The goal conflict theory of eating behavior offers a theoretical explanation for why restrained eaters often fail in their attempts to control their weight.

Most analyses of goal-directed behavior consider it a conscious process that is under volitional control (e.g., Bandura, 1986; Fishbein & Ajzen, 1975). Prime examples of such theories are the theories of reasoned action (Fishbein & Ajzen, 1975) and planned behavior (Ajzen, 2005). These theories assume that behavior is a function of a deliberate intention formed by individuals on the basis of their evaluation of the expected consequences of that behavior, their subjective norms with regard to performing the behavior, and, in the case of the theory of planned behavior, their assessment of the ease or difficulty of performing that behavior. Thus, according to the theory of planned behavior, individuals might form the intention to go on a diet if they think that dieting is likely to result in positive consequences (e.g., weight loss), if they expect the people who are important to them will approve of them going on a diet, and if they think that they will be able to restrict their calorie intake in line with their dieting plans.

Similarly, the boundary model of eating assumes that eating restraint is the result of conscious deliberations. Restrained eaters are individuals who have formed the intention to restrict their food intake. They pursue this goal by consciously matching their calorie intake to the intake permitted by their diet boundary. Because the boundary model was developed to explain not why people diet but why they often fail to maintain their diet, it contains a number of assumptions about processes that result in a breakdown of self-regulation. However, even these processes imply conscious deliberation. Thus, the experience of having violated one's diet is expected to result in "what-the-hell" cognitions, which restrained eaters use to justify abandoning their dietary restrictions. Distress experiences, at least according to the original explanation of Herman and Polivy (1984), undermine the restrained individual's motivation to diet because the dieting goal loses its importance in light of the experience that caused the distress.

Recent research and theorizing on goal pursuit has questioned the assumption that consciousness is always essential in goal pursuit and suggested the possibility that goal-directed behavior can be activated and guided by environmental cues (Bargh & Chartrand, 1999; Custers & Aarts, 2005; Strack & Deutsch, 2004). This notion is not a new one but dates back to behaviorist analyses that conceived of behavior as determined by past reinforcement (e.g., Hull, 1943; Skinner, 1953). However, modern cognitive analyses of nonconscious goal pursuit differ from behaviorist theories in that the "black box" has been replaced by a set of measurable cognitive constructs assumed to mediate the impact of environmental cues on behavior, such as cognitive representations, cognitive accessibility, and cognitive associations (Bargh & Ferguson, 2000; Custers & Aarts, 2005). These constructs, together with experimental methods such as priming procedures, allow the study of the cognitive processes that mediate nonconscious goal pursuit.

Theories of nonconscious goal pursuit share with theories of conscious goal pursuit the basic assumption that goals are mentally represented as desirable future states that the individual wants to attain through action (Custers & Aarts, 2005; Shah, Friedman, & Kruglanski, 2002; Shah & Kruglanski, 2002). Thus, goals are characterized by a discrepancy between some less desirable present state and a more desirable future state (Custers & Aarts, 2005). However, theories of nonconscious goal pursuit assume further that goals are knowledge structures that can be activated by cues in the environment without the individual being aware that any knowledge structure has increased in cognitive accessibility (Moskowitz, Li, & Kirk, 2004). *Cognitive accessibility* refers to the ease and speed with which information stored in memory can be retrieved. The triggering stimuli that increase the accessibility of cognitive constructs are usually referred to as *primes*.

Priming refers to the phenomenon that exposure to an object or a word in one context increases not only the accessibility of the mental representation of that object or concept in a person's mind but also the accessibility of related objects or concepts. As a result, the activated concept exerts for some time an unintended influence on the individual's behavior in subsequent unrelated contexts without the individual being aware of this influence (Bargh & Chartrand, 1999). Goals can be activated (primed) outside of awareness by exposing individuals to relevant semantic concepts (e.g., the words *tasty* and *appetizing* for the goal of eating enjoyment) or to situational cues that in the past were frequently associated with the pursuit of a goal. Thus, seeing palatable food items displayed in the shop window of a fine food store might activate the goal of having an enjoyable dinner at a fine restaurant this weekend, whereas seeing one's protruding stomach reflected in the same window might activate the goal of going on a diet.

There is ample evidence that goal priming can automatically affect goal setting and activate goal-directed behavior (for reviews, see Bargh & Ferguson, 2000; Custers & Aarts, 2005). In a recent demonstration of the impact of goal priming on goal setting, Holland, Hendriks, and Aarts (2005) exposed participants to the odor of an all-purpose cleaner (i.e., the prime) without participants being aware of the presence of this scent. This scent increased not only the accessibility of the concept of cleaning but also the likelihood of cleaning featuring prominently in participants' descriptions of future home activities.

Effects of goal priming on goal adoption were shown in a study by Bargh, Gollwitzer, Lee-Chai, Barndollar, and Trötschel (2001). To prime participants with the goal of cooperation, researchers unobtrusively exposed participants in this study to words such as *cooperative* and *share*. Afterward, they had to engage in a resource dilemma task in which they could keep profits for their own benefit or use them to replenish the common source. Findings indicated that participants who had been primed with words related to cooperation behaved more cooperatively in the game (i.e., replenished the common source more often) than did participants in the control group. In another study, Bargh et al. (2001) demonstrated that participants who had been primed with the achievement goal showed behavior (e.g., increased persistence and effort) consistent with achievement motivation.

The impact of unconscious influences on behavior in general had of course been shown much earlier. For example, Berkowitz and LePage (1967) demonstrated that the presence of a gun while an individual was giving electric shocks to another person significantly increased the number of shocks given (the so-called "weapons effect"). As is now known, this effect occurred because the presence of a handgun primed aggressive thoughts (C. A. Anderson, Benjamin, & Bartholow, 1998), and the priming of aggressive thoughts induced more aggressive behavior. With regard to eating behavior, stimuli that signal or symbolize palatable food are likely to activate thoughts about eating enjoyment in restrained eaters. Thus, the smell or sight of palatable food or the display in the window of a delicatessen shop should prime eating enjoyment in restrained eaters and induce overeating.

Given that goals can be primed unconsciously, one may wonder how people manage to pursue highly valued goals in the face of competing attractive alternative goals. In his analysis of how organisms manage multiple action systems, Shallice (1972) suggested that only one action system can be dominant at any given time. Usually the action system that is highly activated will be translated into action. However, if two action systems are highly activated, the one with the lower activation level will be inhibited. In elaborating these ideas, Shah et al. (2002) argued that the inhibition of alternative goals is so indispensable for effective self-regulation that it is applied automatically and without conscious awareness. They also provided empirical evidence that individuals manage to pursue goals they are highly committed to by inhibiting alternative goals (Shah et al., 2002).

In line with these arguments, the goal conflict theory of eating assumes that for restrained eaters, the goal of dieting is chronically accessible and constitutes the focal goal. Even though the eating enjoyment goal is more desirable than the goal of dieting, it is usually much less accessible. Thus restrained eaters can operate for a long time without ever thinking about eating enjoyment. For example, when focusing on some involving task in their work environment, restrained eaters are unlikely to think about eating enjoyment, and they therefore have no need to shield the weight control goal by inhibiting thoughts about eating palatable food. Unfortunately, however, our environment is rich in stimuli symbolizing or signaling palatable food, and restrained eaters are very sensitive to such stimulation (Papies et al., 2007a, 2007c). Thus, walking past the window of a bakery displaying delicious-looking pastry or inhaling appetizing smells of cooking wafting out of a house window will prime the goal of eating enjoyment. It is likely that initially these temptations will activate automatic attempts to shield the goal of weight control by inhibiting thoughts about the pleasures of eating (Fishbach, Friedman, & Kruglanski, 2003). However, continued exposure to palatable food (or to symbols representing or signaling palatable food) is likely to increase the cognitive accessibility of the goal of eating enjoyment to an extent that it gains dominance over the goal of weight control, resulting in inhibited access to the mental representation of the weight control goal (Shah et al., 2002). In other words, because it interferes with the selection and subsequent production of eating enjoyment goal-responses, the accessible goal of eating control is inhibited, rendering the goal of eating enjoyment more focal (for a discussion of these topics, see, e.g., M. C. Anderson & Spellman, 1995; Norman & Shallice, 1986). Furthermore, this inhibition process can occur outside conscious awareness (e.g., Shah et al., 2002).

Goal Conflict and Ambivalence

According to the goal conflict theory of eating, eating enjoyment and weight control are both highly desirable end states for restrained eaters. One way to assess this goal conflict is to measure ambivalence. *Ambivalence* can be defined as a psychological state in which a person holds both positive and negative feelings toward some psychological object (Jonas, Broemer, & Diehl, 2000). There are two strategies to measure ambivalence: experienced ambivalence and structural ambivalence (Jonas et al., 2000). Measures of experienced ambivalence ask participants to rate the degree to which they experience ambivalence in their attitude toward a given attitude object. Structural measures of ambivalence are based on evaluations of the positive and negative aspects of the attitude object and are thus directly related to the definition of ambivalence as the coexistence of positive and negative evaluations of the same object (Jonas et al., 2000).

My colleagues and I (Stroebe et al., 2008) assessed experienced ambivalence toward eating with a self-constructed scale consisting of 12 items (e.g., "I would enjoy tasty food more, if it would not contain any calories"; "A good meal tastes better, if you forget that it makes you gain weight"). Participants had to indicate the extent to which each of these items applied to them. We assessed structural ambivalence with the split-semantic differential procedure developed by K. J. Kaplan (1972). Participants were supplied with two unipolar semantic differential rating scales. On one scale, they had to evaluate the positive aspects of palatable food, disregarding all negative aspects; on the other, they had to consider only negative aspects of palatable food, disregarding all positive aspects. Ambivalence is high if the two attitude

TABLE 7.1

Correlations Between Restrained Eating
and the Two Measures of Ambivalence

Measure	1	2	3	4	5
1. Structural ambivalence	—				
2. Experienced ambivalence	.46**	—			
3. Restraint total	.35**	.56**	—		
4. Restraint (concern for dieting)	.34**	.65**	.91**	—	
5. Restraint (weight fluctuation)	.27**	.26	.81**	.50**	—

Note. From "Why Dieters Fail: Testing the Goal Conflict Model of Eating," by W. Stroebe, W. Mensink, H. Aarts, H. Schut, and A. W. Kruglanski, 2008, *Journal of Experimental Social Psychology, 44,* p. 30. Adapted with permission.
**$p < .01$, two-tailed.

components are similar in value and of at least moderate intensity.[1] Retrained eating was assessed with the Dutch translation of the Restraint Scale (RS; Jansen, Oosterlaan, Merckelbach, & van den Hout, 1988).

Table 7.1 presents the correlations between these three measures. With a correlation of .46, the magnitude of the association between experienced and structural ambivalence is typical for the relationship that has been reported between these two types of measures (e.g., Jonas et al., 2000). Furthermore, both measures of ambivalence are significantly related to the total RS score, with experienced ambivalence being more closely related to restrained eating than is structural ambivalence. Finally, an inspection of the association between measures of ambivalence and the two subscales of the RS indicates that ambivalence is much more closely related to the measure of Concern for Dieting (RS-CD) than is the measure of Weight Fluctuation (RS-WF). To investigate this further, we conducted two multiple regressions, with the RS-CD and RS-WF subscales as predictors and the two measures of ambivalence as criteria. Both measures of ambivalence were significantly related to the RS-CD but not to the RS-WF. These results are plausible because concern for dieting is one of the two goals involved in the goal conflict according to our goal conflict theory. In view of this pattern and given the low correlation between the two subscales, we decided to rely only on the RS-CD in further tests of our goal conflict theory.

---

[1]To compute the degree of ambivalence, we used a formula suggested by Griffin: $(P + N)/2 - |P - N|$, where P refers to the ratings of positive aspects, and N to the ratings of negative aspects (M. M. Thompson, Zanna, & Griffin, 1995). The first part of the formula results in high scores if the average intensity of the two attitudes is high; the second results in small scores if the two ratings are similar. Thus, high scores reflect greater ambivalence.

The Impact of Eating Enjoyment Primes on Dieting Thoughts

Having supported the first hypothesis derived from our theory, namely that the experience of ambivalence is a reflection of the conflict between the goals of eating control and eating enjoyment, we then tested the second hypothesis, namely that priming of eating enjoyment would result in an inhibition of thoughts about eating control in restrained but not unrestrained eaters (Stroebe et al., 2008). In everyday life, individuals are primed with eating enjoyment by exposure to palatable food or symbols representing such food items. In psychological studies, a variety of procedures have been used to prime concepts. These include asking participants to read synonyms of the concept or asking them to unscramble sentences that are related to the concept. Such procedures are considered *supraliminal priming* because individuals are aware of the concepts they are being primed with, even though they are unlikely to be aware of the impact these concepts have on further judgments. With *subliminal priming*, concepts are presented so briefly that participants see only a flash of light and are unable to recognize the concepts. We used a subliminal priming procedure for the stimulation of eating enjoyment to ensure that our participants remained unaware of the priming of this goal, which thus prevented strategic control over their eating control thoughts.

In our first priming study, we primed participants either with words reflecting eating enjoyment (e.g., *tasty*, *appetizing*) or with neutral primes (e.g., *neither*, *over*, *about*) by presenting these words for 23 milliseconds on a computer screen (Stroebe et al., 2008). To assess whether priming eating enjoyment influenced the accessibility of eating control concepts, we used a lexical decision task (Bargh & Chartrand, 1999; Dijksterhuis, Aarts, & Smith, 2005). In a lexical decision task, participants are presented with either words or nonword letter strings and must decide as quickly as possible whether they have seen a word or a letter string. The idea behind this procedure is that the more accessible these words are in the individuals' minds, the faster they recognize them. Thus, if restrained eaters are frequently thinking about dieting and weight loss, they are likely to recognize words related to dieting and weight loss faster than would unrestrained eaters who rarely think about controlling their weight. We presented five critical words that reflected the concept of weight control (*slim*, *weight-loss*, *weight*, *diet*, *dieting*) interspersed among a great number of irrelevant words. Following previous work we assumed that the time taken to recognize these behavioral concepts presented in this task would reflect the relative accessibility of representations of eating control behavior (e.g., Aarts & Dijksterhuis, 2003; Neely, 1991).

Figure 7.1 presents the mean reaction times of unrestrained and restrained eaters (median split) who had been primed with either neutral or eating enjoyment words. Consistent with predictions from goal conflict theory, there was a significant interaction between eating restraint and

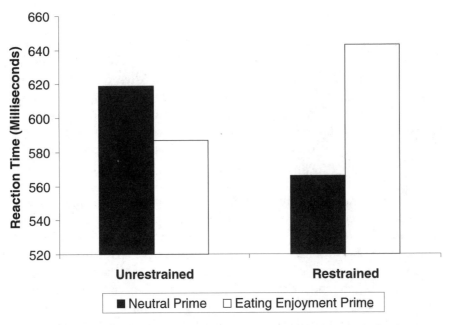

Figure 7.1. Mean reaction time to diet targets of restrained and unrestrained eaters primed with eating enjoyment (category) or neutral words. From "Why Dieters Fail: Testing the Goal Conflict Model of Eating," by W. Stroebe, W. Mensink, H. Aarts, H. Schut, and A. W. Kruglanski, 2008, *Journal of Experimental Social Psychology, 44,* p. 31. Adapted with permission.

priming condition. Simple effect analyses indicated that for restrained (but not unrestrained) eaters, the mean reaction time in the condition with eating enjoyment primes was significantly higher than in the neutral condition. Thus, the findings from this study supported our prediction that increasing the accessibility of thoughts about eating enjoyment through subliminal priming decreases the accessibility of dieting concepts in restrained but not unrestrained eaters. Furthermore, consistent with our theory, restrained eaters in the neutral prime control condition, at least descriptively, had shorter recognition times for diet-related words than did the unrestrained eaters in this condition. In light of the fact that individuals with a high concern for dieting think of dieting much more frequently than do individuals for whom dieting is not an issue, it makes sense that these words are more highly accessible for them.

One might argue, however, that this experiment did not constitute an optimal test of our model because we primed eating enjoyment directly with adjectives such as *tasty* or *appetizing*. In everyday life, these thoughts would be activated through exposure to one's favorite food. Thus, seeing the phrase *French fries* on a menu would activate the goal of eating enjoyment in restrained eaters (make them think of the pleasure they would derive from eating a plate of French fries), and this activation should result in inhibition of the eating control goal. To test this assumption, we replicated the earlier experiment but with an added condition, in which we used words referring to palatable food (e.g., *chocolate, French fries, ice cream*) to activate eating enjoyment thoughts. As in the previous study, the priming of eating enjoyment significantly increased the time that participants with high scores on the RS-CD needed to recognize diet-related words. Furthermore, it did not make a difference whether eating enjoyment was primed directly with adjectives denoting eating enjoyment or more indirectly with object words referring to palatable food items. Replicating the pattern obtained in our first study, restrained eaters in the control condition again had shorter recognition times for diet-related words than did the unrestrained eaters in this condition. Thus, the findings of these two studies are supportive of our goal conflict theory.

Although we demonstrated that priming of eating enjoyment reduced the accessibility of the eating control goal in restrained eaters, we did not assess whether this type of priming would also result in overeating. However, I have already reviewed a number of findings supportive of this assumption (chaps. 5 and 6, this volume). For example, Jansen and van den Hout (1991) found that merely smelling a preload induced overeating in a subsequent taste test in restrained but not in unrestrained eaters. Because smelling a tasty preload is likely to prime eating enjoyment in restrained eaters, these findings are consistent with our goal conflict theory. Similarly, the finding of Fedoroff, Polivy, and Herman (1997) that priming respondents with either the smell of pizza or thoughts about pizza increased the pizza consumption of restrained (but not unrestrained) eaters was another illustration of this phenomenon. Finally, Tom and Rucker (1975), who primed individuals who were obese with eating enjoyment by asking them to rate the appeal of various palatable food items shown to them on slides, found that food-primed individuals ate more crackers in a subsequent taste test than did individuals who had been exposed to neutral primes. These findings go some way in explaining the difficulties restrained eaters experience in keeping to their diet. They might have the best intentions, but when they study the menu in a restaurant offering some of their favorite dishes or when they inhale the delicious smell of home cooking, the goal of eating enjoyment becomes dominant and thoughts about dieting are "forgotten."

Eating Restraint and the Evaluation of Palatable Food

Why should palatable food items have a more positive incentive value for restrained than for unrestrained eaters? One explanation, and one that appeared of obvious validity to us initially (e.g., Stroebe, 2000), was in terms of differences in liking of palatable food. It seemed plausible that compared with unrestrained eaters, restrained eaters would hold more positive attitudes toward palatable food. However, when we asked restrained and unrestrained eaters to evaluate different palatable food items on evaluative semantic differential scales, we not only failed to support our hypothesis but found restrained eaters to be even slightly more negative about these food items than were unrestrained eaters (Mensink, 2005).

At first, these findings did not disturb us because we interpreted them as yet another indication of the ambivalence toward palatable food experienced by restrained eaters. We assumed that restrained eaters had so thoroughly internalized their goal conflict that they had become unable to distinguish the pleasure they might derive from palatable food from the threat these foods posed for their weight control goal. Thus, we assumed that the immediate affective reaction of restrained eaters might have been positive but that their dieting thoughts might have kicked in later, leading them to devalue the high-calorie food items.

Fortunately, social psychologists have developed methods of implicit attitude measurement that allow one to assess the immediate and automatic affective reaction of a respondent to a stimulus (e.g., De Houwer, 2003 [Extrinsic Affective Simon Task (EAST)]; Fazio, Sanbonmatsu, Powell, & Kardes, 1986 [affective priming]; Greenwald, McGhee, & Schwartz, 1998 [Implicit Association Test]). With these procedures, respondents are unaware that their attitude is being measured, so they are also unable to strategically control their responses. Roefs, Herman, MacLeod, Smulders, and Jansen (2005) used the affective priming procedure to assess attitudes of restrained and unrestrained eaters to high-fat, palatable foods (Experiment 1). *Affective priming* refers to the phenomenon that processing of a target word that is positively or negatively valued (e.g., *vacation*) is facilitated when it is preceded by an evaluative consistent prime word (e.g., *love*) rather than an evaluative inconsistent prime word (e.g., *pain*). Roefs et al. (2005) used 16 high-fat (e.g., *chocolate, bacon, chips*) and 16 low-fat (e.g., *melon, banana, broccoli*) food words as primes. These foods were also categorized as palatable or not palatable on the basis of ratings by participants. On any given trial, one of these words was presented as prime followed immediately by a positive or negative target word (e.g., *love, paradise, pleasure; killer, torture, failure*). Participants were instructed to judge as quickly as possible whether the target word was positive or negative. Positive targets should be evaluated faster if they are preceded by positive primes, and negative targets should be evaluated faster if they are preceded by negative primes (Fazio et al., 1986). Response times should be increased if primes and targets are evaluated differently (i.e., evaluative incongruent trials).

Participants responded faster when positive targets were preceded by palatable food items and negative targets by unpalatable food items. This result indicated that the affective priming task constituted a valid measure of attitudes toward these food items. However, there was no evidence for the expected interaction with eating restraint. Thus, there was no evidence that restrained eaters liked palatable food any better than did unrestrained eaters. These findings were replicated by Mensink (2005), who also used the affective priming task, and by Roefs et al. (2005, Experiment 2), who used a different measure of implicit attitudes in their second experiment (EAST; De Houwer, 2003). Thus, there is no evidence for a difference between restrained and unrestrained eaters in their attitudes toward palatable food.

The same conclusion emerged from recent research on differences in food attitudes between individuals with obesity and those of normal weight. Roefs and Jansen (2002), who used the Implicit Association Test (Greenwald et al., 1998) to assess the attitudes of individuals with obesity and those of normal weight toward fatty food, found that individuals with obesity had an even more negative attitude toward fat food than did individuals of normal weight. Unfortunately, palatability was not varied in this study. However, Cox, Perry, Moore, Vallis, and Mela (1999), who had individuals with obesity and those of normal weight rate the palatability of the food they ate at home for 4 days, found no difference either in overall pleasantness ratings or in liking for food with different predominant taste qualities.

The Difference Between Wanting and Liking

These findings posed a puzzle. That there was no difference between restrained and unrestrained eaters in the incentive value of the pleasure of eating palatable food seemed inconsistent with the basic assumption of the goal conflict model. If the goal of eating enjoyment did not have greater incentive value for restrained than for unrestrained eaters, why would restrained eaters find it so much more difficult than unrestrained eaters to regulate their food intake? Recent developments in the theoretical analysis of motivational processes in addiction suggest a solution to this puzzle (Berridge, 1995; T. E. Robinson & Berridge, 2000). With their incentive sensitization theory, T. E. Robinson and Berridge (2000) introduced an important distinction between *liking* and *wanting*. Liking refers to the hedonic preference for food and corresponds closely to the concept of palatability. However, liking does not determine the incentive value of food. The incentive value of food is reflected by wanting. Wanting corresponds to the motivation to obtain food and to engage in eating. Wanting is reflected by appetite or craving (Berridge, 1995). Liking can be inferred from ratings of the palatability of food. Wanting, on the other hand, can be assessed through behavioral measures of how hard a person will work to obtain food. The two dimensions are obviously not unrelated.

There is physiological and psychological evidence to support the distinction between liking and wanting. The physiological evidence indicates that different neurotransmitter systems mediate changes in hedonic and incentive value. The fact that opioid antagonists such as naltrexone block hedonic reactivity to foods but do not suppress general energy intake is consistent with the assumption that the hedonic value of food (but not the incentive value) is mediated by the opioid neurotransmitter system (Berridge, 1995; Epstein,

Truesdale, Wojcik, Paluch, & Raynor, 2003; T. E. Robinson & Berridge, 2000). In contrast, the incentive value of food seems to be mediated by the dopaminergic system; dopamine antagonists reduce the reinforcement value of food but do not alter hedonic reactivity (Berridge, 1995; Epstein et al., 2003).

Psychological evidence for the distinction between liking and wanting comes from a series of studies by Epstein and colleagues (e.g., Raynor & Epstein, 2003; Saelens & Epstein, 1996) that demonstrated that liking and wanting are influenced by different factors. Liking was measured with rating scales after individuals had sampled the food items and performed the sedentary activities. Wanting was assessed with an ingenious measure: Participants could choose between earning points to be traded for attractive snack food (e.g., chocolate bars, ice cream) or earning time to engage in an attractive sedentary activity (e.g., playing a computer game, watching a comedy video). Over several trials, the experimenters kept the price for the sedentary activity constant, but increased the price for the snack food by doubling the number of points that had to be earned for a given amount of snack food on each subsequent trial. This procedure allows one to measure what economists call the *price elasticity of demand*, that is, how easily demand is affected by changes in price.[2] After completion of several trials, participants were allowed to eat the snack food they had earned and to engage in the sedentary activity for the length of time they had earned.

Comparisons of individuals who were obese with those of normal weight support the assumption that liking and wanting are determined by different factors. Saelens and Epstein (1996) reported that participants with obesity showed lower price elasticity for snack foods than did participants of normal weight and also consumed more calories. These findings replicated those of a study by Johnson (1974) described in chapter 5 (this volume), which demonstrated that individuals with obesity were willing to work harder than individuals of normal weight to obtain palatable food (at least when the food was made salient). Saelens and Epstein found no difference between individuals with obesity and those of normal weight as regards their liking for the various snack foods. As mentioned earlier, Roefs and Jansen (2002) even found individuals with obesity to evaluate high-fat foods more negatively than did individuals of normal weight.

Evidence is less consistent for the impact of food deprivation on liking and wanting. Raynor and Epstein (2003) demonstrated that food deprivation affected wanting. The price elasticity for snack foods was lower for food-deprived than for nondeprived individuals: Food-deprived individuals were willing to pay a higher price for snack foods than were individuals who had

---

[2]The price elasticity of demand is expressed quantitatively as a ratio of the percentage change in price and the percentage change in demand. The smaller the percentage decrease in demand for snack foods that results from a given percentage increase in the price of snack foods, the lower the price elasticity of demand for snack food. Thus, the price elasticity of food reflects the incentive value of food.

been fed recently, and they also consumed more calories. Although Raynor and Epstein did not test whether food-deprived participants differed in their liking of these snack foods from nondeprived individuals, Epstein et al. (2003), who replicated the findings for the association between food deprivation and wanting using a questionnaire measure of wanting, observed no association between food deprivation and liking for these snack foods. However, a recent set of studies by Seibt, Häfner, and Deutsch (2007) found that food words were evaluated more positively by food-deprived individuals than by nondeprived individuals. They even found hours of food deprivation positively correlated with evaluation.

Epstein and colleagues (Raynor & Epstein, 2003; Saelens & Epstein, 1996) did not assess whether the price elasticity of snack foods, as measured with their paradigm, correlated with eating restraint. In fact, in several of their studies, they particularly mentioned that their participants were unrestrained eaters (e.g., Epstein et al., 2003; Goldfield, Epstein, Davidson, & Saad, 2005, Study 2). Although Epstein and colleagues did not discuss why they did not include restrained eaters in their sample, one suspects that they realized that their explicit measure of wanting would not work with restrained eaters. After all, restrained eaters have the intention to diet and are able to act in line with their intention unless their ability or motivation to diet is impaired. Because the snack food offered in the experimental paradigm of Epstein and colleagues constituted forbidden food and because the task allowed restrained eaters sufficient time to ponder the consequences of dietary violations, they would probably not have exerted much effort to earn points for calorific snack foods. In our research on restrained eaters, my colleagues and I therefore had to develop other measures to test our hypothesis that wanting and eating restraint are positively related.

Wanting and Incentive Salience

T. E. Robinson and Berridge (2000; Berridge, 1995) argued that "craved" stimuli become especially attractive and attention grabbing through a process of "incentive salience attribution":

> The active attribution of incentive salience by the brain confers upon a representation the ability to capture attention, to directly elicit orientation and approach, to instigate instrumental and cognitive strategies directed towards it as the goal, and potentially to become manifest in subjective awareness as an object of desire. Each of these manifestations has its own appropriate executive systems: sensorimotor systems for orientation and approach, instrumental learning and goal-directed cognitive procedures for instrumental behavior, and cognitive generating systems for translating elemental sensory processes into conscious awareness of subjective desire. (Berridge, 1995, p. 15)

Thus, whereas Epstein and colleagues (Raynor & Epstein, 2003; Saelens & Epstein, 1996) used a measure of instrumental behavior to assess wanting, Berridge (1995) suggested that the incentive salience of wanted stimuli should also be reflected by other cognitive systems, as he illustrated with an example: "When attributed to the smell emanating from a bakery, incentive salience can rivet a person's attention and trigger sudden thoughts of lunch" (Berridge, 2001, p. 257). My colleagues and I therefore began to entertain the possibility that restrained eaters differ from unrestrained eaters in the way they cognitively represent palatable food items and in the extent to which such food draws their attention and that these differences contribute to their problem in resisting palatable food.

The importance of these factors as determinants of individuals' ability to resist temptation had already been demonstrated by Mischel and colleagues in research on delay of gratification in children (e.g., Metcalfe & Mischel, 1999; Mischel & Ayduk, 2004; Mischel, Shoda, & Rodriguez, 1989). Mischel and colleagues examined the ability of children to delay gratification with tasks in which they could have either a less preferred outcome (e.g., one marshmallow, one penny, one cookie) immediately or a preferred outcome (e.g., two marshmallows, two pennies, two cookies) later. Research with this paradigm demonstrated that leaving the rewards available for viewing during the delay period shortened the delay, whereas covering the rewards lengthened it (Peake, Hebl, & Mischel, 2002). Furthermore, if rewards were present during the waiting period, long-delaying children diverted attention from the reward. They looked around or otherwise attended to activities or objects that distracted them from the pull of the rewards. In contrast, children who fixed their attention on the reward during the delay period were typically unable to delay gratification.

Subsequent research demonstrated that activities or instructions that affected the child's cognitive representation of the reward influenced the length of the delay period. A focus on the "hot" features of food stimuli (e.g., imagining the taste of the cookies and the enjoyment one would derive from eating them) made delay of gratification more difficult. In contrast, delay became easier when children distanced themselves psychologically from the consummatory, hot qualities of the reward (e.g., Mischel & Moore, 1973). This distancing could be achieved either by focusing on "cool," cognitive cues about the stimulus (e.g., shape and color of the cookies) or by distracting oneself (e.g., thinking fun thoughts). Although this research did not show that children used distraction or distancing as an effective coping strategy on their own accord, correlational evidence suggests that differences in waiting are associated with children's spontaneous use of these strategies (Peake et al., 2002). Thus, as Baumeister, Heatherton, and Tice (1994) concluded, "Managing attention is not only the most common technique of self-regulation, [but] it may well be the most generally effective one" (p. 25).

There are obvious parallels between the situation of children in the studies of Mischel and colleagues (e.g., Metcalfe & Mischel, 1999; Mischel & Ayduk, 2004; Mischel et al., 1989) and that of restrained eaters. Restrained eaters would like to delay the immediate gratification gained from enjoying palatable food in order to achieve the gratifying long-term goal of weight loss (or at least the avoidance of weight gain). It therefore appears plausible that the problems of restrained eaters are due to (or at least aggravated by) the way they cognitively represent palatable food and by their inability to divert attention from palatable food items. These assumptions suggest two hypotheses: (a) Restrained eaters are more likely than unrestrained eaters to access hot representations of palatable food stimuli, reflecting the arousing, consummatory features of the food (i.e., its taste and smell), whereas unrestrained eaters use cool, informational representations of food items, and (b) restrained eaters are less able than unrestrained eaters to divert their attention from palatable food items. In the following sections I discuss research that supports these hypotheses.

Eating Restraint and the Cognitive Representation of Palatable Food

Indirect support for the hypothesis that restrained eaters are more likely to think of the hot, consummatory qualities of palatable food than are unrestrained eaters comes from studies of physiological and behavioral reactions to the perception of food. The presence or even the smell of palatable food induces more salivation in restrained than unrestrained eaters (e.g., Brunstrom, Yates, & Witcomb, 2004; LeGeoff & Spigelman, 1987; Tepper, 1992). Furthermore, olfactory and cognitive food cues elicit stronger cravings in restrained eaters to eat palatable food (Fedoroff et al., 1997) and also greater consumption (Fedoroff et al., 1997; Jansen & van den Hout, 1991).

A more direct test of this hypothesis was conducted by Papies, Stroebe, and Aarts (2005, 2007c). In their first study, Papies et al. (2005) used the probe recognition paradigm of McKoon and Ratcliff (1986) to test whether spontaneous activation of thoughts about the hot features of the food is more likely to be stimulated upon exposure to palatable food in restrained than in unrestrained eaters. The probe recognition paradigm allows one to assess the spontaneous thoughts of restrained and unrestrained eaters who are exposed to palatable food. We hypothesized that restrained eaters who were, for example, exposed to the word *pizza* (or to a real pizza) would be more likely than unrestrained eaters to automatically think how good a slice of that pizza would taste.

To test this hypothesis, Papies et al. (2005)exposed research participants to a number of behavior descriptions, each description immediately followed by a probe word. Participants were asked to respond to the probe word as quickly and as accurately as possible by indicating whether it had been part of the preceding sentence. In the critical trials, the probe word was implied in the preceding sentence without being explicitly mentioned. Reading these sentences should have increased the accessibility of the implied concept, which should have interfered with the correct response (i.e., "No"). The critical trials in the study of Papies et al. were sentences that described the consumption of palatable food items (e.g., "Jim eats a warm slice of pizza," "Jack eats a piece of apple cake"). In the critical trials, participants had to decide whether words such as *tasty* or *delicious* were contained in these sentences. (In control trials, sentences referring to nonfood objects were used as well as eating-relevant sentences that contained the probe word.) If one's first thought on reading about Jim's pizza was "tasty," one would take slightly longer to decide that this word was not really part of the sentence than when one did not entertain such hedonic thoughts.

The findings of Papies et al. (2005) supported our hypothesis that exposure to cues symbolizing or signaling palatable food triggers spontaneous hot representations of the food and anticipatory pleasure of eating in restrained but not in unrestrained eaters. Restrained eaters were significantly slower than unrestrained eaters to decide that words reflecting eating enjoyment (e.g., tasty, palatable) were not part of critical sentences (see Figure 7.2). No

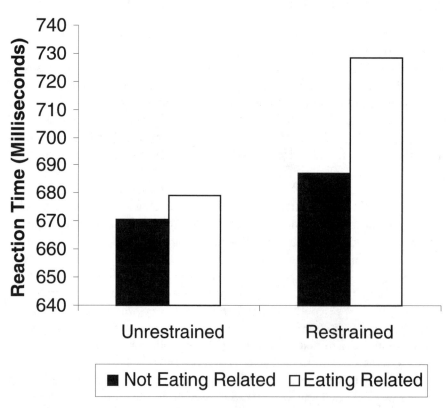

Figure 7.2. Mean response latencies as a function of restraint and sentence type. From Papies, Stroebe, and Aarts (2005, p. 317).

such difference occurred in the control conditions. Further experiments demonstrated that this effect emerged with words reflecting palatable, but not with words reflecting unpalatable, food items (Papies et al., 2007c).

A study by Harvey, Kemps, and Tiggeman (2005) also found evidence for differences in the cognitive representation of food stimuli between restrained and unrestrained eaters. Harvey et al. used current dieting as a proxy for eating restraint and assessed whether differences in the cognitive representation of food were related to food cravings. Participants were asked to imagine either a food-related or a control (holiday) scene. After that, their craving for food was measured, and then they had to perform an imagery task that required them to imagine either several visual scenes or several auditory cues. The goal of requiring a visual or auditory imagery task unrelated to food was to test whether these food cravings were mediated by visual images of favorite food. The main findings of this study were consistent with predictions: (a) Food induction resulted in a significantly greater increase in craving than did the holiday scenario; (b) the increase in food cravings was greater for dieters than for nondieters; (c) food cravings were significantly correlated with the vividness of the food imagery; and (d) food cravings were reduced much more after the visual imagery task than after the auditory imagery task. The latter two findings support the assumption that the imagery underlying food cravings is visual.

In summary, then, the studies of Papies et al. (2005, 2007c) support the assumption that exposure to palatable food items is more likely to activate hot thoughts about the great taste of these items in restrained than in unrestrained eaters. The findings of Harvey et al. (2005) showed that these hot cognitions are stimulated by, or at least associated with, vivid visual representations of the food items. Thus, Harvey et al. showed that imagining eating their favorite food induced higher levels of craving in dieters than in nondieters. They further demonstrated that this type of food imagery was visual and that the vividness of these food images was positively associated with food craving. Individuals who had vivid images of their favorite food were likely to experience a more intense desire to eat this food. Most important, however, the study also showed that interference with the visual imagery (by asking participants to engage in a competing visual imagery task) reduced food cravings.

Eating Restraint and Deployment of Attention

Attentional bias is another factor mentioned by Berridge (1995) as a consequence of incentive salience attribution. It was identified by Mischel and his colleagues as a process that plays an important role in impairing the ability of children to delay gratification (e.g., Metcalfe & Mischel, 1999; Mischel & Ayduk, 2004; Mischel et al., 1989). Children who fixed their attention on the reward during the delay period were typically unable to delay gratification. Applying this finding to the situation of restrained eaters, one would expect that palatable food "grabs" and "holds" the attention of restrained eaters and aggravates their difficulties in controlling their food intake. The attention-grabbing nature of eating-relevant stimuli was actually the basic explanation offered by externality theory for the problems individuals with obesity have in weight control. The evidence reviewed in chapter 5 (this volume) provides ample support for this assumption.

It is instructive to note that evidence for attentional bias has also been found in many addiction-related disorders, including alcohol dependence, nicotine dependence, cocaine dependence, and opiate dependence (for a review, see Franken, 2003). Franken (2003) suggested three processes through which attentional bias contributes to drug use and the maintenance of addiction. First, there is an increased likelihood of detecting and becoming aware of a drug cue and of the fact that these cues may elicit drug craving. Second, once a drug cue is detected, it is automatically processed, and individuals find it difficult to draw their attention away from this cue. Third, because attentional resources are limited, focusing on the drug-related cue might result in a subsequent failure to process competing cues.

Similar processes might operate in the case of restrained eaters, even though I am not arguing that restrained eaters suffer from food addiction. Extrapolating from research conducted in the context of externality theory, one can assume that restrained eaters are more likely than are unrestrained eaters to attend to eating-relevant cues in their environment (Schachter, 1971; Schachter & Rodin, 1974). Once the food-relevant cue has been detected, it will be processed and activate hot cognitions about the great taste of that food in restrained eaters (Papies et al., 2005, 2007c). Repeated exposure to palatable food stimuli is likely to raise the accessibility of the eating enjoyment goal to an extent that it will gain dominance over the goal of weight control. As a result of this priming, restrained eaters are less able to withdraw their attention from these eating-relevant cues. And the research on delay of gratification has shown that attending to food cues makes delay of gratification difficult (e.g., Metcalfe & Mischel, 1999; Mischel & Ayduk, 2004; Mischel, Shoda, & Rodriguez, 1989).

Despite the importance of attentional biases for assessing motivational processes in eating behavior, only a few studies have addressed the association between dietary restraint and attentional bias, and these studies resulted in inconsistent findings. Dobson and Dozois (2004) concluded from their meta-analytic review of attentional bias in individuals with eating disorders that there was no reliable evidence of attentional bias for dieting or eating restrictive samples. However, as Boon, Vogelzang, and Jansen (2000) suggested in an earlier review of this literature, the negative findings of these studies could have been due to their exclusive reliance on the Stroop task to detect attentional bias. With the Stroop task, individuals are presented with neutral as well as eating-relevant words printed in different colors, and they are required to name the color in which the word is printed rather than the word. It is assumed that if an individual's attention is grabbed by the food word, his or her response to the color-naming task will slow down. Thus, an increased latency in naming colors would be considered as evidence for selective hyperattention to the food cues. However, as Boon et al. (2000) argued, a slowing of color naming could also be caused by an avoidance of the food words because, for example, restrained eaters look away or close their eyes.

To avoid these problems, Boon et al. (2000) decided to use the dot probe paradigm developed by MacLeod, Mathews, and Tata (1986) to assess attentional bias with food stimuli. With this task, participants are confronted with two stimuli presented simultaneously—for example, a food word and a neutral word. A probe is subsequently presented beneath one of the two stimuli, and participants are requested to press the key that corresponds to the location of the probe (e.g., right or left) as quickly as possible. If selective attention is in fact biased toward the food word as the critical cue, the key-pressing response should be facilitated if the probe appears in the same location as the critical cue, and it should be impaired if it appears below the neutral cue. The critical words in Boon et al.'s (2000) experiment were 24 food words (e.g., *butter, cake, chips, chocolate*). Because there had also been evidence of biased attention with regard to words reflecting body shape, Boon et al. included 24 body shape words (e.g., *legs, bottom, slimming, stomach, belly*) as additional critical cues. Contrary to their expectations, the latencies in the dot probe task revealed no evidence for biased attention for either the food or the body shape words. However, the goal conflict theory of eating can account for this failure to uncover evidence for biased attention. The body shape words are likely to have acted as dieting primes and thus strengthened the dieting goal. Because these body shape words were interspersed among the food words, their priming effect likely eliminated the tendency of restrained eaters to selectively attend to the food words.

According to the goal conflict theory of eating, restrained eaters shield their weight control goal by suppressing or avoiding thoughts about palatable food. If even the most fleeting exposure to stimuli symbolizing or signaling palatable food would break down this shield, their attempts at dieting would be totally ineffective. Papies et al. (2007a) therefore reasoned that restrained eaters would need some preexposure to palatable food stimuli before they displayed a tendency to selectively attend to food stimuli. To test these hypotheses, they assessed biased attention after priming half of the participants with food cues. They expected that biased attention would emerge only for those participants who had been exposed to food cues. Exposure to food cues was manipulated with a lexical decision task that preceded the visual probe task. For half the participants, the lexical decision task contained 20 food words (food cue condition); for the other half, it contained 20 neutral words. After the lexical decision task, participants had to perform the visual probe task with pairs of words being presented for 200 milliseconds. The critical words were the same 20 food words used in the lexical decision task. The neutral words were words referring to office contents. After the visual probe task, participants had to fill in the RS and were also asked to rate the palatability of the 20 food items that had been used in the critical trials. The main dependent variable was the time it took participants to identify the position of the probe. Attentional bias scores were obtained by subtracting the reaction times on congruent trials (i.e., when the probe was underneath the food word) from reaction times at incongruent trials. The differences were computed separately for food and control items.

Papies et al.'s (2007a) findings supported their hypotheses. Attentional bias emerged only for those restrained eaters who had been exposed to food cues in the lexical decision task. In the food cue condition there was a significant relationship between palatability ratings and attentional bias for restrained but not for unrestrained eaters. For restrained eaters, attention to food items increased with increased liking of the food. Thus, the more palatable they found a given food item, the more their attention was drawn toward it. For unrestrained eaters, palatability did not influence attentional bias. This Palatability × Restraint interaction could not be observed in the neutral cue condition.

The findings of this study support the assumption that the attention of restrained (but not of unrestrained) eaters is drawn toward palatable food words. The results also suggest that their eating restraint protects these individuals, at least temporarily, from the allure of palatable food. At first, they appear to manage to shield their eating control goal against attractive food stimuli. However, their shield seems to weaken after repeated priming with food stimuli, and their attention becomes drawn toward the palatable food stimuli. These findings go some way toward explaining why previous research has failed to find evidence for selective attention processes in restrained eaters. The null effects of these studies may not have been due to their use of the Stroop task, as suggested by Boon et al. (2000), but to their failure to overcome the initial resistance of restrained eaters trying to shield their weight control goal. By interspersing body shape stimuli between the food stimuli in their own study and thus priming individuals with dieting thoughts, Boon et al. likely reestablished the "shield."

To test this interpretation and to examine whether priming individuals with dieting thoughts will eliminate the selective attention bias in restrained eaters, Papies et al. (2007a) conducted a second experiment in which they replicated their previous study but added a second priming manipulation. Half of the participants in the food exposure condition received a version of the visual probe task in which diet-related words were presented subliminally before the food words. Thus, Papies et al. first "switched on" the eating enjoyment goal of restrained eaters by exposing them to food stimuli, but turned it off again for half of the participants by subliminally priming them with dieting thoughts.

The other participants were presented with neutral prime words in the visual probe task. As expected, the visual probe task with the neutral primes had the same results as did the first experiment: Attention to palatable food in the probe task increased with increased liking of this food for restrained but not for unrestrained eaters. However, priming individuals with dieting words eliminated the Restraint × Palatability interaction. Thus, the attentional bias of restrained eaters was eliminated once Papies et al. helped them to reestablish their shield by increasing the accessibility of dieting thoughts.[3]

Can Restrained Eaters Be Successful in Controlling Their Weight?

The moderate correlation between eating restraint and body mass index allows for the possibility that some restrained eaters are successful in controlling their weight. This possibility raises the question that if such individuals exist, how do they manage to be successful? Although not much is known about their weight-control strategies, one can make a number of educated guesses on the basis of what is known about successful weight control (see chap. 8, this volume). First and foremost, these individuals are likely to have started controlling their food intake before they had gained too much weight because weight loss becomes more difficult the more one needs to lose. Psychologically more interesting is how they keep themselves from overeating. Gollwitzer (1999), Mischel (e.g., Mischel & Ayduk, 2004), and Trope and Fishbach (2000) have identified several cognitive, affective, and motivational mechanisms that help individuals resist temptations in their pursuit of a high-priority goal. Individuals might form implementation intentions regarding the goal (Gollwitzer, 1999; Gollwitzer & Sheeran, 2006), bolster the value of the goal by thinking of reasons why reaching the goal is important (Trope & Fishbach, 2000), or use various cognitive strategies to keep the high-priority goal the focus of attention (e.g., Mischel & Ayduk, 2004). However, these self-control efforts can be laborious and demanding of cognitive resources, and, as I have discussed, exposure to palatable food can make people "forget" their good intentions without them even being aware of what is happening (Stroebe et al., 2008).

Fishbach et al. (2003) recently suggested that with repeated and successful attempts at self-control in a given domain, facilitative associative links can be formed between specific temptations and the overriding goal with which they interfere. For these individuals, the activation of a temptation,

---

[3]Because restrained eaters are assumed to reduce their food intake, it would seem plausible that many of the effects described in this and the previous section could be due to more intense hunger feelings of restrained eaters. We found no evidence for this assumption. Self-rated hunger among our participants did not correlate with their RS scores. Furthermore, statistically controlling for self-rated hunger had no effect on any of the findings reported in these sections. We also found no correlation between RS and hours of food deprivation.

even if it occurs without their awareness, might suffice to activate the higher order goal. In terms of the paradigm used in the Stroebe et al. (2008) study, this would mean that for a subgroup of successful restrained eaters, priming the eating enjoyment goal with tempting food stimuli would not result in the suppression of dieting thoughts and might even lead to a slight increase in their accessibility.

Fishbach et al. (2003) found support for this hypothesis in a study in which they measured concern for dieting and perceived regulatory success. Concern for dieting was assessed by asking participants how much they were concerned about watching their weight and being slim. Self-regulatory success was measured by asking participants to indicate the extent to which they (a) were successful in watching their weight, (b) were successful in losing extra weight, and (c) found it difficult to stay in shape (the last item reverse coded).[4] Otherwise, their experiment was similar to that of Stroebe et al. (2008). In support of their hypothesis, they observed a significant interaction between perceived success and importance of dieting for individuals who were subliminally primed with tempting food words (but not in the neutral prime condition). The more successful participants with high concern for dieting perceived themselves to be in their attempts at weight control, the faster they were in recognizing dieting words.

My colleagues and I originally had some difficulties replicating these findings using the RS. However, these difficulties may have been due to problems with the Dutch translation of the measure of successful dieting (because of the double meaning of staying in shape). In the meantime Papies et al. (2007b) found preliminary support for the assumption that subliminal priming with tempting food stimuli will increase recognition times for diet-related words mainly in unsuccessful but not in successful restrained eaters. Priming successful restrained eaters with dieting words actually decreased the time they needed to recognize diet-related words. Even more interesting, however, were findings of a prospective study in which eating restraint (CD) and perceived regulatory success were measured at intake (Papies et al., 2007a). Participants were also asked to indicate their intention not to eat five extremely attractive food items during the next 2 weeks. When participants, who did not expect to be contacted again, were asked 2 weeks later whether they had eaten any of these food items, an interesting pattern emerged. For unrestrained eaters, there was only a main effect of intention on the frequency of eating these food items. The more they intended not to eat them, the less likely they were to do so. The success measure did not predict eating. However, for restrained eaters, a significant interaction between success and intention emerged, with inten-

---

[4]In the study of Papies et al. (2007b), the success measure correlated negatively with body mass index (−.48). It also correlated negatively with RS-CD (−.42).

tion predicting abstention from eating the palatable food items for successful but not for unsuccessful dieters.

The study of successful restrained eaters is obviously in its early stages, and our findings need replication and extension. However, the findings of an association between successful dieting and a measure of self-reported eating particularly indicate that successful restrained eaters might really be better able than unsuccessful restrained eaters to resist the temptation of eating palatable food. The distinction between successful and unsuccessful restrained eaters could also resolve a puzzling inconsistency reported earlier (chap. 6, this volume). The assumption that the group of restrained eaters identified by the Restraint scale of the Three Factor Eating Questionnaire (TFEQ-R; Stunkard & Messick, 1985) and the Restraint scale of the Dutch Eating Behavior Questionnaire (DEBQ-R; van Strien, Frijters, Bergers, & Defares, 1986) contained mainly successful restrained eaters, whereas the Restraint scale (Herman & Polivy, 1980) identified the more unsuccessful restrained eaters would explain the failure of studies that used the TFEQ-R or the DEBQ-R as measure of restraint to find disinhibitory effects of strong emotions or preload manipulations (chap. 6, this volume). Once the findings of the Papies et al. (2007b) study have been confirmed, one would hope to develop intervention strategies that would enable researchers to establish or strengthen the associative link between temptations and dieting thoughts in restrained eaters.

CONCLUSIONS

According to the goal conflict theory of eating, the difficulty of restrained eaters in regulating their food intake is not due to their inability to recognize bodily cues but to a conflict between two incompatible goals, namely, the goal to control their weight and the goal to enjoy palatable food. Weight control is normally the dominant goal for chronic dieters, who can operate for a long time without ever thinking about eating enjoyment. Unfortunately, however, the environment is rich in stimuli symbolizing or signaling palatable food, and chronic dieters are sensitive to such stimulation. These temptations activate automatic attempts to shield the goal of weight control by inhibiting thoughts about the pleasures of eating. However, continued exposure to palatable food (or symbols representing or signaling palatable food) is likely to continue to bring to mind the goal of eating enjoyment to an extent that it gains dominance over the goal of weight control. Once this happens, all thoughts about eating control will temporarily be "forgotten" (i.e., inhibited), and people are likely to overeat.

Although our goal conflict model shares the assumption of the boundary model that restrained eaters try to control their food intake, it does not assume that this control always requires conscious monitoring. Restrained eaters probably use a few simple heuristics rather than complex dieting rules to regulate their food intake. Examples are such rules of thumb as "No snacks between meals,"

"No second portions," and "No butter, but low-calorie margarine." Although the application of these heuristics may sometimes be guided by conscious intentions, they are often applied automatically. Whether restrained eaters will apply these heuristics depends on a stream of restraint-facilitating and inhibiting environmental cues that affect the individual. Thus, the smell of palatable food, the display in the window of a fine food store, and the text in the menu of a restaurant all can prime the eating enjoyment motive and result in the inhibition of eating-control thoughts. The impact of these eating-relevant cues, which operate outside the awareness of the individual, is mediated by the activation of hedonic (hot) cognitions and biased allocation of attention. All of these are automatic processes that eventually might influence the decision of the individual to order a high-calorie dish or to have a second portion.

With so much food-relevant stimuli in the environment, restrained eaters could not engage in eating restraint if they were swayed by even the most cursory exposure to palatable food stimuli. Two processes increase the likelihood that restrained eaters will manage to control their eating in a food-rich environment. First, as the study of Papies et al. (2007a) demonstrated, extended exposure to palatable food stimuli is required to "switch on" the eating enjoyment goal. Thus there is at least an initial resistance against palatable food stimuli. Second, the presence of dieting-relevant cues is likely to interfere with the priming of eating enjoyment, at least temporarily. Thus, a restrained eater who on passing the display in the window of a bakery shop decided to enjoy a cup of coffee and a piece of tart might change his mind after seeing the reflection of his protruding stomach in the shop window.

The goal conflict theory of eating agrees with the boundary model that experiences that require a great deal of cognitive resources result in overeating of palatable food because they interfere with the controlled processing needed for eating control. However, there are major differences between the two models. First, the goal conflict model emphasizes the importance of anticipatory eating enjoyment, a factor that, although central to most popular accounts of human food consumption and overweight, plays no role in the boundary model. Second, as noted earlier, the two theories differ in the cognitive processes assumed to lead to overeating.

With these assumptions, the goal conflict theory cannot only offer plausible alternative explanations for all of the findings that have been interpreted in terms of the boundary model but can also explain findings that were inconsistent with that model. Let me illustrate the first point with the boundary model explanations of the impact of preloads and of emotional arousal on eating. Although it is possible that drinking a milkshake before an ice cream tasting session induces restrained eaters to consciously abandon all thoughts about weight control, the fact that no evidence of such "what-the-hell" cognitions has ever been found speaks against this explanation (e.g., Jansen et al., 1988). The goal conflict model would suggest that drinking a tasty milkshake is likely to prime eating enjoyment in restrained eaters. As a consequence, they pay less attention to controlling their food intake in subsequent taste tests. Because this whole process operates below individuals' awareness, it will not be reflected by measures of conscious cognition.

The goal conflict theory can also deal with findings that were inconsistent with boundary theory. Because overeating following a preload is attributed to the inhibition of thoughts about weight control, this theory can explain nonregulation as well as counterregulation. It can also account for the fact that merely smelling a preload results in counterregulation (Jansen & van den Hout, 1991). Smelling a preload of palatable food can be considered a priming procedure that increases the accessibility of the eating enjoyment goal. As a consequence, the eating control goal should become inhibited (or at least less accessible), which would explain the overeating. More problematic for the goal conflict theory are the findings of the impact of the perceived calorie content of the preload. Because it is the taste of the preload rather than the fact that it has calories that primes eating enjoyment, one would not expect perceived calorie content to make a difference. However, because people tend to associate low-calorie content with less taste, the low-calorie preload might have been a less effective prime of eating enjoyment.

The goal conflict theory can also account for the findings that experiencing strong emotions results in overeating of palatable food. According to the theory, restrained eaters shield their eating control goal by suppressing thoughts about eating enjoyment. In line with the cognitive investment hypothesis suggested earlier, I would argue that restrained eaters invest more cognitive resources in regulating their eating than do unrestrained eaters. As a result, they are more likely than unrestrained eaters to be affected by cognitive capacity restrictions. Because coping with strong emotions requires a great deal of attentional resources, we would expect restrained eaters to be less able to inhibit thoughts about eating enjoyment when exposed to palatable food stimuli. This theoretical reasoning could thus also account for the findings reported earlier that any kind of distraction induces overeating in restrained eaters.

Finally, the goal conflict theory could account for the findings of Schachter and colleagues (e.g., Goldman, Jaffa, & Schachter, 1968; Nisbett, 1968; L. Ross, 1974; Schachter, Goldman, & Gordon, 1968; Schachter & Gross, 1968) on the impact of external cues on the eating behavior of individuals with obesity. According to goal conflict theory, food-relevant external cues are likely to prime the goal of eating enjoyment and induce overeating in individuals with obesity, or at least in those with obesity who score high on eating restraint. Thus, the palatability or cue salience of food, and even the approach of dinner time are likely to prime individuals with thoughts of eating enjoyment and reduce the motivation to control food intake. However, like the boundary theory, our theory would have to assume that these effects are mediated by higher levels of concern for dieting among individuals with obesity.

8

TREATMENT AND PREVENTION OF OVERWEIGHT AND OBESITY

In view of the negative consequences of overweight and obesity for a person's health and social life, it is understandable that these individuals try to lose weight. Given the steep increase in the prevalence of overweight and obesity in the United States during the 1980s, it is hardly surprising that the prevalence of weight-loss attempts has more than tripled since 1960 (Bish et al., 2005; Williamson, Serdula, Anda, Levy, & Byers, 1992). Compared with the general population, dieters are more likely to be women, young to middle aged, and better educated (Levy & Heaton, 1993). Men are far more likely than women to diet only when they are obese (Serdula et al., 1999), probably because for women, weight dissatisfaction is a stronger motive for dieting and sets in at a lower body mass index (BMI). After all, physical attractiveness is a stronger determinant of men's attraction to women than of women's attraction to men (Stroebe, Insko, Thompson, & Layton, 1971).

The fact that of people of normal weight, 8.6% of men and 28.7% of women report that they are trying to lose weight (Serdula et al., 1999) is often considered a reflection of unhealthy vanity, a consequence of the unrealistic ideals of slimness propagated by the media. This may be the case for some people, but most dieters are likely to be individuals who have difficulties in keeping their weight stable and are trying to lose weight they may have gained recently. If one adds individuals who report that they are trying to maintain their present weight to those who say that they are presently trying to lose weight, more than half the U.S. population are weight-concerned citizens (Serdula et al., 1999). Although these surveys do not report how many of those who are currently trying to lose weight participate in structured weight-loss programs, a U.S. survey conducted by Brownell (1994) among 20,000 readers of *Consumer Reports* magazine indicated that at that time, two thirds of dieters lost weight on their own, 20% subscribed to commercial programs, and only 5% participated in hospital- or university-based programs. No data are available on rates of participation in nondieting programs. The aim of nondieting programs is to reduce people's fear about deviating from the culturally ideal body shape, to teach them to stop trying to control their weight according to diet rules, and to listen to their own bodily needs.

In this chapter, I review the effectiveness of these different strategies in achieving weight maintenance or weight loss. In line with the focus of this volume on psychological aspects of obesity, the review is limited to a discussion of the efficacy of lifestyle modifications. Drug and surgical treatments of obesity are not covered. Because the nondieting programs were developed out of the conviction that dieting is harmful and long-term weight loss impossible, I also discuss the justification for these two assumptions. In light of the undisputable fact that weight loss is difficult and maintaining weight loss even more so, interventions aimed at preventing overweight and obesity are greatly needed. In the last section of this chapter, therefore, I focus on the primary prevention of overweight and obesity.

DIETING

The concept of *dieting* is used here to refer to the conscious restriction of food intake in order to lose weight or, at least, to avoid gaining weight. Although there is some overlap with the concept of *restrained eating*, the terms are not synonymous. Not all restrained eaters will be currently dieting and not all people who are dieting at any given moment will be chronically concerned about their body weight. I begin this section with a review of behavioral treatment approaches used by hospital- or university-based programs. I then review commercial weight loss programs and finally discuss the do-it-yourself diets most people engage in when they are trying to lose weight.

Behavioral Treatment Approaches

The basic assumptions underlying the behavioral treatment of overweight and obesity are (a) that eating and exercising are learned behaviors; (b) that therefore it should be possible to modify them; and (c) that for a long-term modification of these behaviors, the environment that influences them needs to be changed (Wing, 2004). The goal of most behavioral programs is to achieve a weight loss of 0.5 kilograms (1.1 pounds) to 1 kilograms (2.2 pounds) per week. To achieve this goal, patients must change their calorie intake, their level of physical activity, or both.

Components of Most Current Behavioral Programs

Before specific goals for behavior change can be set, the particular behavioral problem areas for the individual must be diagnosed. The key strategy for diagnosing problem areas is self-monitoring. Patients are asked to monitor their eating and exercise behaviors to identify specific problem areas that can be targeted in treatment (Wing, 2004). Thus, patients in behavioral weight-loss programs are taught to list everything they eat as well as the calories these foods contain. Once patients have learned how to keep a food diary and how to assess calorie content, self-monitoring of physical activity is added. They have to monitor either the minutes they spend on each physical activity or the calories they expend during the activity. These records should help patients to identify problem behaviors that need to be changed. For some people this might be their sedentary lifestyle, for others their overindulgent calorie intake. Usually change in both of these areas will be necessary.

Feedback is a second function of self-monitoring. Dieters regularly weigh themselves, at least weekly, often daily. This gives them some, albeit imprecise, indication of the effectiveness of their diets, and it also serves as a reward if weight loss has occurred.

Goal setting is the next important step in a behavioral treatment. To achieve their intended weight loss, patients usually set goals for total calories (1,000 to 1,500 kilocalories per day) and for physical activity (1,000 kilocalories per week). Substantial behavior change is required to achieve these goals. Subgoals will be defined, specifying the behaviors that need changing and the extent to which they have to be changed. Thus, if self-monitoring identified frequent visits to fast food restaurants and between-meals snacking as major contributors to total energy intake, a specific subgoal could be to reduce or stop snacking and eating fast food. With regard to exercise, the goal could be walking 10 miles per week (2 miles per day for 5 days of the week).

Training patients in the skills required to achieve weight loss is an important aspect of behavioral programs. Patients not only have to learn how to self-monitor their calorie intake and exercise behavior; they also need to learn how to change these behaviors. Thus, nutrition education is one important component of most behavioral approaches to the treatment of overweight and obesity. Patients are taught to recognize the fat and calorie content of what they are eating. They are also taught the skills required to consume a low-fat diet, such as reading food labels, modifying recipes to cut down on fat, and learning types of special cooking such as stir-frying (Wing, 2004). Instruction on exercising is another essential component of behavioral weight-control strategies. Behavioral programs typically advise individuals on the specific skills required to become more active and on how to deal with barriers that make exercising more difficult (Wing, 2004). Because individuals who are overweight or obese are typically physically inactive and do not enjoy exercising, goals for physical activity are initially set low and are increased over time. According to Wing (2004) most behavioral programs increase goals to an energy cost of 1,000 kilocalories per week. For a 70-kilogram (154-pound) adult, this would involve 4 hours of walking at a moderate pace. Some of this walking might be achieved by walking to shops or one's workplace instead of driving (i.e., lifestyle exercise), but some of it will have to be programmed as extra activities. Thus, patients will need to set aside specific times for going on walks, jogging, or using home exercise equipment.

Setting goals for behavior change and acquiring skills on how to achieve these goals are not enough. Patients also have to stay motivated to want to achieve the goals they set themselves. The two main strategies used in behavioral programs to keep patients motivated are stimulus control and cognitive restructuring. Patients are taught to change the environment they live in, to increase cues that elicit appropriate behavior, and to reduce cues for inappropriate behavior. Thus, they are advised to stock up on healthy food and to place these foods prominently in their refrigerator. They are also discouraged from purchasing and stocking snack foods and other unhealthy food items. The main function of stimulus control within the behavioral program is to direct patients toward the food they are supposed to eat and to prevent them from eating the wrong food by discouraging them from buying it. Another function of stimulus control, according to the goal conflict theory of eating, is to reduce the presence of stimuli that activate eating enjoyment thoughts and to increase the presence of stimuli that remind the individuals of their weight-control goal. For example, individuals who are dissatisfied with their weight could display in strategic locations (e.g., refrigerator, food cabinets) photos that show them in a particularly unfavorable light. Because people might often forget their weight-control intentions once they are exposed to the food-rich environment of their local supermarket, they are also advised to shop only from a list prepared at home and to avoid shopping while hungry.

Because it is not only the sight and smell of palatable food that might tempt people into overeating but also their "faulty" thought processes, lessons on identifying and modifying these faulty cognitions are included in most behavioral weight-control programs. One of the faulty thought processes is the division of calorie intake into daily units and the idea that if diet goals have been violated on a given day, any additional violation would not really matter. These ideas should be replaced by the knowledge that every calorie ingested counts because it will either contribute to fat stores or have to be worked off in some way. Other faulty thought processes are the use of food for mood repair (e.g., "I had a terrible day, I need some enjoyment") or as a reward (e.g., "I did great today; I must be allowed to reward myself"). Behavioral programs teach participants to recognize these thoughts and the impact they have on their eating. Participants are also taught to counter these faulty cognitions with more helpful thoughts.

Cognitive restructuring could also be used to address spontaneous thoughts about the taste of palatable food and the pleasure one would derive from eating it. According to the goal conflict theory of eating, these thoughts are major problems people face in exercising restraint (Papies, Stroebe, & Aarts, 2007c). Patients therefore need to be taught strategies of cognitive distancing to counter these tempting thoughts. One such strategy is anticipated regret, that is, thinking about how one would feel soon after the meal if one had violated one's dietary goal and eaten the extra cake or ice cream. Another cognitive strategy suggested by the goal conflict theory would be to strengthen the cognitive accessibility and desirability of the weight-control goal by reminding oneself why losing weight is important.

In line with the relapse process theory of Marlatt (e.g., 1985) and to keep patients from abandoning the program after some minor violation of their diet or exercise rule, behavioral weight-control programs now emphasize that lapses are a natural part of the weight-loss process. On the basis of information from self-monitoring diaries, patients are taught to identify situations that tempt them into overeating and to develop strategies to cope with these situations.

The Effectiveness of Behavioral Treatment Programs

Behavioral programs can result in substantial weight loss during treatment. For example, in a review of recent weight-loss trials that prescribed diet plus exercise and lasted for an average of 23 weeks, Wing (2004) calculated average weight loss at the end of treatment at 10.4 kilograms (22.9 pounds). A review of studies with particularly long follow-up periods arrived at an even higher estimate (14 kilograms [30.8 pounds] lost at end of treatment; Mann et al., 2007). Unfortunately, most of the weight loss was regained within 5 years after the treatment (Jeffery et al., 2000; Mann et al., 2007; L. H. Powell, Calvin, & Calvin, 2007). One and a half years after treatment, participants in the studies reviewed by Wing (2004) had regained 2.3 kilograms (5.0 pounds). Four to 7 years after treatment, participants in the studies reviewed by Mann et al. (2007) had regained 7.4 kilograms (16.3 pounds), leaving them with an actual weight loss of only 3.0 kilograms (6.6 pounds).

This is depressing news. In view of the deprivation involved in weight-loss treatment, having lost 3.0 kilograms (6.6 pounds) seems hardly worth the effort. Furthermore, these estimates are typically based on individuals who completed the weight-loss treatment and would be lowered by the inclusion of participants who dropped out of the treatment. However, even if people regained all the lost weight 5 years after their diet, they might still be better off than they would have been without dieting. On the basis of a 10-year follow-up of a population study conducted in the 1970s and 1980s, Williamson (1991) estimated that the average American aged 20 to 50 gains 0.5 kilograms (1.1 pounds) to 1.0 kilogram (2.2 pounds) per year. Similarly, in a low-intensity intervention to prevent weight gain, Jeffery and French (1998) reported a weight gain of 1.8 kilograms (4.0 pounds) for their control group over a 3-year period. People in the untreated control group in a recent study by Rothacker (2000) gained 6.5 kilograms (14.3 pounds) over the 5-year period of the follow-up. Less weight gain was observed by Jeffery and Wing (1995), whose untreated control group increased their weight by 0.6 kilograms (1.3 pounds) over a 30-month period. If a weight gain of 0.6 kilograms per year is taken as baseline for untreated individuals, participants with a weight loss of 3.0 kilograms (6.6 pounds) 5 years after treatment ended would be 6.0 kilograms (13.2 pounds) lighter than they would have been without the treatment.

This crude estimate is inconsistent with the results reported by L. H. Powell et al. (2007) in their review of nine lifestyle interventions that included randomized control groups and follow-up periods that ranged from 2½ to 10 years. The net difference between intervention and control groups at follow-up was 3.3 kilograms (7.2 pounds) for interventions that combined dietary treatment with exercise and 3 kilograms (6.7 pounds) for interventions that relied on dietary treatment only. However, most of the participants in these trials either were at high risk for diabetes or suffered from hypertension. It is therefore likely that even participants in the control groups were highly motivated to eat healthily and to control their weight. This would explain why even participants in some of the control groups in these studies lost weight. However, regardless of whether 3.0 kilograms (6.6 pounds) or 6.0 kilograms (13.2 pounds) is taken as the net weight loss maintained after 5 years, such an outcome is insufficient to move individuals with obesity, who are typically more than 20.0 kilograms (44.0 pounds) above normal weight, into the normal-weight category. Thus, behavioral programs may improve weight problems, but they are unlikely to "cure" obesity.

If one takes the position that an obesity treatment should help people reach normal weight, behavioral treatment of childhood obesity has yielded more promising results than obesity treatment for adults. In a report of 10-year treatment outcomes for children with obesity in four randomized treatment studies, Epstein, Valoski, Wing, and McCurley (1994) reported that 30% of these children were not obese 10 years after the treatment. These changes were substantially greater than were those of various control groups included in these studies. The children had been between 20% and 100% overweight when 6 to 12 years old at intake. Treatment was family based and included weekly meetings for 8 to 12 weeks, with monthly meetings continuing for

6 to 12 months from the start of the program. A great deal of evidence indicates that including parents in treating pediatric obesity increases treatment effects (Epstein, Paluch, Roemmich, & Beecher, 2007; Goldfield, Raynor, & Epstein, 2002). For example, Israel, Stolmaker, and Andrian (1985) reported that a short course in general behavior management had significantly greater effects on weight control of children at 1-year follow-up if their parents participated in the course. Similarly, a comparison of a family-based treatment approach, in which parents served as the exclusive agent of change, with that of the traditional approach, treating only children, showed that the family approach resulted in significantly greater reduction of obesity at 12 months posttreatment (Golan, Weizman, Apter, & Fainaru, 1998).[1]

Strategies Aimed at Improving the Effectiveness of the Dietary Component

One such dietary strategy has been the use of very low-calorie diets (VLCDs). VLCDs are total diet replacements with no more than 800 kilocalories per day. They are designed to spare lean body mass through the provision of 70 to 100 grams of protein a day. These diets are safe only if patients are carefully selected and medically monitored (Wing, 2004). In combination with behavioral treatment, VLCDs can produce weight losses of up to 20.0 kilograms (44.0 pounds) in 12 weeks. Thus, VLCDs produce greater short-term weight losses than do low-calorie diets (LCDs) that provide 800 to 1,200 kilocalories per day (J. W. Anderson, Konz, Frederich, & Wood, 2001; Tsai & Wadden, 2006). Two meta-analyses conducted to assess the long-term effectiveness of VLCDs arrived at discrepant conclusions. A meta-analysis based on 29 observational studies (14 trials that used VLCDs and 15 trials that used typical LCDs) concluded (a) that patients lost more weight initially after a VLCD than after an LCD and (b) that both groups regained weight at the same rate during follow-up (J. W. Anderson et al., 2001). Thus, the percentage of body weight lost during treatment and follow-up was significantly greater at all years after VLCDs than after LCDs (see Figure 8.1). However, a more recent meta-analysis based only on randomized controlled trials agreed with the first but not the second conclusion (Tsai & Wadden, 2006): VLCDs induced significantly greater short-term weight losses than did LCDs but induced similar long-term losses because of greater weight regain. It therefore remains unclear whether or not patients undergoing a VLCD are able to maintain their weight-loss advantage. The fact that VLCDs replace normal meals with liquid formulas or other types of replacement food may be both

---

[1]It is interesting to note, however, that the parents with obesity who were treated in the same program studied by Epstein et al. (1994) showed initial weight loss followed by relapse. After 5 years, all had regained their baseline weight, and after 10 years, parents in all groups were more heavily overweight than they had been at the beginning of the study.

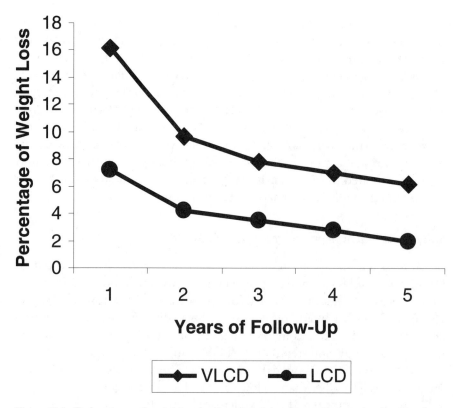

Figure 8.1. Percentage of weight reduction maintained over 5 years in structured weight loss programs. Weight reduction calculated as [(initial body weight – weight at follow-up)/average initial body weight] × 100. Data from J. W. Anderson et al. (2001, p. 580). VLCD = very low-calorie diet; LCD = low-calorie diet.

the strength and the weakness of this type of diet. It prevents patients from overeating while they are on the diet, but it does not teach them to change their eating habits. Once patients stop the diet and are left to buy and pre-pare their own food, they are likely to revert to the diet that resulted in their overweight in the first place.

Meal plans and meal replacements constitute a second strategy aimed at improving the effectiveness of the dietary component. If dieters succeed in preparing low-calorie meals that are tasty, they have to resist the temptation to eat more of that meal than their daily calorie allowance permits. Meal replacements reduce this risk because patients are provided with prepackaged meals in exactly the portion sizes they should consume. Meal replacements consist of a wide range of food products that include beverages, prepackaged shelf-stable and frozen entrees, and meal or snack bars. These foods can be used alone or in combination with other foods. In a study with men and women who were overweight or obese, Jeffery et al. (1993) combined state-of-the-art behavior therapy with a condition in which patients received prepackaged meals for five breakfasts and five dinners each week for an 18-month program. The behavioral intervention program was conducted in group sessions led by trained interventionists. The groups met weekly for the first 20 weeks and monthly thereafter. The prepackaged breakfasts consisted primarily of cereal, milk, juice, and fruit; dinners consisted of lean meat, potato or rice, and vegetables. As Figure 8.2 indicates, adding meal replacements to standard behavioral therapy resulted in greater weight loss than did standard therapy by itself during the 18-month treatment period. A meta-analysis of six randomized controlled studies that compared the effects of partial meal replacements dur-

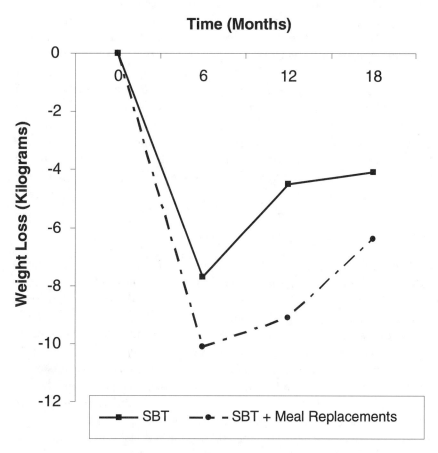

Figure 8.2. Weight loss after 6, 12, and, 18 months of treatment. Adapted from "Strengthening Behavioral Intentions for Weight Loss: A Randomized Trial of Food Provision and Monetary Incentives," by R. W. Jeffery, R. R. Wing, C. Thorson, L. R. Burton, C. Raether, J. Harvey, and M. Mullen, 1993, *Journal of Consulting and Clinical Psychology, 61,* p. 1041. Copyright 1993 by the American Psychological Association. SBT = standard behavioral treatment.

ing a 1-year period with that of a traditional reduced-calorie diet also showed superior effects of partial meal replacements. Whereas patients lost 2.61 kilograms (5.74 pounds) to 4.36 kilograms (9.59 pounds) over 1 year with the traditional diet, partial meal replacements resulted in a weight loss that ranged from 6.97 kilograms (15.33 pounds) to 7.31 kilograms (16.08 pounds).

The problem with these diets is again weight maintenance. A follow-up of the Jeffery et al. (1993) study conducted 1 year later found that patients had regained most of the weight they had lost, and that the advantage of the meal replacement treatment had disappeared (Jeffery & Wing, 1995). When patients stopped eating prepackaged meals, they probably returned to their old eating habits, increasing the portion size and the fat content of their meals. In a study conducted in Germany, participants who stayed on a meal replacement diet for 4 years were able to maintain a weight loss of 8.4% of their body weight (Flechtner-Mors, Ditschuneit, Johnson, Suchard, & Adler, 2000). Good weight-loss maintenance with meal replacements over a 5-year period was also reported by Rothacker (2000). It is important to note, however, that in both studies replacement meals were provided for free by the researchers. When participants have to pay for these meals themselves, the costs can be prohibitive. Evidence suggests that if researchers merely provided patients with the opportunity to purchase and use portion-controlled meals as a maintenance strategy but did not pay for them, patients would choose not to buy them and consequently fail in their attempt at weight-loss maintenance (Wing, Jeffery, Hellerstedt, & Burton, 1996).

Strategies Aimed at Improving the Effectiveness of the Exercise Component

During the past few decades, exercise has become a standard component of behavioral treatment programs. However, because weight-loss trials that use only exercise typically have reported very moderate weight losses of 1.0 to 2.0 kilograms (2.2 to 4.4 pounds; e.g., Garrow & Summerbell, 1995), it was generally believed that exercise was more important for weight-loss maintenance than for the initial weight loss. This was probably a misconception. As W. C. Miller and Wadden (2004) pointed out, most trials based on exercise alone prescribe only very moderate forms of exercise, usually walking three to four times a week for 20 to 40 minutes. This exercise would increase participants' calorie expenditure by only 300 to 900 kilocalories per week, an energy deficit that compares poorly with the 500 to 1,000 kilocalories per day reduction prescribed even by the less extreme low-energy diets.

When energy deficits induced by exercise are equal to those induced by calorie reduction, exercise and diet result in the same weight loss, at least for men. This was first demonstrated in a randomized controlled study by Sopko et al. (1985), who induced weight loss in their two experimental groups of men who were overweight or obese either by reducing energy intake by

500 kilocalories per day through a weight-reducing diet or by increasing energy output through supervised exercise (treadmill walking) by 500 kilocalories per day. Great care was taken that the diet-only group did not increase their level of physical activity during the intervention period and similarly that the exercise-only group did not change their diet. At the end of the 12-week intervention, both groups had lost approximately 6.0 kilograms (13.2 pounds). Similar results were reported by R. Ross et al. (2000), who compared a group of men who were overweight or obese and had an exercise-induced energy deficit of 700 kilocalories per day with a group for whom the same energy deficit was induced through a reduced-calorie diet. Both groups lost on average 0.6 kilograms (1.3 pounds) per week and ended up with a nearly identical weight loss of more than 7.0 kilograms (15.4 pounds) during the 12-week treatment period.

These studies show, at least for men, that a weight-loss treatment based only on exercise leads to the same results as one based only on calorie reduction, if the two treatments are matched with regard to the energy deficit they induce. However, a recent study by Donnelly et al. (2003) raises doubts about whether the same conclusion can be drawn for women. In this study, men and women who were overweight or obese participated in a 6-month program of supervised exercise, gradually achieving an energy equivalent of 400 kilocalories per day. Energy intake was measured during several 2-week periods, when participants ate ad libitum in the university cafeteria. At 16 months, men had lost 5.2 kilograms (11.4 pounds) of body weight, but women had gained 0.6 kilograms (1.3 pounds). Although the weight gain of women in the exercise group was significantly lower than that of a nonexercise control group of women, who gained 2.1 kilograms (4.6 pounds), it is still puzzling that despite an increase in energy expenditure achieved in supervised exercise sessions (and also checked by the doubly labeled water method over a 12-day period at baseline and after 16 months), these women did not lose weight. Unless these results are embodying an exception to the first law of thermodynamics, these women must have somehow increased their energy intake during the course of the study.

However, even if exercise programs are assumed to have similar effects for men and women, the problem remains that to induce a deficit of 500 kilocalories per day by exercise alone, individuals have to walk nearly 2 hours a day (more or less depending on their weight). Even if people had the inclination to do this, few would have the time. This lack of time and inclination is probably why modern behavioral weight-loss programs combine calorie reduction with more moderate levels of exercise. Studies that compare "diet only" with "diet plus exercise" conditions typically demonstrate that participants in the combined conditions lose more weight than do those in the diet-only groups. A recent meta-analysis based on six randomized controlled studies that directly compared diet plus exercise with diet-only conditions found a significantly greater weight loss (20%) in the diet plus exercise group immediately after the intervention and 1 year later (Curioni & Lourenco, 2005). However, weight regain after 1 year was similar in both groups.

Although it is widely believed that exercise is important for weight-loss maintenance, the evidence on this point is ambiguous. Thus, the meta-analysis of Curioni and Lourenco (2005) found no support for this assumption: Those in the diet plus exercise groups were no more successful in maintaining the weight loss than were those in the diet-only groups. In contrast, studies of individuals who were overweight and who had successfully maintained a weight loss of more than 10% of their body weight for several years found that these individuals not only consumed a low-fat, low-calorie diet but also engaged in comparatively high levels of physical activity (McGuire, Wing, & Hill, 1999; Wing & Hill, 2001). Explaining this discrepancy between intervention and observational studies, W. C. Miller and Wadden (2004) argued that the level of exercise in intervention studies tends to decrease during the follow-up period (as does the adherence to dieting rules).

Why should exercise increase weight-loss maintenance? One reason is that the calories one burns up by exercising do not need to be reduced by calorie restriction. A second reason could be that it is easier to maintain moderate levels of exercising than moderate levels of calorie reduction because exercising may be more rewarding than calorie reduction. Whereas the only rewards of calorie reduction are in the weight one might lose (or not gain in the case of weight maintenance), people might enjoy walking, cycling, or even jogging after having done it for a while. Thus, exercising can become intrinsically motivating.

As a reluctant jogger myself, I am aware of the multiple barriers one has to overcome to exercise regularly. Often there is no time, and when there is time, weather conditions are sometimes sufficiently uninviting to deter one from running. One strategy aimed at addressing the time problem by replacing long bouts of exercise with short bouts that could be more easily integrated into people's daily schedule has not been successful (Jakicic, Winters, Lang, & Wing, 1999), but lowering time costs by allowing people to exercise at home rather than at an exercise center does seem to increase adherence. Results of comparisons of home-based versus away-from-home (supervised) exercise consistently show that home-based exercise programs result in greater weight loss and better weight maintenance (e.g., R. E. Andersen et al., 1999; Perri, Martin, Leermakers, Sears, & Notelovitz, 1997).

Commercial Weight-Loss Programs

Commercial weight-loss programs are big business in Europe as well as in the United States. Although there are differences between these programs, their common feature is that they focus on diet, exercise, and lifestyle modifications and apply some of the same techniques that are used in the clinical programs. Weight Watchers International is the commercial weight-loss program that so far has been most thoroughly evaluated (Dansinger, Gleason, Griffith, Selker, & Schaefer, 2005; Djuric et al., 2002; Heshka et al., 2003; Rippe et al., 1998; Truby et al., 2006), even though Jenny Craig, the second major U.S. commercial program, has now also begun to encourage and financially support scientific studies (Finley et al., 2007; Rock, Pakiz, Flat, & Quintana, 2007).

Clients ("members") of Weight Watchers attend weekly group meetings, led by "lifetime members" who have been trained by the parent organization. Lifetime members are successful program-completers who have reached their personal weight-loss goal (a weight goal determined by the member and usually within a BMI of 20–25) and maintained it for at least 6 weeks. The nutrition advice given at these meetings centers on a Flex Plan, which assigns point values to all food items. Members have to stay within their allotted points for the day but typically prepare their own meals. With point values available for 27,000 foods, they have great freedom in their food choice. If they follow the plan correctly, members will eat a moderately reduced-calorie diet of 1,200 to 1,500 kilocalories per day. This should result in a weight loss of 0.5 kilogram (1.1 pounds) to 1.0 kilogram (2.2 pounds) per week. Explicit exercise goals are not given, but members receive instruction on how to develop a program that suits their needs (Womble, Wang, & Wadden, 2002). Members can also get information through the Internet that complements the weekly group meetings (eTools). If they choose to, they can also follow the whole program online, rather than attending group meetings.

During the past few years, the efficacy of the Weight Watchers program has been evaluated in several randomized controlled studies (Dansinger et al., 2005; Djuric et al., 2002; Heshka et al., 2003; Rippe et al., 1998; Truby et al., 2006). Heshka et al. (2003) randomly assigned 423 men and women who were overweight or obese either to Weight Watchers or to a self-help program. Participants assigned to the self-help program received a 20-minute consultation with a dietitian at intake and were given publicly available printed material about dieting and exercising. Participants assigned to Weight Watchers were given vouchers that entitled them to attend sessions. After 2 years, approximately 25% of the original participants had dropped out in either condition. Analyses were conducted on an intention-to-treat basis (last available weight value for dropouts carried forward). Throughout the 2 years, participants in the commercial group lost more weight than did those in the self-help group. Those in the self-help group lost 1.3 kilograms (2.9 pounds) to 1.4 kilograms (3.1 pounds) during the 1st year but returned to baseline after 2 years. Those in the commercial group lost 4.3 kilograms (9.5 pounds) to 5.0 kilograms (11.0 pounds) during the 1st year and were still 2.7 kilograms (5.9 pounds) to 3.0 kilograms (6.6 pounds) below their initial weight at the end of the 2-year period.

A 12-month randomized controlled trial of 48 women who had had breast cancer assigned these women to one of four conditions: a no-treatment control group, individual counseling with a dietitian, Weight Watchers, or individual counseling combined with Weight Watchers (Djuric et al., 2002). Attrition rate across the four conditions was 19% at 12 months. Whereas those in the control group had gained 0.9 kilogram (1.9 pounds), all participants in the other conditions had lost weight (2.6 kilograms [5.7 pounds] with Weight Watchers; 8.0 kilograms [17.6 pounds] with individualized counseling; 9.4 kilograms [20.7 pounds] with combined conditions). Only the individualized and the combined conditions differed significantly from the control group. However, for the two conditions that included Weight Watchers meetings, frequency of attendance was significantly correlated with weight loss ($r = .42$). A 12-week randomized controlled trial with 80 women compared Weight Watchers with a no-treatment control group (Rippe et al., 1998). At 12 weeks, attrition rates were 25% and 65%, respectively. The Weight Watchers group lost 6.1 kilograms (13.4 pounds), and the control group gained 1.3 kilograms (2.9 pounds), a difference that was significant.

Two other randomized trials compared the efficacy of Weight Watchers with that of popular diet programs (Dansinger et al., 2005; Truby et al., 2006). Dansinger et al. (2005) assigned 160 adults who were overweight or obese to either Weight Watchers, the Atkins diet (carbohydrate restriction), the Ornish diet (fat restriction), or the Zone diet (macronutrient balance) in a 12-month trial. Dietary advice in all conditions was administered in small group meetings by two of the authors of the study. Groups met for 1 hour on four occasions during the first 2 months. After 1 year, attrition was highest in the Atkins (48%) and the Ornish (50%) diets and somewhat lower for Zone (35%) and Weight Watchers (35%). After 12 months, all diets had resulted in a modest but statistically significant weight loss, with no significant differences between conditions. If one assumes that having small group meetings with experts is a more effective way of dispensing dietary advice than is reading a diet book, this study might have overestimated the effects of the popular diets by having researchers organize group meetings for all four conditions.

A 6-month randomized controlled trial conducted in Great Britain compared Weight Watchers with three other programs, namely Slim-Fast, Rosemary Conley, and the Atkins diet (Truby et al., 2006). Participants were 292 men and women who were overweight or obese who applied in response to a BBC advertising campaign. This study also included a waiting-list control group. Rosemary Conley is a group-based program similar to Weight Watchers. Like Weight Watchers, it offers a low-fat diet, but unlike Weight Watchers, it includes an exercise session in every class. Slim-Fast provides a program of replacement meals, and the Atkins diet is a well-known low-carbohydrate diet described in a diet book. For the group-based programs, participants were reimbursed for participation in regular meetings. For Slim-Fast, two meal replacements per day were paid for. Participants in the Atkins condition received a copy of *Dr. Atkins' New Diet Revolution* (Atkins, 2002). After 6 months, 82 participants had dropped out of the study (17 Atkins; 11 Weight Watchers; 16 Slim-Fast; 17 Rosemary Conley; 21 control group). An analysis on an intention-to-treat basis, with baseline values carried forward to replace missing values, did not yield significant differences between the different treatment conditions. However, weight loss in all treatment conditions was significantly greater than that in the control group.

In the meantime, other commercial weight-loss programs have recognized the value of scientific assessments of the efficacy of their programs. The first randomized controlled trial of the Jenny Craig program was published recently (Rock et al., 2007). Participants were 70 women with obesity who were randomly assigned to the Jenny Craig program or to a normal-care control condition. The Jenny Craig program is similar to Weight Watchers, the major differences being that weekly meetings are on a one-to-one basis with a trained consultant and that the diet consists of prepackaged Jenny Craig meals, which provide the core of a prescribed meal plan. In addition, counseling is provided for making appropriate food choices in situations apart from the context of prepackaged food (e.g., restaurants). Specific goals are also set for exercising (30 minutes of physical activity 5 or more days per week). Participants in the control group were provided with two consultations with a research staff dietitian, who also provided publicly available printed guidelines for weight loss and exercise strategies. Data collection occurred at three clinic visits: at baseline and after 6 and 12 months. At each clinic visit, blood samples were taken to assess plasma cholesterol and triglycerides. All of the women completed the baseline and 6-month clinic visit, and 65 completed the 12-month visit (32 intervention, 33 control). At 12 months the women in the intervention group had lost 7.3 kilograms (16.1 pounds) and 9.0 centimeters (3.6 inches) of waist circumference, whereas the women in the control group had lost only 0.7 kilogram (1.5 pounds) and 0.2 centimeter (0.1 inch) of waist circumference. In addition, high-density lipoprotein cholesterol levels had significantly increased in the intervention group. There was no change in triglyceride concentration.

A second evaluation of Jenny Craig was based on a large observational study of 65,154 men and women who had enrolled in the program between May 2001 and May 2002 (Finley et al., 2007). The study is interesting because in addition to information about weight loss, it also provides adherence data under naturalistic conditions. Attrition rates were 27% after 1 month, 58% after 3 months, 78% after 6 months, and 93% after 1 year. Thus, less than half of the clients remained in the program for more than 3 months. The longer participants remained in the program, the more weight they lost. The 7% of participants who remained in the program for the whole year lost 12.3% of their body weight.

For Weight Watchers, information is now also available regarding weight-loss maintenance of those participants who successfully completed the program (lifetime members). The self-reported weight of a sample of lifetime members who had successfully completed the Weight Watchers program between 1992 and 1996 was assessed in 1997 (Lowe, Miller-Kovach, & Phelan, 2001). For a subsample of those interviewed, weight was also measured. Based on the discrepancy between measured and self-reported weight, a correction factor was applied to all self-reports. Overall, participants reported initially losing 12.2 kilograms (26.8 pounds) to reach their goal weight. With an average weight regain of 7.4 kilograms (38.3 pounds) over the 5-year period, these individuals were still 4.8 kilograms (10.6 pounds) below their initial weight 5 years later.

What can be concluded from these studies? Participants in commercial weight-loss programs manage to lose moderate amounts of weight, and the weight loss is greater the longer they participate. For the Weight Watchers program, members who are successful in reaching their goal weight are also successful in maintaining a proportion of their weight loss over a 5-year period. The magnitude of weight loss and weight loss maintained is relatively small compared with the weight individuals with obesity would need to lose to reach normal weight. However, if one takes into account that without the intervention, these individuals would probably have continued to gain weight, even a relatively small weight loss is definitely worthwhile.

The fact that in one study (Truby et al., 2006) participants who merely read a diet book lost as much weight as did those who participated in Weight Watchers raises the question of whether using a diet book is as effective as participation in a commercial program. On the other hand, participants in the control condition of the Heshka et al. (2003) study lost hardly any weight, even though they had two consultations with a dietitian and were given "publicly available printed material orienting them to dietary principles and exercise guidelines" (p. 1793). There is indication that written material that is well structured can sometimes be even more effective than customized advice. Thus, a 16-week randomized controlled study that assigned 47 women who were overweight or obese to either a condition with a weight-loss manual (*The LEARN Program for Weight Control*; Brownell, 1997) or a condition with a popular commercial Internet weight-loss program found the Internet program less effective than the weight-loss manual, even though participants in the Internet program received customized meal plans and had access to online meetings moderated by a professional (Womble et al., 2004).

Dieting Without Professional Help

The majority of dieters try to lose weight without professional help. It is therefore unfortunate that few observational studies have followed cohorts of these dieters to assess the effectiveness of their dieting attempts. Most of what is known about the weight-loss practices of the ordinary dieter is based on surveys such as the 1992 Weight Loss Practices Survey (WLPS; Levy & Heaton, 1993), the Behavioral Risk Factor Surveillance System (BRFSS; Bish et al., 2005), and the National Health Interview Survey (NHIS; Kruger, Galuska, Serdula, & Jones, 2004). Table 8.1 summarizes the weight-loss practices reported by a nationally representative NHIS sample of 9,419 adults who were trying to lose weight (Kruger et al., 2004). The top three strategies were eating fewer calories, eating less fat, and exercising more. Thirty-four percent of respondents used the recommended strategy of combining exercise with calorie restriction. Only a small proportion of adult dieters reported (or admitted to) engaging in unhealthy weight-loss practices strategies such as fasting; skipping meals; taking diet pills, diuretics, or laxatives; or inducing vomiting. The latter finding is consistent with results of other surveys (e.g., French, Jeffery, & Murray, 1999; French, Perry, Leon, & Fulkerson, 1995; Levy & Heaton, 1993; Wardle, Griffith, Johnson, & Rapoport, 1999; Williamson et al., 1992). However, some evidence suggests that unhealthy weight-loss practices may be much more frequent among adolescents (Neumarkt-Sztainer et al., 2006).

Data on the effectiveness of different weight-loss strategies for adults were collected by French et al. (1999) as part of the Pound of Prevention Study, a 4-year weight-gain prevention study in which participants received monthly newsletters recommending regular self-weighing, increased physical activity, increased intake of fruits and vegetables, and decreased intake of high-fat food as strategies for weight-gain prevention. Because the general

TABLE 8.1
Specific Weight-Loss Practices Among Adults Trying to Lose Weight

Practice	Percentage
Eating fewer calories	61.0
Eating less fat	53.2
Exercising more	53.0
Skipping meals	9.8
Nothing	8.7
Eating food supplements	5.8
Joining a weight-loss program	4.5
Taking diet pills	2.5
Taking water pills or diuretics	1.7
Fasting for ≥24 hours[a]	0.7
Taking laxatives[a]	0.4
Vomiting[a]	0.1

Note. Weight-loss practices reported by a National Health Interview Survey sample of 9,419 adults. From "Attempting to Lose Weight: Specific Practices Among U.S. Adults," by J. Kruger, D. A. Galuska, M. K. Serdula, and D. A. Jones, 2004, *American Journal of Preventive Medicine, 26,* p. 404. Copyright 2004 by Elsevier. Adapted with permission from Elsevier.
[a]Estimates may be unstable.

population is likely to be exposed to similar information, the findings of this study are probably representative for the general population. At annual assessment points, participants' weight was measured, and they had to report their weight-control practices during the past year. Analyses that related weight-control behaviors to weight change found calorie reduction, increased fruit and vegetable intake, elimination of sweets, and reduction of the amount of food eaten associated with less weight gain over the 4-year period. Increased physical activity, decreased alcohol consumption, or participating in a weight-loss group surprisingly were not associated with weight change over 4 years. Unhealthy weight-loss practices (vomiting or use of laxatives, diuretics, appetite suppressants, and diet pills), liquid diet supplements, and eating low-calorie diet food were also not related to weight change. With regard to diet pills, a study conducted in Denmark reported a negative association with weight loss and weight-loss maintenance (Bendixen et al., 2002).

Additional information on the effectiveness of various weight-loss practices comes from a 2-month prospective study of 132 female students who were on a weight-loss diet and available at follow-up (Knäuper, Cheema, Rabiau, & Borten, 2005). These students were asked to write down the rules they were following in their present diet, and researchers evaluated not only the type of rule listed but also whether the same rules were listed at both points in time. Dieting rules could be categorized into five categories: reducing calories, changing what one eats, increasing exercise, changing attitudes and making plans, and changing eating habits. Adherence to dieting rules was low, with only 27.6% of the sample reporting the same dieting rules at both times. Weight loss after 2 months was modest (1.01 kilograms [2.22 pounds]). Consistent with all other studies, dieters reported mainly healthful dieting rules. Analysis relating the number of practices used in each category to self-reported weight loss found that the more individuals reported rules relating to exercising or to reducing calories, the more likely they were to lose weight, with calorie restriction being more effective than exercising. None of the other practices appeared to be effective.

With weight-loss practices merely slowing down weight gain in the Pound of Prevention Study (French et al., 1999) or resulting only in an extremely modest weight loss in the study of Knäuper et al. (2005), these findings are not very encouraging for the do-it-yourself dieter. However, the goal in the Pound of Prevention Study was weight maintenance rather than loss. Furthermore, the weight loss reported by individuals on a weight-loss diet is usually greater than that of participants in the Knäuper et al. (2005) study. Dieters interviewed in 1992 for the WLPS reported an average weight loss of just over 6.0 kilograms (13.2 pounds) in 6 months (Levy & Heaton, 1993). Similar weight loss was reported in the 1989 BRFSS (Williamson et al., 1992). In that survey, average weight loss was 4.54 kilograms (9.99 pounds) for men and 3.63 kilograms (7.99 pounds) for women during a weight-loss attempt lasting 4 to 6 weeks.

Yet, the results of the Knäuper et al. (2005) study may give a more realistic estimate of the likely result of diet plans than the weight loss reported in the various surveys. The low adherence to dieting rules in Knäuper et al.'s study suggests that many of their dieters abandoned their diet during the course of the study. In contrast, the outcomes in the survey data are based on individuals who maintained their weight-loss attempts for the reported period of time.

NONDIETING: THE NEW PARADIGM

The new paradigm is based on three basic premises, namely that mild to moderate overweight is not unhealthy and that dieting is not only ineffective but also harmful (Cogan & Ernsberger, 1999; Polivy & Herman, 1992). The health problems found to be associated with overweight are attributed to other factors such as lack of exercise, crash dieting, and weight cycling. Dieting is ineffective because body weight is largely determined genetically and bodies defend their "natural weight" against attempts at weight loss. To force success against poor odds, dieters often adopt unhealthy dieting strategies that only aggravate their problems. According to the nondieting approach, overweight dieters have to stop dieting and learn to accept their body weight. They have to accept that being overweight is neither unhealthy nor ugly. They are taught to stop worrying about calories and "forbidden food," and they are also instructed to adopt a healthier eating style and to increase physical activity. The goals of the nondieting approach are improvement in psychological well-being and a reduction in the risk of weight gain. However, modest weight loss might occur as a result of lifestyle changes, even though it is not a primary aim of this treatment (Rapoport, Clark, & Wardle, 2000).

Randomized controlled studies that compared nondieting treatments with behavioral treatment programs have had mixed results (Ciliska, 1998; Goodrick, Poston, Kimball, Reeves, & Foreyt, 1998; Hetherington & Davies, 1998; Rapoport et al., 2000; Sbrocco, Nedegaard, Stone, & Lewis, 1999; Tanco, Linden, & Earle, 1998; Wadden et al., 2004). The all-female participants in the nondieting conditions of these studies were explicitly instructed not to diet. In an attempt to encourage them to give up dieting, they were asked to list all the diets they had tried and the weight loss and regain they had experienced. However, they were encouraged to adopt a healthier eating style and to stop eating when full. Typically, they were also instructed to increase their level of physical activity. Finally, social and political influences regarding bodily appearances were discussed to make participants aware that present-day body ideals are a social construction heavily influenced by the media.

Nondieting interventions produce improvements in emotional well-being and eating pathology, but these improvements are generally no greater than those achieved with the groups exposed to regular behavioral weight-loss treatment (e.g., Goodrick et al., 1998; Rapoport et al., 2000; Sbrocco et al., 1999; Wadden et al., 2004). The one exception occurred in a study with women who were morbidly obese by Tanco et al. (1998), who compared an 8-week nondieting approach to a standard weight-loss treatment and a waiting-list control. Over the course of the treatment, participants in the nondieting condition showed improvements in depression, anxiety, and self-control scores, whereas individuals in the behavioral treatment and the control group did not. However, the fact that there was no improvement in psychological well-being of the group that received behavioral treatment is inconsistent with the findings of most other studies and could have been specific to the morbid-obesity status of this group. Because weight loss was minimal, the main factor impacting psychological well-being could have been the questioning of conventional weight ideals.

In the majority of studies, the nondieting approach achieved no significant weight loss at posttreatment (e.g., Ciliska, 1998; Goodrick et al., 1998; Hetherington & Davies, 1998; Rapoport et al., 2000; Wadden et al., 2004). In the few cases in which the nondieting treatment resulted in significant weight loss (Sbrocco et al., 1999; Tanco et al., 1998), the posttreatment effects were significantly smaller than those of traditional treatment. However, two studies showed some indication that rather than decreasing after treatment, the nondieting treatments might even show continuing weight loss during follow-up. For example, participants in the nondieting condition of the study of Rapoport et al. (2000) achieved a nonsignificant weight loss of 1.3 kilograms (2.9 pounds) at the end of the 10-week treatment, compared with a significant loss of 3.9 kilograms (8.6 pounds) in the behavioral treatment group. However, when the 52-week follow-up data were included in the analysis, a significant Time × Treatment interaction on weight loss emerged. Whereas the participants in the standard treatment had gained a small amount of weight, participants in the nondieting condition had continued to lose weight, and weight loss had become significant in both conditions (nondieting: 2.1 kilograms [4.6 pounds]; standard treatment: 3.8 kilograms [8.4 pounds]). Sbrocco et al. (1999) reported even more marked effects, with participants under traditional treatment regaining weight during follow-up, whereas participants in the nondieting conditions continued to show substantial weight loss. At the 12-month follow-up, the nondieting group had lost more than twice as much weight (10.06 kilograms [22.13 pounds]) as the group under traditional treatment (4.29 kilograms [9.44 pounds]). However, Wadden et al. (2004) found no indication of such posttreatment effects. In this study, the nondieting group lost no weight during and after treatment.

There is little support for the claim that nondieting treatment results in greater improvement in psychological well-being than does the traditional behavioral approach. Similarly, studies of eating pathology have found no differences in the impact of both types of treatment on eating pathology (e.g., Goodrick et al., 1998; Wadden et al., 2004). Thus, the two forms of treatment can be considered equally effective with regard to those two criteria. With regard to weight loss achieved at the end of treatment, the behavioral approach achieved clearly superior results. However, the fact that the nondieting treatment appeared to have superior long-term effects in one of the studies reviewed (Sbrocco et al., 1999) deserves further investigation.

IS LONG-TERM WEIGHT LOSS POSSIBLE?

As I have shown, the main problem in weight-loss research is not that people do not manage to lose weight, but that they fail to keep it off. However, there are reasons to argue that data based on individuals who participate in clinical weight-loss trials might paint too gloomy a picture. First, as Schachter (1982) pointed out many years ago, these conclusions are based on single attempts at weight loss, and individuals with weight problems typically make multiple attempts to lose weight. Whereas any single attempt at weight loss might have a low probability of success, the cumulative probability of repeated attempts could be considerably higher. Thus, to take stopping smoking as an example, the probability of a smoker quitting successfully is very low for any individual attempt but is cumulatively quite high. After all, in the United States alone, millions have stopped successfully over the years.

Second, there is consistent evidence that persons with obesity who enroll in weight-loss programs may represent the most severe cases and may be more resistant to successful treatment (e.g., Fitzgibbon, Stolley, & Kirschenbaum, 1994; French et al., 1995). For example, a study that compared a group of individuals with obesity who had sought treatment with one that had not sought treatment found that the treatment seekers not only had more extreme forms of obesity but also reported greater psychopathology on a symptoms checklist and more binge eating than did those who had not sought treatment (Fitzgibbon et al., 1994). Similarly, French et al. (1995) reported that compared with the girls in their sample who did not use weight-loss programs, those who did had a higher BMI and a more severe dieting and weight-loss history.

Information on weight loss and weight-loss maintenance in the general population allows slightly more optimism. McGuire, Wing, and Hill (1999) found that of a random sample of 474 individuals, 228 reported being overweight at their maximum weight. Of these 228 individuals, 95 (42%) said they intentionally lost at least 10% of their maximum weight. Forty-nine percent of these 95 individuals were successful weight-loss maintainers according to the 1-year criterion and 26% according to the stricter 5-year criterion (maintaining a 10% weight loss). Thus, the prevalence of weight loss and weight-loss maintenance among the members of this small sample was higher than that reported in clinical samples.

Further information on a nonclinical sample is available from the 3,000 members of the National Weight Control Registry (NWCR) in the United States (Wing & Hill, 2001). Although the NWCR cannot provide information about the prevalence of successful weight loss or weight-loss maintenance in the general population, it allows one to study the strategies used by individuals who were successful in maintaining substantial amounts of weight loss. To enroll in the registry, participants must have lost at least 13.6 kilograms (29.9 pounds) and maintained this loss for at least 1 year. The members of the registry who responded to the survey had lost an average of 30.0 kilograms (66.0 pounds) and maintained the required minimum loss for 5 years. The overwhelming majority of members of the registry are White (95%) and female (77%; Hill, Wyatt, Phelan, & Wing, 2005). Members of the registry had been considerably overweight before they engaged in their weight-loss attempt (maximum lifetime BMI: 35), and nearly 90% reported previous weight-loss attempts that had been unsuccessful.

Members used many different strategies to lose weight, but the one commonality is that 89% combined diet with exercise to achieve weight loss (Hill et al., 2005). The most popular weight-loss practices were to restrict certain foods (88%), limit quantities (44%), and count calories or fat grams (25%). More than half of these members reported receiving some type of help with their weight loss (commercial program, physician, nutritionist), a percentage that is considerably higher than that in the general population (Wing & Phelan, 2005). They now maintain a body weight that is on average 10 BMI units lower than their pre-weight-loss BMI (Wing & Hill, 2001). On average, members reported consuming 1,381 kilocalories per day, with 24% of calories from fat, 19% from protein, and 56% from carbohydrates. They also engage in high levels of physical activity comparable to approximately 1 hour of brisk walking per day.

Thus, registry members seem to engage in three strategies to help them to maintain their weight loss (Wing & Hill, 2001): (a) high levels of physical activity, (b) a diet that is low in fat and high in carbohydrates, and (c) regular self-monitoring of weight. More than 44% reported weighing themselves at least once a day. All of this evidence suggests that these individuals are chronic dieters who adjust their eating to avoid weight gain. By continuously monitoring their weight, they are able to reduce their calorie intake immediately to counteract any weight gain.

Are those successful weight-loss maintainers individuals with an iron will? There is reason to doubt this. Many studies indicate that self-control is a limited resource that is easily depleted (e.g., Baumeister, Bratslavsky, Muraven, & Tice, 1998; Muraven, Tice, & Baumeister, 1998). Even though these studies tested depletion only in the short run, there is no reason to believe that these effects would not also occur in the long run. Weight-loss strategies that rely mainly on self-control are therefore likely to fail. I would speculate that compared with unsuccessful weight-loss maintainers, successful individuals (a) have a somewhat lower propensity toward obesity, (b) lost weight with a diet that with slight modifications could be continued for weight-loss maintenance, (c) changed their food preferences and attitudes toward exercising, and (d) are flexible restrained eaters (Westenhoefer, Stunkard, & Pudel, 1999).

The barriers against substantial changes in food preferences, eating habits, and exercise habits are very high. There is general agreement that permanent weight loss is achievable only if "a person is willing to totally restructure behavior patterns in relation to food and activity" (Ikeda et al., 2005, p. 203). Self-control motivation is likely to be highest during the early phase of a weight-loss attempt and becomes depleted as time goes on. Dramatic changes in behavior patterns therefore need to be made during these early phases, when people trying to lose weight are still sufficiently motivated to deny themselves the food they like, to eat food they dislike, and to go on long dull walks they hate. Because they are unlikely to maintain this level of motivation, their resolve is likely to break down unless they manage to change their food preferences and attitudes toward exercising during the period of high motivation. With regard to food preferences, some chronic dieters may manage to devalue the fatty food they previously loved. More likely, however, chronic dieters who lose weight on a varied diet of low-calorie food might discover that some of this less familiar food (e.g., grilled fish, salads, chicken) is tasty. They might therefore begin to enjoy eating it, at least some of the time.

Similarly, with regard to exercising, people might discover that walking, jogging, or another sport can be fun. Exercising can be enjoyable, once one is in good physical shape. It would seem plausible that individuals who increase their level of physical exercise begin to enjoy being physically active much more after they have done it for a while and improved their physical condition. Furthermore, people might manage to integrate a substantial proportion of their physical exercise into their daily activities by walking to shops or to their workplace. Because these changes need to be made during the early phases of a weight-loss attempt, when motivation is still high, it is important that people trying to lose weight engage in the same, only more intense, dietary and exercise practices during weight loss as during weight-loss maintenance. For this reason, one would expect that weight loss achieved with an extreme and one-sided diet such as Atkins or some liquid formula is less easily maintained than is weight loss achieved by eating a varied low-calorie diet that can be continued into the weight-loss maintenance phase.

Finally, in light of the important work of Westenhoefer and colleagues (e.g., Westenhoefer et al., 1999), one would expect that individuals who engage in flexible rather than rigid control of their eating are more likely to be successful in maintaining substantial weight loss. Westenhoefer et al. (1999) suggested that there are two types of restrained eaters: those who control their eating rigidly and engage in an all-or-nothing approach to dieting and those who engage in flexible control, who allow themselves to eat a little bit more one day and then make up for it by eating less the next day. These flexible dieters do not totally deny themselves the pleasure of the high-calorie food they love, but they eat it within reason and make up for the overconsumption by eating less the next day.

There is some, albeit limited, empirical support for these speculations. A 1-year prospective study of 714 members of the NWCR found that 35% had regained 2.3 kilograms (5.1 pounds) during that period (Klem, Wing, Lang, McGuire, & Hill, 2000). A comparison of these weight gainers with weight-loss maintainers showed that weight gainers had been heavier initially than had weight maintainers, had been more likely to lose weight with a structured program, had used a liquid-formula diet for their weight loss, and had higher scores on the Disinhibition subscale of the Three Factor Eating Questionnaire. These findings tend to support the assumption that compared with individuals who fail to maintain their weight loss, weight-loss maintainers have a somewhat lower propensity toward weight gain (i.e., lower initial weight, lower disinhibition scores) and are less likely to have engaged in a diet that does not help to change eating habits (liquid formula). Similarly, individuals who lost weight with a diet of meal replacements are unlikely to maintain their weight loss unless they keep on buying meal replacements, which they are unlikely to do (Wing et al., 1996).

The prospective study of members of the NWCR found no support for the assumption that individuals who had maintained their weight loss for longer periods of life enjoyed exercising or a low-fat diet any more than did those who had maintained their weight loss for a shorter period (Klem, Wing, et al., 2000). However, members with longer durations reported that significantly less effort was required to diet and to maintain weight. A potential reason for the failure of this study to find duration differences in enjoyment could be that the minimum duration of weight-loss maintenance was 1 year for all participants (NWCR membership criteria). It is possible that changes in enjoyment occur relatively early during weight-loss maintenance.

Support for the assumption that successful weight-loss maintainers are flexible rather than rigid restrained eaters comes from the finding that successful weight-loss maintainers had lower scores on the Disinhibition subscale of the Three Factor Eating Questionnaire than did unsuccessful individuals (McGuire, Wing, Klem, Lang, & Hill, 1999). Westenhoefer et al. (1999) found increasing flexible control associated with lower disinhibition scores, whereas increasing rigid control was associated with higher disinhibition scores. Flexible control was also associated with lower BMI, less frequent and severe binge eating, and higher probability of successful weight loss during a 1-year weight-loss program. Finally, Westenhoefer, von Falck, Stellfeldt, and Fintelmann (2004) reported that participants in a weight-loss program who were successful in maintaining their weight loss over a 3-year period were more likely than those unsuccessful in maintaining weight loss to have increased their flexible control during the treatment phase and maintained this improvement during follow-up.

Weight regain is a slippery slope. Unless one takes corrective action as soon as one has gained a few pounds, one's weight tends to creep up, with the extra weight becoming more and more difficult to lose. It is therefore a matter of concern that according to a 2-year longitudinal study of 1,483 members of the NWCR, most of them seemed to slowly regain weight (Phelan, Hill, Lang, Dibello, & Wing, 2003). During the 2-year period, 65.7% of the sample had gained some weight in the 1st year and only 11.0% had managed to shed this weight a year later. Whether individuals managed to return to their baseline weight depended on the amount of weight they had gained in the 1st year. Of those who gained between 1% and 3% of their initial weight, 17.5% were able to return to baseline compared with 14.4% of those who had gained 3% to 5% of their body weight during the 1st year. Amount of initial weight gain was the only predictor of success in losing the gained weight. If this trend continues, the members of the NWCR are doomed in the long run to regain most of the weight they originally lost.

IS DIETING HARMFUL?

Because obesity is unhealthy, it would seem plausible that losing weight should improve the health of individuals with obesity. Thus, why should dieting or weight loss in general be harmful? That this question is being asked at all reflects the changing attitude toward dieting. However, during the past few decades, some researchers have become worried that dieting, aside from being of doubtful efficacy, may also have potentially harmful effects. There are several concerns about dieting, namely that weight cycling or yo-yo dieting has negative consequences for the physical and psychological health of the dieters, particularly that dieting and weight concerns increase the risk of depression and of the development of eating disorders. There can be little doubt that extreme weight-control behaviors such as use of laxatives, diuretics, induced vomiting, diet pills, or crash starvation diets are health impairing. However, as discussed earlier, most of these practices are used relatively infrequently, at least by adult dieters. The question to be addressed in this section is whether even healthy dieting involving a moderate calorie reduction (e.g., consuming 1,500 kilocalories per day) and exercise can be harmful.

Dieting and Physical Health

There is evidence that weight loss improves physiological risk factors such as glucose tolerance, hyperlipidemia, and blood pressure, at least in the short run (Gregg & Williamson, 2002; L. H. Powell et al., 2007). Furthermore, several lifestyle intervention studies demonstrated that modest weight loss can reduce diabetes incidence among those at high risk for the disease (e.g., Eriksson & Lindgärde, 1998; Sjöström, Peltonen, Wedel, & Sjöström, 2000; Tuomilehto et al., 2001). For example, in the Malmö Prevention Trial (Eriksson & Lindgärde, 1998), individuals with impaired glucose tolerance (a risk factor for diabetes) who were exposed to a diet plus exercise intervention had less than half the diabetes incidence 6 years later (11%) than did the nonrandomized control group of people with impaired glucose tolerance who had not been exposed to the lifestyle intervention (29%).

Similar effects were observed in the Swedish Obese Subjects Study (Sjöström et al., 2000), in which surgically treated patients with a BMI of 41.6 at baseline were compared with a matched control group who had received nonsurgical treatment. Eight years later, the surgically treated participants, who had lost 20 kilograms (44 pounds), had a diabetes incidence of 3.6% compared with 18.5% in the control group. Finally, the Finnish Diabetes Prevention Study, a randomized control trial of individuals with obesity and impaired glucose tolerance who were either given individualized counseling aimed at reducing weight and increasing activity or assigned to a control group, found a 58% reduction in the cumulative incidence of diabetes 4 years later (Tuomilehto et al., 2001). Diabetes incidence was 11% in the intervention group and 23% in the control group.

Given these positive effects of weight loss for morbidity, one would have expected that epidemiological studies that monitor the longevity of individuals who lost weight would demonstrate substantial benefits. It was therefore puzzling that early reviews of epidemiological studies of individuals who lost weight typically indicated that the greatest benefits with regard to longevity were associated with life-long weight stability and that repeated weight loss and regain (i.e., weight cycling) may be detrimental (e.g., Andres, Muller, & Sorkin, 1993; I. Lee & Paffenbarger, 1996). These early reviews were based on studies that did not account for the fact that people lose weight for different reasons and that these reasons have important implications for the interpretation of the weight loss–longevity association. Thus, if people lose weight because of a serious health problem, their shortened life span is likely to be due to this disease rather than the loss of weight. In studying the association between weight loss and longevity, it is therefore important to distinguish between intentional and unintentional weight loss. *Intentional weight loss* refers to weight loss resulting from intentional calorie restriction or increased physical activity, or both. *Unintentional weight loss* typically reflects weight loss resulting from some illness. When this distinction is applied, unintentional weight loss is found to be consistently associated with increased mortality (Wannamethee, Shaper, & Lennon, 2005). However, it is disappointing that the results of studies of intentional weight loss have been equivocal. According to a review by

Fontaine and Allison (2001), "results indicate that intentional weight loss appears to neither increase nor decrease mortality rates" (p. 87).

A potential solution to this puzzle has been suggested by Wannamethee et al. (2005), who pointed out that even intentional weight loss could be health-related. People might lose weight intentionally on their doctors' advice or to ameliorate some health problem. The male participants in a large-scale prospective study conducted in Britain who reported a recent intentional weight change were therefore asked to specify whether the change was due to personal choice, ill health, or the advice of their physician. When mortality was assessed 12 years later, unintentional weight loss was found to be associated with increased mortality. For intentional weight loss, there was neither an increase nor a decrease in mortality risk. However, when intentional weight loss was separated into weight loss motivated by ill health or medical advice versus weight loss resulting from personal choice, weight loss as a result of personal choice was associated with a significant reduction in all-cause mortality, largely owing to a significant reduction in non-cardiovascular-disease mortality. These benefits were most apparent in men who were overweight and in younger men (aged 56 to 64 years). In contrast, intentional weight loss because of health reasons or medical advice was associated with increased mortality risk.

It is obvious that the findings of Wannamethee et al. (2005) need to be replicated. However, because most studies of intentional weight loss did not differentiate reasons for the weight-loss intention, the Wannamethee et al. findings offer a plausible explanation for the conflicting findings that emerged from this research.[2] It is highly probable that further research on the effects of intentional weight loss will reveal additional moderating factors. One potential set of moderators consists of lifestyle variables that are associated with weight-loss intentions. Thus, individuals who try to lose weight are likely to be aware of the benefits of a healthy lifestyle and might therefore also engage in other health-enhancing behaviors. Consistent with this assumption, Gregg, Gerzoff, Thompson, and Williamson (2003) found in a prospective study of 20,439 adults that weight-loss intention reduced mortality, even if it did not result in actual weight loss. Unfortunately, this study lacked data that would have allowed one to test whether the association between weight-loss intention and longevity was partially mediated by other health behaviors. However, these findings suggest the need to control for other health-enhancing behaviors in

---

[2]It is important to note, however, that Wannamethee et al.'s (2005) findings should not be misinterpreted as showing that weight loss has no benefits for individuals who lose weight for medical reasons. It should be kept in mind that these researchers compared the mortality risk of individuals who lost weight for medical reasons with the risk of those who had no medical reason to lose weight. Thus, their findings merely indicate that with weight loss kept constant, individuals with a medical problem have a shorter life expectancy. Lifestyle intervention studies that assess the impact of weight-loss interventions on groups with medical risk factors typically find that weight loss reduces risk of health problems, particularly for individuals at high risk for the development of non-insulin-dependent diabetes (Diabetes Prevention Program Research Group, 2002; Tuomilehto et al., 2001).

future studies of the association between intentional weight loss and health or longevity.

Initial body weight and body composition are also likely to moderate the health effects of moderate weight loss. It seems plausible that individuals who are overweight or obese derive greater health benefits from weight loss than do individuals with a BMI of less than 25 (Allison et al., 1999; Fine et al., 1999). Thus, Fine et al. (1999) found weight loss associated with positive health effects for women who were overweight but with negative effects for women who were of normal weight or underweight. Because this study did not differentiate among weight-loss intentions, the negative health consequences of weight loss for women who were normal weight or underweight could have been due to the fact that their weight loss was mostly unintentional and resulted from some underlying health disorder. However, Allison et al. (1999) found weight loss associated with increased mortality, but fat loss (i.e., reduction in skin fold thickness) associated with decreased mortality. This finding suggests that the health benefits of a weight-loss attempt will be greatest if the weight loss is due mainly to loss of fat rather than lean body mass. Because individuals with obesity have much more body fat to lose, they should on average profit more from weight loss than would individuals of normal weight. This last finding also has implications for the type of weight-loss practices that should be used. There is some indication that the combination of calorie reduction with physical exercise results in greater loss of fat mass than does calorie reduction alone (W. C. Miller & Wadden, 2004).

All in all, there is no evidence that healthy weight-loss practices that combine dieting with exercise can impair physical health. Furthermore, there is evidence that weight loss due to such healthy weight-loss practices is beneficial, particularly for individuals who are overweight or obese, and that a loss of 5% of body weight is associated with substantial health benefits (Institute of Medicine, 2002). It is important to note, however, that this conclusion applies only to healthy weight-loss practices. Extended use of VLCDs (less than 800 kilocalories per day and insufficient protein content) has been associated with cardiac arrhythmias and even acute cardiac arrest (Gregg & Williamson, 2002). Intentional weight loss exceeding 1.5 kilograms per week (3.3 pounds) has also been found to increase the risk of gallstone formation among individuals with obesity (e.g., Weinsier, Wilson, & Lee, 1995). Finally, weight-loss practices such as the use of over-the-counter diet pills, appetite suppressants or laxatives, and vomiting for weight-control purposes are not only unhealthy but also unlikely to result in weight loss.

Dieting and Psychological Health

As I mentioned earlier, concerns about the consequences of dieting have not been limited to physical health impairment. It has also been suspected that dieting might have deleterious psychological consequences. In the following I review evidence as to whether dieting increases the risk of depression and of eating disorders.

Depression

In light of the fact that people go on diets because they are unhappy with their present weight, why should dieting and losing weight cause even more distress? There are at least two plausible reasons: first, that some dieters do not manage to lose weight and, second, that most of those who do lose weight regain it in the years following their diet attempt. However, in an exhaustive review of the relevant literature, the National Task Force on the Prevention and Treatment of Obesity (2000b) concluded that participants in behavioral weight-loss programs typically experience improvements in symptoms of depression and anxiety. Furthermore, in a review of the findings of several cross-sectional studies of weight cycling as well as of their own longitudinal study, Foster, Wadden, Kendall, Stunkard, and Vogt (1996) found no evidence that individuals who had regained the weight they had lost reacted with increased depression.

It has even been suggested that successful weight-loss maintenance could increase the risk of depression. According to set-point theory, weight suppression can result in distress because the body actively defends against changes in weight and attempts to return to its original weight or set point (Keesey, 1986). However, research that compared depression levels of the successful weight-loss maintainers of the NWCR with those of nondepressed community control participants found no indication of increased levels of depression (Wing & Hill, 2001).

Eating Disorders

Studies of the association of weight concerns and dieting with eating disorders have resulted in conflicting findings: Prospective studies of adolescents, particularly young girls, find such a relationship; randomized controlled interventions do not. Numerous longitudinal studies of samples of adolescents have indicated that dieting and weight concerns at intake predict disordered eating and even obesity at follow-up (e.g., Field et al., 2003; Killen et al., 1996; Neumarkt-Sztainer et al., 2006; Patton, Selzer, Coffey, Carlin, & Wolfe, 1999; Stice, Cameron, Killen, Hayward, & Taylor, 1999; Stice, Presnell, Shaw, & Rhode, 2005; Stice, Presnell, & Spangler, 2002). For example, Killen et al. (1996) measured weight and shape concerns in a sample of 877 ninth-grade high school girls (average age 14.9 years). The measure of weight concern assessed participants' fear of weight gain, worry over weight gain, and importance of weight and diet history. Eating disorder symptoms were assessed 4 years later in structured clinical interviews. To be classified as symptomatic, girls had to manifest bulimic episodes; compensatory behaviors such as the use of laxatives, diuretics, or overexercise; and overconcern with body weight. By age 17, four percent of these girls had become symptomatic. Weight concern at entry was the best predictor of the development of the eating disorder syndrome: None of the girls in the lowest quartile of the Weight Concern subscale had become symptomatic, but 10% of the girls in the highest quartile had. Similarly, Stice et al. (2002) found in a sample of 231 girls (mean age at intake 14.9 years) that eating restraint (Dutch Restrained Eating Scale [DRES]; van Strien et al., 1986), BMI, and appearance overevaluation at intake were significant predictors of binge eating 2 years later. Further analyses suggested that eating restraint was a risk factor mainly for girls who were heavier at intake and placed greater importance on their appearance. In a large Australian sample (mean age at intake 14.9 years), Patton et al. (1999) found girls who dieted severely to be considerably more likely to develop an eating disorder.

There is also consistent evidence from longitudinal studies of adolescents that eating restraint or dieting at intake is a risk factor for obesity at follow-up (e.g., Field et al., 2003; Neumarkt-Sztainer et al., 2006; Stice et al., 1999, 2002; Stice, Presnell, Shaw, & Rhode, 2005). In a 3-year longitudinal study of 692 female high school students (age at intake 14.9 years), Stice et al. (1999) found dietary restraint (Restraint Scale), self-labeled dieting, appetite suppressant or laxative use, vomiting for weight-control purposes, and binge eating predictive of obesity onset at follow-up. Stice, Presnell, Shaw, and Rhode (2005) replicated most of these findings in a 4-year longitudinal study of a sample of 496 girls (mean age at intake 13.5 years). They found dietary restraint (DRES; van Strien et al., 1986), radical weight-control behaviors, depressive symptoms, and perceived parental obesity predictive of obesity onset 5 years later. Similar results were reported by Neumarkt-Sztainer et al. (2006) in a 5-year longitudinal study of 2,516 boys and girls. These authors found that boys and girls who reported dieting at intake had substantially higher BMIs at follow-up (27.5 and 25.1) than did participants who did not engage in dieting behavior at intake (23.6 and 22.5). These authors also found dieting, and particularly unhealthy dieting behavior, predictive of binge eating at follow-up.

In contrast to findings from observational studies, results of randomized controlled trials testing behavioral weight-loss interventions consistently show substantial weight loss and either improvement or no change in symptoms of eating disorders. A review of five pediatric behavior modification programs concluded that "professionally administered weight loss programs for overweight children did not increase symptoms of eating disorders and were associated with significant improvements in psychosocial status" (Butryn & Wadden, 2005, pp. 289–290). All of these treatments also resulted in substantial weight loss, and follow-up periods varied from 6 months to 10 years. There is also ample evidence that professionally administered weight-control programs do not increase (and sometimes even decrease) the risk of eating disorders for adults (for reviews, see Butryn & Wadden, 2005; National Task Force on the Prevention and Treatment of Obesity, 2000b; Stice, 2002).[3]

Three potential explanations for the contradictory findings of prospective and intervention studies have been discussed (e.g., Stice, Presnell, Groesz, & Shaw, 2005). First, the inconsistency might have occurred because measures of dietary restraint do not assess dieting behavior. As discussed earlier (see chap. 6, this volume), studies have repeatedly demonstrated that measures of dietary restraint are at best weakly related to observational measures of dietary behavior. However, this assumption could not account for the findings of Neumarkt-Sztainer et al. (2006) who reported a relationship between a measure of dieting behavior and disordered eating. A second explanation for these contradictory findings, which suggests that behavioral interventions promote healthy dieting behavior whereas eating restraint scales might reflect unhealthy dieting behavior, is therefore more consistent with existing evidence. The fact that weight-loss practices performed by the weight-concerned adolescents in the prospective studies resulted in weight gain rather than weight loss strongly indicates that the adolescents either did not engage in any weight-loss practices at all or used unhealthy and ineffective weight-loss practices. That eating disorder prevention programs with adolescents not only reduce eating pathology but also reduce the risk of weight gain would be consistent with this assumption (Stice & Shaw, 2004). However, the findings of Neumarkt-Sztainer et al. (2006) give no indication that individuals who engaged in healthy dieting practices ran a lower risk of weight gain than did those who practiced unhealthy dieting behaviors. Thus, the third explanation needs to be considered: namely, that the association between dieting and binge eating in observational studies is due to a third factor that increased the risk of both variables. As Stice (2002) suggested, "a tendency toward caloric overconsumption may lead to both self-reported dieting and eventual onset of binge eating and bulimic pathology" (p. 836). If this were the case, "dieting would be a proxy risk factor for binge eating and bulimic symptoms solely because it is a marker for overconsumption" (Stice, 2002, p. 836).

Although it would be scientifically satisfying to have sufficient data to resolve the inconsistency between the findings of longitudinal and prospective studies, one can draw practical conclusions without such a resolution. The findings of intervention studies have demonstrated that if adolescents engage in healthy dieting practices, not only can they lose weight without risk of developing eating disorders, but their dieting might even improve their disordered eating (Stice, 2002). There is also evidence that children with obesity can reach and maintain normal weight if they change their eating habits

---

[3]Since publication of these reviews, at least two further studies with adults found that dieting intervention resulted in significant weight loss and significant decreases in bulimic symptoms (Presnell & Stice, 2003; Wadden et al., 2004).

(e.g., Epstein et al., 1994). Children and adolescents are therefore an important target group for weight-loss interventions. However, in light of the magnitude of the obesity problem, there is no hope of solving this problem with clinical interventions alone. Public health interventions aimed at children are needed to persuade them to change poor eating habits and to help them to develop healthy weight-loss and weight-maintenance practices. Because parents control what children eat at home, these prevention efforts should also target parents and educate them in the importance of providing healthy food for their children.

PREVENTION OF OVERWEIGHT AND OBESITY

What are the implications of the research reviewed in this chapter? Probably the most consistent and least disputed finding of the weight-loss studies reviewed in this chapter is that weight loss is difficult and that maintaining weight loss is even more difficult. Furthermore, the difficulty of weight loss and of weight-loss maintenance increases steeply with the amount of weight that needs to be lost. These findings lead to the inescapable conclusion that the war against obesity can be won only with effective primary prevention: People should be prevented (or prevent themselves) from becoming overweight or obese in the first place (Crawford & Jeffery, 2005). There are two strategies to achieve this: namely, health education and environmental changes (Stroebe, 2000). The aim of health education is to persuade individuals to change unhealthy eating and exercising habits and to adopt a healthier lifestyle. To be effective, health education campaigns need to make people realize that they are engaging in a lifestyle that makes them vulnerable to serious negative health consequences. Unless people are made to feel vulnerable, they will not change their health behavior (de Hoog, Stroebe, & de Wit, 2005, 2007). This is relatively easy with smoking or drinking too much alcohol because individuals who engage in this behavior are usually aware of the fact that they are damaging their health. However, it poses a major obstacle when one tries to persuade individuals who are normal weight or slightly overweight that their eating pattern and sedentary lifestyle expose them to the risk of obesity. It might therefore be useful to also emphasize other positive health consequences of a healthier diet and increased exercise.

The aim of environmental changes is to reduce or eliminate those factors in today's "toxic environment" that facilitate unhealthy eating and exercising behaviors. This goal can be achieved by changing the costs associated with alternative courses of actions: for example, by increasing the price or the availability of unhealthy options or by reducing the price or availability of healthy options. Children and adolescents are the most promising target for such interventions, not only because their obesity rates are increasing with alarming speed in most industrialized countries, but also because in countries where children also eat in schools, their food environment can be influenced. In the United States and Britain, schoolchildren not only spend a large amount of their time at school but also eat a large share of their daily food while they are there.

Health Education

Health education constitutes an application of social psychology. To be effective, health education campaigns need to use the whole range of persuasive techniques that have been developed by social and health psychologists during the past few decades.

School-Based Programs

The prevention programs in schools focus on improving diet (decreasing consumption of high-fat foods; increasing consumption of fruits and vegetables) and exercise behavior (increasing physical activity; reducing television time). Planet Health, probably one of the most effective school-based prevention programs, was a 2-year interdisciplinary intervention for sixth- to eighth-graders conducted in 10 multiethnic schools in Massachusetts, randomly assigned to intervention and control groups (Gortmaker et al., 1999). Planet Health sessions, which were included in regular sessions within the core subjects, including physical education, focused on decreasing television viewing to 2 hours per day, increasing moderate and vigorous physical activity, decreasing consumption of high-fat foods, and increasing consumption of fruits and vegetables to 5 a day or more. After 2 years, obesity prevalence among female students had decreased from 23.6% to 20.3% in the intervention schools but increased from 21.5% to 23.5% in the control schools. Controlling for baseline obesity, female students in the intervention schools were at a significantly lower risk of becoming obese during the 2-year period of the study than were girls at the control schools. Regression analyses suggested that this reduction was mediated by a reduction in television viewing. None of the other behavior changes emerged as a significant mediator. No significant effects emerged for boys, even though the intervention had also reduced hours of television viewing for them.

A recent meta-analysis of 64 school-based prevention programs found that only 13 of these programs produced significant effects (Stice, Shaw, & Marti, 2006). All studies had control groups, and assignment to intervention or control group was either random or based on matching. With $r = .04$, the average effect size for all prevention programs was exceedingly small but still significantly different from zero. As in the Planet Health study, interventions were typically more effective with girls than with boys. For the 13 interventions that were successful, the effect size was $r = .22$, which would be considered a medium effect size of clinical significance. Because few of these programs included long-term follow-up periods, it is unclear whether these weight-gain prevention effects persisted after the end of the intervention. These effects may seem disappointing, but the average effect size for these interventions was similar to that observed for prevention programs for other public health problems, except for smoking, for which effect sizes are usually somewhat higher (Stice et al., 2006). In view of the effectiveness with children of weight-loss treatment programs that involve their parents (Epstein et al., 1994), one would have expected parental involvement to emerge as a strong moderator of the impact of weight-loss prevention programs. However, this was not the case. In fact, the effect size of parental involvement was nonsignificant and negligible.

It is interesting to note that programs that were specifically developed to target only obesity were more effective than were programs that targeted multiple health behaviors. Stice et al. (2006) suspected that the greater the complexity of the message relayed by the intervention, the more difficult it is for participants to process and remember. An alternative possibility suggested by ego depletion theory (e.g., Baumeister et al., 1998) would attribute this difference to the fact that self-control is a limited resource. Thus, if many different behaviors have to be controlled, less of this scarce resource can be used for the control of dietary and exercise behavior.

Programs for Adults

Few weight-gain prevention programs have been conducted with adults, and their success has been exceedingly modest (Jeffery & French, 1998; Klem, Viteri, & Wing, 2000; Simkin-Silverman, Wing, Boraz, Meilahn, & Kuller, 1998). One of these programs, the Pound of Prevention Study, has already been mentioned. The intervention in this 3-year prospective randomized controlled study of 1,226 male and female participants (aged 20 to 55 years) consisted of educational materials about weight-gain prevention delivered through monthly newsletters (Jeffery & French, 1998). Educational messages emphasized typical themes, such as weighing oneself regularly; eating more fruits and vegetables and less high-fat food; and increasing exercise, particularly walking. After 3 years, the intervention group had gained 10% less weight than did the control group, but this difference was not statistically significant.

Klem, Viteri, and Wing (2000) assigned 102 women of normal weight aged 25 to 34 years to one of three conditions: 100 weekly group meetings, a 10-week correspondence course, or a no-treatment control. Those in the control group received a lifestyle brochure. At the end of the intervention, participants in the group treatment condition had lost significantly more weight (1.9 kilograms [4.2 pounds]) than had those in the control group (0.2 kilograms [0.4 pounds]), and the mean weight loss of the correspondence group (1.1 kilograms [2.4 pounds]) fell midway between the other two conditions. The group treatment condition also had the greatest number of no-shows.

Furthermore, at a 6-month follow-up there were no longer significant differences among the three conditions.

The Women's Healthy Lifestyle Project was an intensive intervention for 435 premenopausal women aged 44 to 50 (Simkin-Silverman et al., 1998). Women in the intervention condition attended a 15-session group program held over a 20-week period followed by fewer meetings spread out over the next few months and finally by regular mail or telephone contact. They were asked to achieve a modest weight loss, an experience that was supposed to help them to avoid future weight gain. After 54 months, the women in the control condition had gained significantly more weight (2.36 kilograms [5.19 pounds]) than did the women in the treatment condition, who had essentially kept their weight constant.

Although it targeted mainly groups with a higher level of overweight and obesity, the "Fighting Fat, Fighting Fit" campaign of the British Broadcasting Corporation (BBC) should be mentioned here because as a radio and TV campaign it had much greater reach than any of these other interventions. A questionnaire survey of a subsample of individuals who had registered with the campaign to receive additional material suggested that approximately 10% were normal weight (Miles, Rapoport, Wardle, Afuape, & Duman, 2001). According to the self-reports of individuals who responded twice to the survey questionnaire, the campaign resulted in significant changes in dietary intake, activity pattern, and weight. Obviously, these were the most highly involved members of the audience, but effects remained significant when analyzing the data on an intention-to-treat basis (assuming no change for nonresponders).

Eating Disorder Prevention Programs

Because disordered eating and unhealthy dieting practices have emerged as risk factors for obesity, prevention programs aimed at these behaviors are also likely to reduce the obesity risk. Because girls and women are at much higher risk for eating pathology than are boys and men, these programs are likely to be more effective for the former than the latter group. These programs typically provide information on eating disorders and the negative consequences of eating disorders. By questioning the culturally held thin ideal, interventions aim at influencing thin idealization and lowering body dissatisfaction. They also provide information on healthy dieting and weight management skills. In a recent meta-analysis of such programs, Stice and Shaw (2004) found that such programs had significant effects in reducing BMI.

Environmental Changes

In light of the modest effects of intervention based on health education, the main hope for stemming the obesity epidemic appears to rest with interventions aimed at changing the obsogenic environment. The findings reported in chapter 4 (this volume) suggest numerous possibilities for environmental interventions: reducing portion sizes in restaurants; forbidding food advertising during children's TV shows; restricting the sales of soft drinks, candy bars, and other high-calorie foods in schools; taxing soft drinks and fast food, with the tax income used to subsidize healthy food and to finance health education programs; and providing incentives for communities to encourage physical activity by developing parks and public sports facilities and by building bicycle paths and sidewalks. The possibilities are endless, but most changes would be difficult to implement for political reasons, not only because they interfere with powerful economic interests but also because many of these measures would have limited popular support.

There is some evidence from the United States that taxing soft drinks and fast food can be effective in reducing the obesity risk (Kim & Kawachi, 2006). Some U.S. states level such taxes, some do not, and some did but repealed them. Analyzing data between 1991 and 1998, Kim and Kawachi (2006) found that states without a soft drink or snack food tax were more than 4 times as likely to undergo a high relative increase in obesity prevalence (defined as at or above the 75th percentile in the relative increase) than were states that taxed soft drinks and snack food. States that had repealed the tax were 13 times more likely than states with a tax to experience a high relative increase (Kim & Kawachi, 2006). These findings are compatible with the assumption that taxes on unhealthy food can influence obesity prevalence. However, as the authors observed, these tax effects were rather large given the small magnitude of the taxes and given the fact that the limited available information suggests that household demand, at least for salty snack food, is relatively inelastic (Kuchler, Tegene, & Harris, 2004).

Pricing strategies would probably be most easily implemented in specific settings such as schools and work sites. In their review of obesity prevention interventions, Schmitz and Jeffery (2002) described several studies that tested the impact of pricing strategies to increase the sales of low-fat food in cafeterias and through vending machines. For example, lowering fresh fruit and salad bar prices by 50% in a work-site cafeteria resulted in a threefold increase in sales (Jeffery, French, Raether, & Baxter, 1994). Another study showed that a price reduction of fresh fruits and baby carrots by 50% resulted in a two- to fourfold increase in sales in a high school cafeteria (French et al., 1997). Whereas sales of fruits and vegetables returned to baseline at the end of the intervention when prices were returned to baseline values, sales of salads remained high in the work-site cafeteria (Jeffery et al., 1994).

Because snack food is frequently sold through vending machines, these machines could be used to implement pricing strategies effectively. In 1998 more than 1.5 million vending machines were situated in U.S. schools and worksites (French, Story, & Jeffery, 2001). Several studies have demonstrated that sales of low-fat snacks at vending machines increase when prices for these snacks are reduced (French et al., 1997, 2001). One of the most stringent studies of the impact of price changes on purchases from vending machines was the Changing Individuals' Purchases of Snacks Study conducted by French et al. (2001). These researchers crossed four levels of price reduction (no change, 10%, 25%, 50%) with three levels of promotional signs for low-fat snack choices (no signs, labels on items, and signs on vending machines encouraging low-fat snack choices) and two settings (work sites and schools). Over the course of 1 year, each of the 12 possible combinations of pricing and signs was tested in each of the 24 test sites in random order for 1 month each. Price reductions of 59%, 25%, and 10% were associated with increases in the sales of low-fat snacks of 93%, 39%, and 9%, respectively. Only the 10% price reduction did not differ significantly from the condition in which prices were equal (i.e., no price change). These substantial price effects on demand may appear inconsistent with the low elasticity previously found for snack foods, but one has to remember that the price manipulation here was aiming at a substitution between low- and high-fat snack food alternatives. Of the informational conditions, only labels plus promotional signs resulted in a significant increase of low-fat snack sales.

Although more information on the sales elasticity of fast food, soft drinks, and snack foods is needed, using taxes and pricing would appear to be an effective strategy in battling the obesity epidemic. Although these strategies lack popular support at present, opinions might change as the obesity epidemic takes its inevitable course. Once people have become convinced of the health damage of obesity and of the fact that these nonnutritious foods are major contributors to the obesity epidemic, they might be more willing to support such changes, particularly if some of the tax income was used to subsidize healthier options.

CONCLUSIONS

Weight loss is possible but becomes increasingly difficult the more weight people want to lose. Furthermore, the need to lose substantial amounts of weight encourages aggressive dieting that is likely to be associated with ill effects. Thus, the most effective strategy would be to not put on weight in the first place and to stay within the range of normal weight. There seem to be people who are fortunate enough to have no need for weight monitoring. It is unclear whether they have a very active metabolism, do not like fatty food, have no interest in food, or are exceedingly physically active, but for whatever reason, their energy intake appears to be in permanent harmony with their energy output. However, the fact that nearly 50% of men of normal weight and 70% of women of normal weight in the United States report that they are either trying to lose weight or trying to maintain their present weight (Serdula et al., 1999) suggests that a great number of individuals of normal weight feel that they need to monitor their weight to maintain it. Unfortunately, not much is known about the weight-control practices of these individuals because, having no serious weight problems, this group has never been studied. However, weight gain is a gradual process, and once it has gotten out of hand is difficult to correct. The most efficient strategy of weight control for those with a tendency to gain weight might therefore be to regularly monitor their weight and either keep it stable or go on short-term diets when their weight creeps up. It is possible that some of the 9% of men of normal weight and 29% of women of normal weight (Serdula et al., 1999) who reported that they were trying to lose weight at the time of the 1996 behavioral risk survey were practicing this strategy.

Once people have become overweight or obese, they have to face the reality that their chances of losing sufficient weight to become normal weight are not very good. If they want to reach this goal, they are in for a very long struggle. The important message of research on weight loss and weight-loss maintenance is that strategies that rely mainly on will power will eventually fail. However motivated, in the long run people prove to be unable to maintain a diet of food they dislike. It is therefore important that they explore low-calorie food alternatives they like. If prepared the right way, salads, grilled fish, and grilled chicken can be tasty. Similarly, a great deal of physical activity can be integrated into most people's daily activities.

Of course, these changes are often difficult, and there are many barriers. With regard to a healthy diet of low-calorie food, one of the barriers, in addition to taste, can be financial. As Drewnowski and Darmon (2005) recently showed, there is an inverse relationship between the energy density of food and its cost. This is probably one of the reasons why the highest rates of obesity and diabetes are found among individuals of low socioeconomic status, even though these differences are decreasing. However, even small changes in diet and physical activity, if maintained, can have sizable impact in the long run. Thus, individuals who are overweight or obese are well advised to take a long-term perspective. A first step would be to stabilize their weight and to stop further weight gain. Once this is achieved, small changes in diet, replacement of some of the high-calorie meals with low-fat options, and eating less high-calorie food on the occasions when one still wants to enjoy it would be likely to result in small weight losses. The problem is that once substantial weight has been lost, a new balance between input and output will be reached and further calorie reduction or increase in physical exercise will be needed to achieve additional weight loss. Losing weight is a long haul, but it is not impossible. More disheartening is the fact that it is a permanent battle but there is no permanent victory. As the study of the NWCR demonstrated, successful weight-loss maintainers have to live with a low-calorie diet and be extremely physically active, but the members of that program appear not to find this a problem. Furthermore, as the research of Westenhoefer et al. (1999) has shown, watching one's weight does not imply that one has to deny oneself all high-calorie food. Flexible dieters who allow themselves to eat more one day and make up for it by eating less the next have a higher probability of weight loss than do individuals who rigidly stick to their diet. Furthermore, as long as one does not eat too much of it, high-calorie food can be integrated into a low-calorie diet. This need to resist temptation is the price one must pay for living in the land of plenty.

REFERENCES

Aarts, H., & Dijksterhuis, A. (2003). The silence of the library: Environment, situational norm, and social behavior. *Journal of Personality and Social Psychology, 84,* 18–28.

Abramson, E. E., & Wunderlich, R. A. (1972). Anxiety, fear and eating: A test of the psychosomatic concept of obesity. *Journal of Abnormal Psychology, 79,* 317–321.

Adair, L. S., & Popkin, B. M. (2005). Are child eating patterns being transformed globally? *Obesity Research, 13,* 1281–1299.

Aisbitt, B. (2007). Obesity—Should we blame our genes? *Nutrition Bulletin, 32,* 183–186.

Ajani, E. U., Lotufo, P. A., Gaziano, J. M., Lee, I. M., Spelsberg, A., Buring, J. E., et al. (2004). Body mass index and mortality among US male physicians. *Annals of Epidemiology, 14,* 731–739.

Ajzen, I. (2005). *Attitudes, personality and behavior.* Maidenhead, England: Open University Press.

Ajzen, I., & Fishbein, M. (1977). Attitude–behavior relation: A theoretical analysis and review of empirical research. *Psychological Bulletin, 84,* 888–918.

Albu, J., & Pi-Sunyer, F. X. (1998). Obesity and diabetes. In G. A. Bray, C. Bouchard, & W. P. T. James (Eds.), *Handbook of obesity* (pp. 697–708). New York: Dekker.

Allender, S., Peto, V., Scarborough, P., Boxer, A., & Rayner, M. (2006). *Diet, physical activity and obesity statistics.* Retrieved October 4, 2007, from http://www.heartstats.org/temp/Dopaspmainspdocspweb06.pdf

Allison, D. B., Zanolli, R., Faith, M. S., Heo, M., Pietrobelli, A., VanItallie, T. B., et al. (1999). Weight loss increases and fat loss decreases all-cause mortality rate: Result from two independent cohort studies. *International Journal of Obesity, 23,* 603–611.

American Psychiatric Association. (1980). *Diagnostic and statistical manual of mental disorders* (3rd ed.). Washington, DC: Author.

American Psychiatric Association. (1994). *Diagnostic and statistical manual of mental disorders* (4th ed.). Washington, DC: Author.

Anderson, C. A., Benjamin, Jr., A. J., & Bartholow, B. D. (1998). Does the gun pull the trigger? Automatic priming effects of weapon pictures and picture names. *Psychological Science, 9,* 308–314.

Anderson, J. W., Konz, E. C., Frederich, R. C., & Wood, C. L. (2001). Long-term weight-loss maintenance: A meta-analysis of US studies. *American Journal of Clinical Nutrition, 74,* 579–584.

Anderson, M. C., & Spellman, B. A. (1995). On the status of inhibitory mechanisms in cognition: Memory retrieval as a model case. *Psychological Review, 102,* 68–100.

Anderson, R. E., Wadden, T. A., Bartlett, S. J., Zemel, B., Verde, T. J., & Franckowiac, S. C. (1999). Effects of lifestyle activity vs. structured aerobic exercise in obese women; a randomized trial. *Journal of the American Medical Association, 281,* 335–340.

Andres, R., Muller, D. C., & Sorkin, J. D. (1993). Long-term effects of change in body weight on all-cause mortality: A review. *Annals of Internal Medicine, 119,* 737–743.

Astrup, A., Beuman, B., Christensen, N. J., & Toubro, S. (1995). Prognostic markers for diet-induced weight loss in obese women. *International Journal of Obesity, 19,* 275–278.

Astrup, A., Gotzsche, P. C., van de Werken, K., Ranneries, C., Toubro, S., Raben, A., & Buemann, B. (1999). Meta-analysis of resting metabolic rate in formerly obese subjects. *American Journal of Clinical Nutrition, 69,* 1117–1122.

Atkins, R. (2002). *Dr. Atkins' new diet revolution.* New York: Avon.

Atkinson, R. L., & Stern, J. S. (1998). Weight cycling: Definitions, mechanisms, and problems with interpretation. In G. A. Bray, C. Bouchard, & W. P. T. James (Eds.), *Handbook of obesity* (pp. 791–804). New York: Dekker.

Baik, I., Ascherio, A., Rimm, E. B., Giavannucci, E., Spiegelman, D., Stampfer, M. J., & Willett, W. C. (2000). Adiposity and mortality in men. *American Journal of Epidemiology, 152,* 264–271.

Bak, H., Petersen, L., & Sorensen, T. I. A. (2004). Physical activity in relation to development and maintenance of obesity in men with and without juvenile onset obesity. *International Journal of Obesity, 28,* 99–104.   ·

Bandura, A. (1986). *Social foundations of thought and action.* Englewood Cliffs, NJ: Prentice Hall.

Bargh, J. A. (1996). Automaticity in social psychology. In T. Higgins & A. Kruglanski (Eds.), *Social psychology: Handbook of basic processes* (pp. 169–183). New York: Guilford Press.

Bargh, J. A., & Chartrand, T. L. (1999). The unbearable automaticity of being. *American Psychologist, 54,* 462–479.

Bargh, J. A., & Ferguson, M. J. (2000). Beyond behaviorism: On the automaticity of higher mental processes. *Psychological Bulletin, 126,* 925–945.

Bargh, J. A., Gollwitzer, P. M., Lee-Chai, A., Barndollar, K., & Trötschel, R. (2001). The automated will: Nonconscious activation and pursuit of behavioral goals. *Journal of Personality and Social Psychology, 81,* 1014–1027.

Barlow, C. E., Kohl, H. W., III, Gibbons, L. W., & Blair, S. N. (1995). Physical fitness, mortality and obesity. *International Journal of Obesity, 19*(Suppl. 4), S41–S44.

Baron, R. M., & Kenny, D. A. (1986). The moderator–mediator variable distinction in social psychological research: Conceptual, strategic and statistical considerations. *Journal of Personality and Social Psychology, 51,* 1173–1182.

Basdevant, A., Craplet, C., & Guy-Grand, B. (1993). Snacking pattern in obese French women. *Appetite, 21,* 17–23.

Batterham, R. L., Heffron, J. L., Kapoor, S., Chivers, J. E., Chandaran, K., Herzog, H., et al. (2006). Critical role for peptide YY in protein-mediated satiation and body weight regulation. *Cell Metabolism, 4,* 223–233.

Baucom, D. H., & Aiken, P. A. (1981). Effect of depressed mood on eating among obese and nonobese dieting and nondieting persons. *Journal of Personality and Social Psychology, 41*, 577–585.

Baumeister, R. F., Bratslavsky, E., Muraven, M., & Tice, D. M. (1998). Ego depletion: Is the active self a limited resource. *Journal of Personality and Social Psychology, 74*, 1252–1265.

Baumeister, R. F., Heatherton, T. F., & Tice, D. M. (1994). *Losing control: How and why people fail at self-regulation.* New York: Academic Press.

Bell, A. C., Ge, K., & Popkin, B. M. (2002). Weight gain and its predictors in Chinese adults. *International Journal of Obesity, 25*, 1079–1086.

Bendixen, H., Madsen, J., Bay-Hansen, D., Boesen, U., Ovesen, L. F., Bartels, E. M., & Astrup, A. (2002). An observational study of slimming behavior in Denmark in 1992 and 1998. *Obesity Research, 10*, 911–922.

Benecke, A., & Vogel, H. (2005). *Übergewicht und Adipositas* [Overweight and adiposity] (Gesundheitsberichterstattung des Bundes, Heft 16). Berlin: Robert Koch-Institut.

Berkowitz, L., & LePage, A. (1967). Weapons as aggression-eliciting stimuli. *Journal of Personality and Social Psychology, 7*, 2002–2007.

Berridge, K. C. (1995). Food reward: Brain substrates of wanting and liking. *Neuroscience and Biobehavioral Reviews, 20*, 1–25.

Berridge, K. C. (2001). Reward learning: Reinforcement, incentive, and expectation. *Psychology of Learning and Motivation, 40*, 223–278.

Bertéus Forslund, H., Torgerson, J. S., Sjöström, L., & Lindroos, A. K. (2005). Snacking frequency in relation to energy intake and food choices in obese men and women compared to a reference population. *International Journal of Obesity, 29*, 711–719.

Bes-Rastrollo, M., Sánchez-Villegas, A., Gómez-Gracia, E., Martinez, J. A., Pajares, R., & Martinez-Gonález, M. A. (2006). Predictors of weight gain in a Mediterranean cohort: The Seguimiento Universidad de Navarra Study. *American Journal of Clinical Nutrition, 83*, 362–370.

Bessenoff, G. R., & Sherman, J. W. (2000). Automatic and controlled components of prejudice toward fat people: Evaluation versus stereotype activation. *Social Cognition, 18*, 329–353.

Bish, C. L., Blanck, H. M., Serdula, M. K., Marcus, M., Kohl, H. W., & Kettel-Khan, L. (2005). Diet and physical activity behaviors among Americans trying to lose weight: 2000 Behavioral Risk Factor Surveillance System. *Obesity Research, 13*, 596–607.

Black, A. E., Goldberg, G. R., Jebb, S. A., Livingstone, M. B. E., Cole, T. J., & Prentice, A. M. (1991). Critical evaluation of energy intake data using fundamental principles of energy physiology: 2. Evaluating the results of published surveys. *European Journal of Clinical Nutrition, 4*, 583–599.

Blair, S. N., & Leermakers, E. A. (2002). Exercise and weight management. In T. A. Wadden & A. J. Stunkard (Eds.), *Handbook of obesity treatment* (pp. 283–300). New York: Guilford Press.

Blass, E. M., Anderson, D. R., Kirkorian, H. L., Pempek, T. A., Price, I., & Koleini, M. F. (2006). On the road to obesity: Television viewing increases intake of high-density foods. *Physiology & Behavior, 88,* 597–604.

Bleau, R. (1996). Dietary restraint and anxiety in adolescent girls. *British Journal of Clinical Psychology, 35,* 573–583.

Blundell, J. E., Burley, V. J., Cotton, J. R., & Lawton, C. L. (1993). *American Journal of Clinical Nutrition, 57*(Suppl.), 772S–778S.

Blundell, J. E., & Stubbs, R. J. (1998). Diet composition and the control of food intake in humans. In G. A. Bray, C. Bouchard, & W. P. T. James (Eds.), *Handbook of obesity* (pp. 243–272). New York: Dekker.

Boon, B. (1998). *Why dieters overeat: On the cognitive regulation of eating behaviour.* Unpublished doctoral dissertation, Utrecht University, Utrecht, the Netherlands.

Boon, B., Stroebe, W., Schut, H., & Ijtema, R. (2002). Reformulating the boundary model: Ironic processes in the eating behaviour of restrained eaters. *British Journal of Health Psychology, 7,* 1–10.

Boon, B., Stroebe, W., Schut, H., & Jansen, A. (1997). Does cognitive distraction lead to overeating in restrained eaters? *Behavioural and Cognitive Psychotherapy, 25,* 319–327.

Boon, B., Vogelzang, L., & Jansen, A. (2000). Do restrained eaters show attention towards or away from food, shape and weight stimuli? *European Eating Disorders Review, 8,* 51–58.

Bouchard, C. (2007a). The biological predisposition to obesity: Beyond the thrifty genotype scenario. *International Journal of Obesity, 31,* 1337–1339.

Bouchard, C. (2007b). BMI, fat mass, abdominal adiposity and visceral fat: Where is the "beef"? *International Journal of Obesity, 31,* 1552–1553.

Bouchard, C., Pérusse, L., Rice, T., & Rao, D. C. (2004). Genetics of human obesity. In G. A. Bray & C. Bouchard (Eds.), *Handbook of obesity: Etiology and pathophysiology* (2nd ed., pp. 157–200). New York: Dekker.

Bouchard, C., & Rankinen, T. (2008). Genetics of human obesity: Exciting advances and new opportunities. In K. Clement & T. I. A. Sorensen (Eds.), *Obesity, genomics, and postgenomics* (pp. 549–562). New York: Informa Healthcare.

Bouchard, C., Tremblay, A., Després, J. P., Thériault, G., Nadeau, A., Lupien, P. J., et al. (1990). The response to long-term overfeeding in identical twins. *New England Journal of Medicine, 322,* 1477–1482.

Bouchard, C., Tremblay, A., Després, J. P., Thériault, G., Nadeau, A., Lupien, P. J., et al. (1994). The response to exercise with constant energy intake in identical twins. *Obesity Research, 2,* 400–410.

Bouchard, C., Tremblay, A., Nadeau, A., Després, J. P., Thériault, G., Boulay, M. R., et al. (1989). Genetic effect in resting and exercise metabolic rates. *Metabolism, 38,* 364–370.

Bowman, S. A., & Vinyard, B. T. (2004). Fast food consumption of US adults: Impact on energy and nutrient intake and overweight status. *Journal of the American College of Nutrition, 23,* 163–168.

Braam, L. A. J. L., Ocké, M. C., Bueno-de-Mesquita, B., & Seidell, J. C. (1998). Determinants of obesity-related underreporting of energy intake. *American Journal of Epidemiology, 147,* 1081–1086.

Bray, G. A. (1998). Classification and evaluation of obesity. In G. A. Bray, C. Bouchard, & W. P. T. James (Eds.), *Handbook of obesity* (pp. 831–834). New York: Dekker.

Bray, G. A. (2004). Classification and evaluation of the overweight patient. In G. A. Bray & C. Bouchard (Eds.), *Handbook of obesity: Clinical applications* (2nd ed., pp. 1–32). New York: Dekker.

Bray, G. A., Bouchard, C., & James, W. P. T. (1998). Definitions and proposed current classification of obesity. In G. A. Bray, C. Bouchard, & W. P. T. James (Eds.), *Handbook of obesity* (pp. 31–40). New York: Dekker.

Bray, G. A., Lovejoy, J. C., Most-Windhauser, M., Smith, S. R., Volaufova, J., Denkins, J., et al. (2002). A 9-mo randomized clinical trial comparing fat-substituted and fat-reduced diets in health obese men: The Ole Study. *American Journal of Clinical Nutrition, 76,* 928–934.

Brenner, M. (1973). The next-in-line effect. *Journal of Verbal Learning and Verbal Behavior, 12,* 320–323.

Briefel, R. R., & Johnson, C. L. (2004). Secular trends in dietary intake in the United States. *Annual Review of Nutrition, 24,* 401–431.

Brownell, K. D. (1994). Whether obesity should be treated. *Health Psychology, 12,* 339–341.

Brownell, K. D. (1997). *The LEARN program for weight control* (7th ed.). Dallas, TX: American Health Publishing Company.

Brownell, K. D. (2002). The environment and obesity. In C. G. Fairburn & K. D. Brownell (Eds.), *Eating disorders and obesity* (pp. 433–438). New York: Guilford Press.

Brownell, K. D., & Horgen, K. B. (2004). *Food fight.* Chicago: Contemporary Books.

Brownell, K. D., Puhl, R. M., Schwartz, M. B., & Rudd, L. (Eds.). (2005). *Weight bias: Nature, consequences and remedies.* New York: Guilford Press.

Bruch, H. (1961). The transformation of oral impulses in eating disorders: A conceptual approach. *Psychiatric Quarterly, 35,* 458–481.

Bruch, H. (1974). *Eating disorders.* London: Routledge & Kegan Paul.

Brunstrom, J. M., Yates, H. M., & Witcomb, G. L. (2004). Dietary restraint and heightened reactivity to food. *Physiology and Behavior, 81,* 85–90.

Bulik, C. M., & Allison, D. B. (2001). The genetic epidemiology of thinness. *Obesity Reviews, 2,* 107–115.

Bundred, P., Kitchiner, D., & Buchan, I. (2001). Prevalence of overweight and obese children between 1989 and 1998: Population-based series of cross sectional studies. *British Medical Journal, 322,* 1–4.

Butryn, M. L., & Wadden, T. A. (2005). Treatment of overweight in children and adolescents: Does dieting increase the risk of eating disorders? *International Journal of Eating Disorders, 37,* 285–293.

Calle, E. E., Thun, M. J., Petrelli, J. M., Rodriguez, C., & Heath, C. W. (1999). Body-mass index and mortality in a prospective cohort of U.S. adults. *New England Journal of Medicine, 341*, 1097–1105.

Campfield, L. A., Smith, F. J., & Jeanrenaud, B. (2004). Central integration of peripheral signals in the regulation of food intake and energy balance: Role of leptin and insulin. In G. A. Bray & C. Bouchard (Eds.), *Handbook of obesity: Etiology and pathophysiology* (2nd ed., pp. 461–479). New York: Dekker.

Canning, H., & Mayer, J. (1966). Obesity—Its possible effect on college acceptance. *New England Journal of Medicine, 275*, 1172–1174.

Carr, T. (2003). *Discovering nutrition*. Blackwell, England: Oxford University Press.

Centers for Disease Control. (1994). *Behavioral Risk Factor Surveillance System: 1994 Behavioral Risk Factor Questionnaire*. Retrieved October 31, 2007, from http://cdc.gov/brfss/questionnaires/pdf-ques/94brfss.pdf

Centers for Disease Control. (2007). *Behavioral Risk Factor Surveillance System: Trends data nationwide (states, DC, and territories) grouped by gender*. Retrieved October 31, 2007, from http://apps.nccd.cdc.gov/brfss/Trends/sexchart.asp?qkey=10020&state=US.

Chamontin, A., Pretzer, G., & Booth, D. A. (2003). Ambiguity of "snack" in British usage. *Appetite, 41*, 21–29.

Chandola, T., Deary, I. J., Blane, D., & Batty, G. D. (2006). Childhood IQ in relation to obesity and weight gain in adult life. The National Child Development (1958) Study. *International Journal of Obesity, 30*, 1422–1432.

Chapelot, D., Pasquet, P., Apfelbaum, M., & Fricker, J. (1995). Cognitive factors in the dietary response of restrained and unrestrained eaters to manipulation of the fat content of a dish. *Appetite, 25*, 155–176.

Ciliska, D. (1998). Evaluation of two nondieting interventions for obese women. *Western Journal of Nursing Research, 20*, 119–135.

Cogan, J. C., & Ernsberger, P. (Eds.). (1999). Dying to be thin in the name of health: Shifting the paradigm [Special issue]. *Journal of Social Issues, 55*(2).

Colditz, G. A., Giovannucci, E., Rimm, E. B., Stampfer, M. J., Rosner, B., Speizer, F. E., et al. (1991). Alcohol intake in relation to diet and obesity in women and men. *American Journal of Clinical Nutrition, 54*, 49–55.

Considine, R. V., & Caro, J. F. (1996). Leptin and the regulation of body weight. *International Journal of Biochemistry and Cell Biology, 29*, 1255–1272.

Cools, J., Schotte, D. E., & McNally, R. J. (1992). Emotional arousal and overeating in restrained eaters. *Journal of Abnormal Psychology, 101*, 348–351.

Coon, K. A., Goldberg, J., Rogers, B. L., & Tucker, K. L. (2001). Relationship between use of television during meals and children's food consumption patterns. *Pediatrics, 107*, 7–10.

Cooper, P. J., Taylor, M. J., Cooper, Z., & Fairburn, C. G. (1987). The development and validation of the Body Shape Questionnaire. *International Journal of Eating Disorders, 6*, 485–494.

Cox, D. N., Perry, L., Moore, P. B., Vallis, L., & Mela, D. J. (1999). Sensory and hedonic associations with macronutrient and energy intakes of lean and obese consumers. *International Journal of Obesity, 23*, 403–410.

Cramer, P., & Steinwert, T. (1998). This is good, fat is bad: How early does it begin? *Journal of Applied Developmental Psychology, 19*, 429–451.

Crandall, C. S. (1991). Do heavyweight students have more difficulty in paying for college? *Personality and Social Psychology Bulletin, 17*, 606–611.

Crandall, C. S., & Biernat, M. (1990). The ideology of anti-fat attitudes. *Journal of Applied Social Psychology, 20*, 227–243.

Crawford, D., & Jeffery, R. W. (Eds.). (2005). *Obesity prevention and public health.* New York: Oxford University Press.

Crespo, C. J., Smit, E., Troiano, R. P., Bartlett, S. J., Macera, C. A., & Andersen, R. E. (2001). Television watching, energy intake, and obesity in US children. *Archives of Pediatric and Adolescent Medicine, 155*, 360–365.

Cross, A. T., Babicz, D., & Cushman, L. F. (1994). Snacking patterns among 1,800 adults and children. *Journal of the American Dietetic Association, 12*, 1398–1403.

Curb, J. D., & Marcus, E. B. (1991). Body fat and obesity in Japanese Americans. *American Journal of Clinical Nutrition, 53*(Suppl.), 1552S–1555S.

Curioni, C. C., & Lourenco, P. M. (2005). Long-term weight loss after diet and exercise: A systematic review. *International Journal of Obesity, 29*, 1168–1174.

Custers, R., & Aarts, H. (2005). Beyond priming effects: The role of positive affect discrepancies in implicit processes of motivation and goal pursuit. In W. Stroebe & M. Hewstone (Eds.), *European review of social psychology* (Vol. 16, pp. 257–300). Brighton, England: Psychology Press.

Cutler, D. M., Glaeser, E. L., & Shapiro, J. M. (2003). Why have Americans become more obese? *Journal of Economic Perspectives, 17*, 93–118.

Dansinger, M. L., Gleason, J. A., Griffith, J. L., Selker, H. P., & Schaefer, E. J. (2005). Comparison of the Atkins, Ornish, Weight Watchers, and Zone diets for weight loss and heart disease risk reduction. *Journal of the American Medical Association, 293*, 43–53.

Dawber, T. R. (1980). *The Framingham Study.* Cambridge, MA: Harvard University Press.

de Hoog, N., Stroebe, W., & de Wit, J. B. F. (2005). The impact of fear appeals on processing and acceptance of action recommendations. *Personality and Social Psychology Bulletin, 31*, 24–33.

de Hoog, N., Stroebe, W., & de Wit, J. B. F. (2007). The impact of vulnerability to and severity of a health risk on processing and acceptance of fear-arousing communications: A meta-analysis. *Review of General Psychology, 11*, 258–285.

De Houwer, J. (2003). The extrinsic affective Simon task. *Experimental Psychology, 50*, 77–85.

De Jonge, L., & Bray, G. A. (1997). The thermic effect of food and obesity: A critical review. *Obesity Research, 5*, 622–631.

Department for Environment, Food and Rural Affairs. (2006). *Data for energy intake 1974–2005. Family food: Report on the Food & Expenditure Survey.* Retrieved September 28, 2006, from http://statistics.defra.gov.uk/esg/publications/efs/default.asp

Després, J.-P. (2002). The metabolic syndrome. In C. G. Fairburn & K. D. Brownell (Eds.), *Eating disorders and obesity* (pp. 477–483). New York: Guilford Press.

Després, J.-P., & Krauss, R. M. (1998). Obesity and lipoprotein metabolism. In G. A. Bray, C. Bouchard, & W. P. T. James (Eds.), *Handbook of obesity* (pp. 651–676). New York: Dekker.

Devine, P. G. (1989). Stereotypes and prejudice: Their automatic and controlled components. *Journal of Personality and Social Psychology, 56,* 5–18.

Diabetes Prevention Program Research Group. (2002). Reduction in the incidence of Type 2 diabetes with lifestyle intervention or metformin. *New England Journal of Medicine, 346,* 393–403.

Diehr, P., Bild, D. E., Harris, T. B., Duxbury, A., Sicovick, D., & Rossi, M. (1998). Body mass index and mortality in nonsmoking older adults: The cardiovascular health study. *American Journal of Public Health, 88,* 623–629.

Dietz, W. H. (1998). Prevalence of obesity in children. In G. A. Bray, C. Bouchard, & W. P. T. James (Eds.), *Handbook of obesity* (pp. 93–102). New York: Dekker.

Dietz, W. H., & Gortmaker, S. L. (1985). Do we fatten our children at the television set? Obesity and television viewing in children and adolescents. *Pediatrics, 75,* 807–812.

Dijksterhuis, A., Aarts, H., & Smith, P. K. (2005). The power of the subliminal: Subliminal perception and possible applications. In R. R. Hassin, J. S. Uleman, & J. A. Bargh (Eds.), *The new unconscious* (pp. 77–106). New York: Oxford University Press.

Diliberti, N., Bordi, P. L., Conklin, M. T., Roe, L. S., & Rolls, B. J. (2004). Increased portion size leads to increased energy intake in a restaurant meal. *Obesity Research, 12,* 562–568.

DiMeglio, D. P., & Mattes, R. D. (2000). Liquid versus solid carbohydrate: Effects on food intake and body weight. *International Journal of Obesity, 24,* 794–800.

Djuric, Z., DiLaura, N. M., Jenkins, I., Darga, L., Jen, C., Mood, D., et al. (2002). Combining weight-loss counseling with the Weight Watchers plan for obese breast cancer survivors. *Obesity Research, 10,* 657–664.

Dobson, K. S., & Dozois, D. J. A. (2004). Attentional biases in eating disorders: A meta-analytic review of Stroop performance. *Clinical Psychology Review, 23,* 1001–1022.

Donnelly, J. E., Hill, J. O., Jacobsen, D. J., Potteiger, J., Sullivan, D. K., Johnson, S. L., et al. (2003). Effects of a 16-month randomized controlled exercise trial on body weight and composition in young, overweight men and women. *Archives of Internal Medicine, 163,* 1343–1350.

Dreon, D. M., Frey-Hewitt, B., Ellsworth, N., Williams, P. T., Terry, R. B., & Wood, P. D. (1988). Dietary fat: Carbohydrate ratio and obesity in middle-aged men. *American Journal of Nutrition, 47,* 995–1000.

Drewnowski, A., & Darmon, N. (2005). Food choice and diet costs: An economic analysis. *Journal of Nutrition, 135,* 900–904.

Dritschel, B., Cooper, P. J., & Charnock, D. (1993). A problematic counter-regulation experiment: Implications for the link between dietary restraint and overeating. *International Journal of Eating Disorders, 13,* 297–304.

Durazo-Arvizu, R., Cooper, R. S., Luke, A., Prewitt, T. E., Liao, Y., & McGee, D. L. (1997). Relative weight and mortality in U.S. Blacks and Whites: Findings from representative national population samples. *Annals of Epidemiology, 7,* 383–395.

Ebbeling, C. B., Sinclair, K. B., Pereira, M. A., Garcia-Lago, E., Feldman, H. A., & Ludwig, D. S. (2004). Compensation for energy intake from fast food among overweight and lean adolescents. *Journal of the American Medical Association, 291,* 2828–2833.

Eldredge, K. L. (1993). An investigation of the influence of dieting and self-esteem on dietary disinhibition. *International Journal of Eating Disorders, 13,* 57–67.

Elgar, F. J., Roberts, C., Moore, L., & Tudor-Smith, C. (2005). Sedentary behaviour, physical activity and weight problems in adolescents in Wales. *Public Health, 119,* 518–524.

Epstein, L. H., Paluch, R. A., Roemmich, J. N., & Beecher, M. D. (2007). Family-based obesity treatment, then and now: Twenty-five years of pediatric obesity treatment. *Health Psychology, 26,* 381–391.

Epstein, L. H., Truesdale, R., Wojcik, A., Paluch, R. A., & Raynor, H. A. (2003). Effects of deprivation on hedonics and reinforcing value of food. *Physiology & Behavior, 78,* 221–227.

Epstein, L. H., Valoski, A., Wing, R. R., & McCurley, J. (1994). Ten-year outcomes of behavioral family-based treatment for childhood obesity. *Health Psychology, 13,* 373–383.

Eriksson, K. F., & Lindgärde, F. (1998). No excess 12-year mortality in men with impaired glucose tolerance who participated in the Malmö Preventive Trial with diet and exercise. *Diabetologia, 41,* 1010–1016.

Ewing, R. (2005). Can physical environment determine physical activity levels. *Exercise and Sport Sciences Reviews, 33,* 69–75.

Ewing, R., Schmid, R., Killingsworth, A., Zlot, K., & Raudenbush, S. (2003). Relationship between urban sprawl and physical activity, obesity, and morbidity. *American Journal of Health Promotion, 18,* 47–57.

Falconer, D. S. (1981). *Introduction to quantitative genetics* (2nd ed.). New York: Ronald Press.

Farooqi, I. S., & O'Rahilly, S. (2007). Genetic factors in human obesity. *Obesity Reviews, 9*(Suppl. 1), 37–40.

Farooqi, I. S., Wangensteen, T., Collins, S., Kimber, W., Matarese, G., Keogh, J. M., et al. (2007). Clinical and molecular genetic spectrum of congenital deficiency of the leptin receptor. *New England Journal of Medicine, 356,* 237–247.

Farooqi, I. S., Jebb, S. A., Langmack, G., Lawrence, E., Cheetham, C. H., Prentice, A. M., et al. (1999). Effects of recombinant leptin therapy in a child with congenital leptin deficiency. *New England Journal of Medicine, 341,* 879–884.

Farrington, G. (2006). *Oliver "sparks school food drop."* BBC radio five live. Retrieved September 28, 2006, from http://news.bbc.co.uk/2/hi/uk_news/education/4243986.stm

Fazio, R. H., Sanbonmatsu, D. M., Powell, M. C., & Kardes, F. R. (1986). On the automatic activation of attitudes. *Journal of Personality and Social Psychology, 69,* 1013–1027.

Fedoroff, I. C., Polivy, J., & Herman, C. P. (1997). The effect of pre-exposure to food cues on the eating behavior of restrained and unrestrained eaters. *Appetite, 28,* 33–47.

Fedoroff, I. C., Polivy, J., & Herman, C. P. (2003). The specificity of restrained versus unrestrained eaters' responses to food cues: General desire to eat, or craving for cued food? *Appetite, 41,* 7–13.

Fehily, A. (1999). Epidemiology of obesity in the UK. In British Nutrition Foundation (Ed.), *Obesity* (pp. 23–36). Oxford, England: Blackwell Science.

Field, A. E., Austin, S. B., Gillman, M. W., Rosner, B., Rockett, H. R., & Colditz, G. A. (2004). Snack food intake does not predict weight change among children and adolescents. *International Journal of Obesity, 28,* 1210–1216.

Field, A. E., Austin, S. B., Taylor, C. B., Malspeis, S., Rosner, B., Rockett, H. R., et al. (2003). Relation between dieting and weight change among preadolescents and adolescents. *Pediatrics, 112,* 900–906.

Fikkan, J., & Rothblum, E. (2005). Weight bias in employment. In K. D. Brownell, R. M. Puhl, M. B. Schwartz, & L. Rudd (Eds.), *Weight bias: Nature, consequences and remedies* (pp. 15–28). New York: Guilford Press.

Fine, J. T., Colditz, G. A., Coakley, E. H., Mosely, G., Manson, J. E., Willett, W. C., & Kawachie, I. (1999). A prospective study of weight change and health-related quality of life in women. *Journal of the American Medical Association, 282,* 2136–2142.

Finley, C. E., Barlow, C. E., Greenway, F. L., Rock, C. L., Rolls, B. J., & Blair, S. N. (2007). Retention rates and weight loss in a commercial weight loss program. *International Journal of Obesity, 31,* 292–298.

Fishbach, A., Friedman, R. S., & Kruglanski, A. W. (2003). Leading us not into temptation: Momentary allurements elicit overriding goal activation. *Journal of Personality and Social Psychology, 84,* 296–309.

Fishbein, M., & Ajzen, I. (1975). *Belief, attitude, intention, and behavior: An introduction to theory and research.* Reading, MA: Addison-Wesley.

Fitzgibbon, M. S., Stolley, M. R., & Kirschenbaum, D. S. (1994). Obese people who seek treatment have different characteristics than those who do not seek treatment. *Health Psychology, 12,* 342–345.

Flatt, J. P. (2007). Exaggerated claim about adaptive thermogenesis. *International Journal of Obesity, 31,* 1626.

Flechtner-Mors, M., Ditschuneit, H. H., Johnson, T. D., Suchard, M. A., & Adler, G. (2000). Metabolic and weight loss effects of long-term dietary intervention in obese patients: Four-year results. *Obesity Research, 8,* 399–402.

Fontaine, K. R., & Allison, D. B. (2001). Does intentional weight loss affect mortality rate? *Eating Behaviors, 2*, 87–95.

Foster, G. D., Wadden, T. A., Kendall, P. C., Stunkard, A. J., & Vogt, R. A. (1996). Psychological effects of weight loss and regain: A prospective study. *Journal of Consulting and Clinical Psychology, 64*, 752–757.

Fox, K. (1999). Aetiology of obesity XI: Physical inactivity. In British Nutrition Foundation (Ed.), *Obesity* (pp. 116–131). Oxford, England: Blackwell Science.

Francis, L. A., Lee, Y., & Birch, L. L. (2003). Parental weight status and girls' television viewing, snacking, and body mass indexes. *Obesity Research, 11*, 143–151.

Franken, I. H. A. (2003). Drug craving and addiction. Integrating psychological and neuropsychopharmacological approaches. *Progress in Neuro-Psychopharmacology and Biological Psychiatry, 27*, 563–579.

Frederiksen, H., & Christensen, K. (2003). The influence of genetic factors on physical functioning and exercise in second half of life. *Scandinavian Journal of Medicine & Science in Sports, 13*, 9–18.

French, S. A. (1992). Restraint, food choice, and cognitions. *Addictive Behaviors, 17*, 273–281.

French, S. A., Harnack, L., & Jeffery, R. W. (2000). Fast food restaurant use among women in the Pound of Prevention study: Dietary, behavioral and demographic correlates. *International Journal of Obesity and Related Metabolic Disorders, 24*, 1353–1359.

French, S. A., & Jeffery, R. W. (1994). Consequences of dieting to lose weight: Effects on physical and mental health. *Health Psychology, 13*, 195–212.

French, S. A., Jeffery, R. W., Forster, J. L., McGovern, P. G., Kelder, S. H., & Baxter, J. E. (1994). Predictors of weight change over two years among a population of working adults: The Healthy Worker Project. *International Journal of Obesity and Related Metabolic Disorders, 18*, 145–154.

French, S. A., Jeffery, R. W., & Murray, D. (1999). Is dieting good for you? Prevalence, duration and associated weight and behaviour changes for specific weight loss strategies over four years in US adults. *International Journal of Obesity and Related Metabolic Disorders, 23*, 320–327.

French, S. A., Jeffery, R. W., Story, M., Breitlow, K. K., Baxter, J. S., Hannan, P., & Snyder, M. P. (1997). A pricing strategy to promote low-fat snack choices through vending machines. *American Journal of Public Health, 87*, 849–851.

French, S. A., Perry, C. L., Leon, G. R., & Fulkerson, J. A. (1995). Dieting behaviors and weight change history in female adolescents. *Health Psychology, 14*, 548–555.

French, S. A., Story, M., & Jeffery, R. W. (2001). Environmental influences on eating and physical activity. *Annual Review of Public Health, 22*, 309–336.

Friedman, M. A., & Brownell, K. D. (1995). Psychological correlates of obesity: Moving to the next research generation. *Psychological Bulletin, 117*, 3–20.

Frieze, I. H., Olson, J. E., & Good, D. C. (1990). Perceived and actual discrimination in the salaries of male and female managers. *Journal of Applied Social Psychology, 20*, 46–67.

Froedevaux, F., Schutz, Y., Christin, L., & Jéquier, E. (1993). Energy expenditure in obese women before and during weight loss, after refeeding, and in the weight-relapse period. *American Journal of Clinical Nutrition, 57*, 35–42.

Frost, R. O., Goolkasian, G. A., Ely, R. J., & Blanchard, F. A. (1982). Depression, restraint and eating behavior. *Behaviour Research and Therapy, 20*, 113–121.

Gallo, A. E. (1997). First major drop in food product introductions in over 20 years. *Food Review, 20*(3), 33–35.

Galst, J. P., & White, M. A. (1976). The unhealthy persuader: The reinforcing value of television and children's purchase influencing attempts at the supermarket. *Child Development, 51*, 935–938.

Garner, D. M., Olmstead, G. A., Bohr, Y., & Garfinkel, P. E. (1982). The Eating Attitude Test: Psychometric features and clinical correlates. *Psychological Medicine, 12*, 871–878.

Garner, D. M., Olmsted, M. P., & Polivy, J. (1983). Development and validation of a multidimensional eating disorder inventory for anorexia nervosa and bulimia. *International Journal of Eating Disorders, 2*, 15–34.

Garrow, J. (1999). Clinical assessment of obesity. In British Nutrition Foundation (Ed.), *Obesity* (pp. 17–22). Oxford, England: Blackwell Science.

Garrow, J. S., & Summerbell, C. D. (1995). Meta-analysis: Effects of exercise, with or without dieting, on the body composition of overweight subjects. *European Journal of Clinical Nutrition, 49*, 1–10.

Gatenby, S., Anderson, A. O., Walker, A. D., Southon, S., & Mela, D. J. (1994). "Meals" and "snacks"—Implications for eating patterns in adults. *Appetite, 23*, 292.

Giammattei, J., Blix, G., Marshak, H. H., Wollitzer, A. O., & Pettitt, D. J. (2006). Television watching and soft drink consumption: Associations with obesity in 11- to 13-year-old schoolchildren. *Archive of Pediatric and Adolescent Medicine, 157*, 882–886.

Gillis, L. J., & Bar-Or, O. (2003). Food away from home, sugar-sweetened drink consumption and juvenile obesity. *Journal of the American College of Nutrition, 22*, 539–545.

Golan, M., Weizman, A., Apter, A., & Fainaru, M. (1998). Parents as exclusive agents of change in the treatment of childhood obesity. *American Journal of Clinical Nutrition, 67*, 1130–1135.

Goldblatt, P. B., Moore, E., & Stunkard, A. J. (1965). Social factors in obesity. *Journal of the American Medical Association, 192*, 1930–1944.

Goldfield, G. S., Epstein, L. H., Davidson, M., & Saad, F. (2005). Validation of a questionnaire measure of the relative reinforcing value of food. *Eating Behaviors, 6*, 283–292.

Goldfield, G. S., Raynor, H. A., & Epstein, L. H. (2002). Treatment of pediatric obesity. In T. A. Wadden & A. J. Stunkard (Eds.), *Handbook of obesity treatment* (pp. 532–556). New York: Guilford Press.

Goldman, R., Jaffa, M., & Schachter, S. (1968). Yom Kippur, Air France, dormitory food, and the eating behavior of obese and normal persons. *Journal of Personality and Social Psychology, 10*, 117–123.

Gollwitzer, P. M. (1999). Implementation intentions: Strong effects of simple plans. *American Psychologist, 54*, 493–503.

Gollwitzer, P. M., & Sheeran, P. (2006). Implementation intentions and goal achievement: A meta-analysis of effects and processes. In M. Zanna (Ed.), *Advances in experimental social psychology* (Vol. 38, pp. 69–120). San Diego, CA: Academic Press.

Goodrick, G. K., Poston, W. S. C., Kimball, K. T., Reeves, R. S., & Foreyt, J. P. (1998). Nondieting versus dieting treatment for overweight binge-eating women. *Journal of Consulting and Clinical Psychology, 66*, 363–368.

Goran, M. I. (1997). Genetic influence on human energy expenditure and substrate utilization. *Behavioral Genetics, 27*, 389–399.

Gordon, T., & Kannel, W. B. (1973). The effects of overweight on cardiovascular disease. *Geriatrics, 28*, 80–88.

Goris, A. H. C., Westerterp-Platenga, M. S., & Westerterp, K. R. (2000). Under-eating and underrecording of habitual food intake in obese men: Selective under-reporting of fat intake. *American Journal of Clinical Nutrition, 71*, 130–134.

Gorman, B. S., & Allison, D. B. (1995). Measures of restrained eating. In D. B. Allison (Ed.), *Handbook of assessment methods for eating behaviors and weight-related problems* (pp. 149–184). Thousand Oaks, CA: Sage.

Gortmaker, S. L., Must, A., Perrin, J. M., Sobol, A. M., & Dietz, W. H. (1993). Social and economic consequences of overweight in adolescence and young adulthood. *New England Journal of Medicine, 329*, 1008–1012.

Gortmaker, S. L., Peterson, K., Wiecha, J., Sobol, A. M., Dixit, S., Fox, M. K., & Laird, N. (1999). Reducing obesity via a school-based interdisciplinary inter-vention among school youth. *Archives of Pediatrics and Adolescent Medicine, 153*, 409–418.

Greenwald, A. G., McGhee, D. E., & Schwartz, J. L. K. (1998). Measuring individ-ual differences in implicit cognition. The Implicit Association Test. *Journal of Personality and Social Psychology, 74*, 115–139.

Gregg, E. W., Gerzoff, R. B., Thompson, T. J., & Williamson, D. F. (2003). Inten-tional weight loss and death in overweight and obese U.S. adults 35 years of age and older. *Annals of Internal Medicine, 138*, 383–390.

Gregg, E. W., & Williamson, D. F. (2002). The relationship of intentional weight loss to disease incidence and mortality. In T. A. Wadden & A. J. Stunkard (Eds.), *Handbook of obesity treatment* (pp. 125–143). New York: Guilford Press.

Grilo, C. M. (2006). *Eating and weight disorders*. Hove, England: Psychology Press.

Grilo, C. M., & Pogue-Geile, M. F. (1991). The nature of environmental influences on weight and obesity: A behavior genetic analysis. *Psychological Bulletin, 115*, 444–464.

Grilo, C., Shiffman, S., & Wing, R. (1989). Relapse crises and coping among dieters. *Journal of Consulting and Clinical Psychology, 57*, 488–495.

Guo, S. S., Zeller, C., Chumlea, W. C., & Siervogel, R. M. (1999). Aging, body com-position and life style: The Fels Longitudinal Study. *American Journal of Clinical Nutrition, 70*, 405–411.

Guthrie, J. F., Biing-Hwan, L., & Frazao, E. (2002). Role of food prepared away from home and the American diet, 1977–78 versus 1994–96: Changes and consequences. *Journal of Nutrition Education and Behavior, 34*, 140–150.

Haapanen, N., Miilunpalo, S., Pasanen, M., Oja, P., & Vuori, I. (1997). Association between leisure time physical activity and 10-year body mass change among working-aged men and women. *International Journal of Obesity, 21*, 288–296.

Halford, J. C. G., Gillespie, J., Brown, V., Pontin, E. E., & Dovey, T. M. (2004). Effect of television advertisements for foods on food consumption in children. *Appetite, 42*, 221–225.

Halkjoer, J., Holst, C., & Sorensen, T. I. A. (2003). Intelligence test score and educational level in relation to BMI changes and obesity. *Obesity Research, 11*, 1238–1245.

Hampl, J. S., Heaton, C. L. B., & Taylor, C. A. (2003). Snacking patterns influence energy and nutrient intakes but not body mass index. *Journal of Human Nutrition and Dietetics, 16*, 3–11.

Hancox, R. J., Milne, B. J., & Poulton, R. (2004). Association between child and adolescent television viewing and adult health: A longitudinal birth cohort study. *Lancet, 364*, 257–262.

Hancox, R. J., & Poulton, R. (2004). Watching television is associated with childhood obesity: But is it clinically important? *International Journal of Obesity, 30*, 171–175.

Harnack, L. J., Jeffery, R. W., & Boutelle, K. N. (2000). Temporal trends in energy intake in the United States: An ecologic perspective. *American Journal of Clinical Nutrition, 71*, 1478–1484.

Harvey, K., Kemps, E., & Tiggemann, M. (2005). The nature of imagery processes underlying food cravings. *British Journal of Health Psychology, 10*, 49–56.

Hastings, G., Stead, M., McDermott, L., Forsyth, A., MacKintosh, A. M., Rayner, M., et al. (2003). Review of research in the effects of food promotion to children. Report prepared for the UK Food Standards Agency. Retrieved November 29, 2007, from http://www.foodstandards.gov.uk/multimedia/pdf/foodpromotiontochildren1/.pdf

Hawkins, R. C. (1979). Meal/snack frequencies of college students: A normative study. *Behavioural Psychotherapy, 7*, 85–90.

Haynes, C., Lee, M. D., & Yeomans, M. R. (2003). Interactive effects of stress, dietary restraint, and disinhibition on appetite. *Eating Behaviors, 4*, 369–383.

Heatherton, T. F., & Baumeister, R. F. (1991). Binge eating as escape from self-awareness. *Psychological Bulletin, 110*, 86–108.

Heatherton, T. F., Herman, C. P., & Polivy, J. (1991). Effects of physical threat and ego threat on eating behavior. *Journal of Personality and Social Psychology, 60*, 138–143.

Heatherton, T. F., Herman, C. P., & Polivy, J. (1992). Effects of distress on eating: The importance of ego-involvement. *Journal of Personality and Social Psychology, 62*, 801–803.

Heatherton, T. F., Herman, C. P., Polivy, J., King, G. A., & McGree, S. T. (1988). The (mis)measurement of restraint. An analysis of conceptual and psychometric issues. *Journal of Abnormal Psychology, 97*, 19–28.

Heatherton, T. F., Polivy, J., Herman, C. P., & Baumeister, R. F. (1993). Self-awareness, task failure, and disinhibition: how attentional focus affects eating. *Journal of Personality, 61,* 49–61.

Heatherton, T. F., Striepe, M., & Wittenberg, L. (1998). Emotional distress and disinhibited eating. *Personality and Social Psychology Bulletin, 24,* 301–313.

Hebl, M. R., & Heatherton, T. F. (1998). The stigma of obesity in women: The difference is black and white. *Personality and Social Psychology Bulletin, 24,* 417–426.

Hebl, M. R., & Mannix, L. M. (2003). The weight of obesity in evaluating others: A mere proximity effect. *Personality and Social Psychology Bulletin, 29,* 28–38.

Heiat, A., Vaccarino, V., & Krumholz, H. M. (2001). An evidence-based assessment of federal guidelines for overweight and obesity as they apply to elderly persons. *Annals of Internal Medicine, 161,* 1194–1203.

Heid, I. M., Vollmert, C., Hinney, A., Döring, A., Geller, F., Löwel, H., et al. (2007). Association of the 1031 MC4R allele with decreased body mass in 7937 participants of two population based surveys. *Journal of Medical Genetics, 42,* e21.

Heitmann, B. L., Kaprio, J., Harris, J. R., Rissanen, A., Korkeila, M., & Koskenvuou, M. (1997). Are genetic determinants of weight gain modified by leisure-time physical activity? A prospective study of Finnish twins. *American Journal of Clinical Nutrition, 66,* 672–678.

Heitmann, B. L., Lissner, L., & Osler, M. (2000). Do we eat less fat, or just report so? *International Journals of Obesity, 24,* 435–442.

Hellerstein, M., Schwarz, J. M., & Neese, R. (1996) Regulation of hepatic de novo lipogenesis in humans. *Annual Review of Nutrition, 16,* 523–557.

Helzer, J. E., & Robins, L. N. (1988). The Diagnostic Interview Schedule: Its development, evolution and use. *Social Psychiatry and Psychiatric Epidemiology, 23,* 6–16.

Hemmingsson, E., & Ekelund, U. (2007). Is the association between physical activity and body mass index obesity dependent? *International Journal of Obesity, 31,* 663–668.

Henderson, V. R., & Kelly, B. (2005). Food advertising in the age of obesity: Content analysis of food advertising on general market and African American television. *Journal of Nutrition Education and Behavior, 37,* 190–196.

Herman, C. P., & Mack, D. (1975). Restrained and unrestrained eating. *Journal of Personality, 43,* 647–660.

Herman, C. P., & Polivy, J. (1975). Anxiety, restraint, and eating behavior. *Journal of Abnormal Psychology, 84,* 666–672.

Herman, C. P., & Polivy, J. (1980). Restrained eating. In A. J. Stunkard (Ed.), *Obesity* (pp. 208–225). Philadelphia, PA: Saunders.

Herman, C. P., & Polivy, J. (1984). A boundary model for the regulation of eating. In J. A. Stunkard & E. Stellar (Eds.), *Eating and its disorders* (pp. 141–156). New York: Raven Press.

Herman, C. P., & Polivy, J. (2004). The self-regulation of eating: Theoretical and practical problems. In R. F. Baumeister & K. D. Vohs (Eds.), *Handbook of self-regulation* (pp. 492–508). New York: Guilford Press.

Herman, C. P., Polivy, J., & Esses, V. M. (1987). The illusion of counter-regulation. *Appetite, 9,* 161–169.

Herman, C. P., Polivy, J., Pliner, P., Threlkeld, J., & Munic, D. (1978). Distractibility in dieters and nondieters: An alternative view of "externality." *Journal of Personality and Social Psychology, 36,* 536–548.

Heshka, S., Anderson, J. W., Atkinson, R. L., Greenway, F. L., Hill, J. O., Phinney, S. D., et al. (2003). Weight loss with self-help compared with a structured commercial program. *Journal of the American Medical Association, 289,* 1792–1798.

Hetherington, M., & Davies, M. (1998). Weight management: A comparison between non-dieting and dieting approaches. *Health Psychology Update, 32,* 33–39.

Heymsfield, S. B., Greenberg, A. S., Fujioka, K., Dixon, R. M., Kushner, T., Lubina, J. A., et al. (1999). Recombined leptin for weight loss in obese and lean adults. *Journal of the American Medical Association, 27,* 1568–1575.

Hibscher, J. A., & Herman, C. P. (1977). Obesity, dieting and the expression of obese characteristics. *Journal of Comparative and Physiological Psychology, 91,* 374–380.

Higgins, M., Kannel, W., Garrison, R., Pinsky, J., & Stokes, J. (1988). Hazards of obesity: The Framingham experience. *Acta Medica Scandinavica, 723*(Suppl.), 23–36.

Hill, J. O., Saris, W. H. M., & Levine, J. A. (2004). Energy expenditure in physical activity. In G. A. Bray & C. Bouchard (Eds.), *Handbook of obesity: Etiology and pathophysiology* (pp. 631–654). New York: Dekker.

Hill, J. O., Wyatt, H. R., Reed, G. W., & Peters, J. C. (2003, February 7). Obesity and environment: Where do we go from here? *Science, 299,* 853–855.

Hill, J. O., Wyatt, H., Phelan, S., & Wing, R. R. (2005). The National Weight Control Registry: Is it useful in helping deal with our obesity epidemic? *Journal of Nutrition Education and Behavior, 37,* 206–210.

Holland, R. W., Hendriks, M., & Aarts, H. (2005). Smells like clean spirit: Nonconscious effects of scent of cognition and behavior. *Psychological Science, 16,* 689–693.

Horgen, K. B., & Brownell, K. D. (2002). Confronting the toxic environment: Environmental public health actions in a world crisis. In T. A. Wadden & A. J. Stunkard (Eds.), *Handbook of obesity treatment* (pp. 95–106). New York: Guilford Press.

Howarth, N. C., Huang, T. T.-K., Roberts, S. B., Lin, B.-H., & McCrory, M. A. (2007). Eating patterns and dietary composition in relation to BMI in younger and older adults. *International Journal of Obesity, 31,* 675–684.

Hu, F. B., Li, T. Y., Colditz, G. A., Willett, W. C., & Manson, J. E. (2003). Television watching and other sedentary behaviors in relation to risk of obesity and type 2 diabetes mellitus in women. *Journal of the American Medical Association, 289,* 1785–1791.

Hu, F. B., Willett, W. C., Li, T., Stampfer, M. J., Colditz, G. A., & Manson, J. E. (2004). Adiposity as compared with physical activity in predicting mortality among women. *New England Journal of Medicine, 351,* 2694–2703.

Huang, T. T.-K., Roberts, S. B., Howarth, N. C., & McCrory, M. A. (2005). Effect of screening out implausible energy intake reports on relationships between diet and BMI. *Obesity Research, 13,* 1205–1216.

Hubert, H. B., Feinleib, M., McNamara, P. M., & Castelli, W. P. (1983). Obesity as an independent risk factor for cardiovascular disease: A 26-year follow-up of participants in Framingham heart study. *Circulation, 67,* 968–977.

Hull, C. L. (1943). *Principles of behavior.* New York: Appleton-Century-Crofts.

Huon, G. F., Wootton, M., & Brown, L. B. (1991). The role of restraint and disinhibition in appetite control. *Journal of Psychosomatic Research, 35,* 49–58.

Ikeda, J., Amy, N. K., Ernsberger, P., Gaesser, G. A., Berg, F. M., Clark, C. A., et al. (2005). The National Weight Control Registry: A critique. *Journal of Nutrition Education and Behavior, 37,* 203–205.

Institute of Medicine. (2002). *Dietary reference intakes for energy, carbohydrate, fiber, fat, fatty acids, cholesterol, protein, and amino acids, Part I.* Washington, DC: National Academy of Sciences.

International Association of Consumer Food Organizations. (2003). *Broadcasting bad health. Why food marketing to children needs to be controlled* (Report to the World Health Organization). Retrieved September 28, 2006, from http://www.foodcomm.org.uk/Broadcasting_bad_health.pdf

Iribarren, C., Sharp, D. S., Burchiviel, C. M., & Petrovitch, H. (1995). Association of weight loss and weight fluctuation with mortality among Japanese American men. *New England Journal of Medicine, 333,* 686–692.

Israel, A. C., Stolmaker, L., & Andrian, C. A. (1985). The effects of training parents in general child management skills on a behavioral weight loss program for children. *Behavior Therapy, 16,* 169–180.

Jakes, R. W., Day, N. E., Khaw, K. T., Luben, R., Oakes, S., Welch, A., et al. (2002). Television viewing and low participation in vigorous recreation are independently associated with obesity and markers of cardiovascular disease risk: EPIC-Norfolk population-based study. *European Journal of Clinical Nutrition, 57,* 1089–1096.

Jakicic, J., Winters, C., Lang, W., & Wing, R. R. (1999). Effects of intermittent exercise and use of home exercise equipment on adherence, weight loss, and fitness in overweight women. *Journal of the American Medical Association, 282,* 1554–1560.

James, J., Thomas, P., Cavan, D., & Kerr, D. (2004). Preventing childhood obesity by reducing consumption of carbonated drinks: Cluster randomized controlled trial. *British Medical Journal, 328,* 1237–1239.

Jansen, A., Oosterlaan, J., Merckelbach, H., & van den Hout, M. A. (1988). Non-regulation of food intake in restrained and emotional external eaters. *Journal of Psychopathology and Behavioral Assessment, 10,* 345–353.

Jansen, A., & van den Hout, M. A. (1991). On being led into temptation: "Counter-regulation" of dieters after smelling a "preload." *Addictive Behaviors, 16,* 247–253.

Janssen, I., Katzmarzyk, P. T., Boyce, W. F., King, M. A., & Pickett, W. (2004). Overweight and obesity in Canadian adolescents and their association with dietary habits and physical activity patterns. *Journal of Adolescent Health, 35,* 360–367.

Janssen, I., Katzmarzyk, P. T., & Ross, R. (2002). Body mass index, waist circumference, and health risk. *Archives of Internal Medicine, 162,* 2074–2079.

Jeffery, R. W., Drewnowski, A., Epstein, L. H., Stunkard, A. J., Wilson, G. T., Wing, R. R., & Hill, D. R. (2000). Long-term maintenance of weight loss. Current studies. *Health Psychology, 19*(Suppl.), 5–16.

Jeffery, R. W., & French, S. A. (1998). Epidemic obesity in the United States: Are fast foods and television viewing contributing? *American Journal of Public Health, 88,* 277–280.

Jeffery, R. W., French, S. A., Raether, C., & Baxter, J. E. (1994). An environmental intervention to increase fruit and salad purchase in a cafeteria. *Preventive Medicine, 23,* 788–792.

Jeffery, R. W., & Wing, R. R. (1995). Long-term treatment for weight loss. *Journal of Consulting and Clinical Psychology, 63,* 793–796.

Jeffery, R. W., Wing, R. R., Thorson, C., Burton, L. R., Raether, C., Harvey, J., & Mullen, M. (1993). Strengthening behavioral intentions for weight loss: A randomized trial of food provision and monetary incentives. *Journal of Consulting and Clinical Psychology, 61,* 1038–1045.

Jéquier, E., & Schutz, Y. (1988). Energy expenditure in obesity and diabetes. *Diabetes Metabolism Reviews, 4,* 583–593.

Johnson, W. G. (1974). Effect of cue prominence and subject weight on human food-directed performance. *Journal of Personality and Social Psychology, 29,* 843–848.

Johnstone, A. M., Shannon, E., Whybrow, S., Reid, C. A., & Stubbs, R. J. (2000). Altering the temporal distribution of energy intake with isoenergetically dense foods given as snacks does not affect total daily energy intake in normal-weight men. *British Journal of Nutrition, 83,* 7–14.

Jonas, K., Broemer, P., & Diehl, M. (2000). Attitudinal ambivalence. In W. Stroebe & M. Hewstone (Eds.), *European Review of Social Psychology* (Vol. 10, pp. 35–74). Chichester, England: Wiley.

Joosen, A., Gielen, M., Vlietinck, R., & Westerterp, K. R. (2005). Genetic analysis of physical activity in twins. *American Journal of Clinical Nutrition, 82,* 1253–1259.

Kaplan, H. I., & Kaplan, H. S. (1957). The psychosomatic concept of obesity. *Journal of Nervous and Mental Disease, 125,* 181–201.

Kaplan, K. J. (1972). On the ambivalence-indifference problem in attitude theory and measurement. A suggested modification of the semantic differential technique. *Psychological Bulletin, 77,* 361–372.

Karnehed, N., Rasmussen, F., Hemmingsson, T., & Tynelius, P. (2006). Obesity and attained education: Cohort study of more than 700,000 Swedish men. *Obesity, 14,* 1421–1428.

Karp, S. H., & Pardes, H. (1965). Psychological differentiation (field dependence) in obese women. *Psychosomatic Medicine, 27,* 238–244.

Katzmarzyk, P. T., Malina, R. M., Song, T. M. K., & Bouchard, C. (1998). Television viewing, physical activity, and health-related fitness of youth in the Québec Family Study. *Journal of Adolescent Health, 23,* 318–325.

Kaur, H., Choi, W. S., Mayo, M. S., & Harris, K. J. (2003). Duration of television watching is associated with increased body mass index. *Journal of Pediatrics, 143,* 506–511.

Keesey, R. E. (1986). A set-point theory of obesity. In K. D. Brownell & J. P. Foreyt (Eds.), *The physiology, psychology, and treatment of the eating disorders* (pp. 63–87). New York: Basic Books.

Keith, S. W., Redden, D. T., Katzmarzyk, P. T., Boggiano, M. M., Hanlon, E. C., Benca, R. M., et al. (2006). Putative contributors to the secular increase in obesity: Exploring the roads less traveled. *International Journal of Obesity, 30,* 1585–1599.

Kenny, D. A., Kashy, D. A., & Bolger, N. (1998). Data analysis in social psychology. In D. T. Gilbert, S. T. Fiske, & G. Lindzey (Eds.), *Handbook of social psychology* (pp. 233–265). Boston, MA: McGraw-Hill.

Keys, A., Brozek, J., Henschel, A., Mickelson, O., & Taylor, H. L. (1950). *The biology of human starvation.* Minneapolis: University of Minnesota Press.

Killen, J. D., Taylor, C. B., Hayward, C., Haydel, K. F., Wilson, D. M., Kraemer, H., et al., (1996). Weight concerns influence the development of eating disorders: A 4-year prospective study. *Journal of Consulting and Clinical Psychology, 64,* 936–940.

Kim, D., & Kawachi, I. (2006). Food taxation and pricing strategies to "thin out" the obesity epidemic. *American Journal of Preventive Medicine, 30,* 430–437.

Kimm, S. Y. S., Glyn, N. W., Obarzanek, E., Kriska, A. M., Daniels, S. R., Barton, B. A., & Liu, K. (2005). Relation between the changes in physical activity and body-mass index during adolescence: A multicentre longitudinal study. *Lancet, 366,* 301–307.

Klem, M. L., Viteri, J. E., & Wing, R. R. (2000). Primary prevention of weight gain for women aged 25–34: The acceptability of treatment formats. *International Journal of Obesity, 24,* 219–225.

Klem, M. L., Wing, R. R., Lang, W., McGuire, M. T., & Hill, J. O. (2000). Does weight loss maintenance become easier over time? *Obesity Research, 8,* 438–444.

Klem, M. L., Wing, R. R., McGuire, M. T., Seagle, H. M., & Hill, J. O. (1998). Psychological symptoms in individuals successful at long-term maintenance of weight loss. *Health Psychology, 17,* 336–345.

Knäuper, B., Cheema, S., Rabiau, M., & Borten, O. (2005). Self-set dieting rules: Adherence and prediction of weight loss success. *Appetite, 44,* 283–288.

Knight, L. J., & Boland, F. J. (1989). Restrained eating: An experimental disentanglement of the disinhibiting variables of perceived calories and food type. *Journal of Abnormal Psychology, 98,* 412–420.

Koh-Banerjee, P., Chu, N. F., Spiegelman, D., Rosner, B., Colditz, G., Willett, W., & Rimm, E. (2003). Prospective study of the association of changes in dietary intake, physical activity, alcohol consumption, and smoking with 9-y gain in waist circumference among 16587 US men. *American Journal of Clinical Nutrition, 78,* 719–727.

Kruger, J., Galuska, D. A., Serdula, M. K., & Jones, D. A. (2004). Attempting to lose weight: Specific practices among U.S. adults. *American Journal of Preventive Medicine, 26*, 402–406.

Kruglanski, A. W., Shah, J. Y., Fishbach, A., Friedman, R., Chun, W. Y., & Sleeth-Keppler, D. (2002). A theory of goal systems. In M. Zanna (Ed.), *Advances in experimental social psychology* (Vol. 34, pp. 331–378). San Diego, CA: Academic Press.

Kuchler, F., Tegene, A., & Harris, J. M. (2004). Taxing snack foods: Manipulating diet quality or financing information programs? *Review of Agricultural Economics, 27*, 4–20.

Kuczmarski, R. J., Flegal, K. I. M., Campbell, S. M., & Johnson, C. L. (1994). Increasing prevalence of overweight among US adults: The National Health and Nutrition Examination Surveys 1960–1992. *Journal of the American Medical Association, 272*, 205–211.

Labriola, M., Lund, T., & Burr, H. (2006). Prospective study of physical and psychosocial risk factors for sickness absence. *Occupational Medicine, 56*, 469–474.

Laessle, R. G., Tuschl, R. J., Kotthaus, B. C., & Pirke, K. M. (1989). A comparison of the validity of three scales for the assessment of dietary restraint. *Journal of Abnormal Psychology, 98*, 504–507.

Lapidus, L., Bengtsson, C., & Lissner, L. (1990). Distribution of adipose tissue in relation to cardiovascular and total mortality as observed during 20 years in a prospective population study of women in Gothenburg, Sweden. *Diabetes Research and Clinical Practice, 10* (Suppl.), S185–S189.

Larson, D. E., Ferraro, R. T., Robertson, D. S., & Ravussin, E. (1995). Energy metabolism in weight-stable postobese individuals. *American Journal of Clinical Nutrition, 62*, 735–739.

Larson, D. E., Tataranni, P. A., Ferraro, R. T., & Ravussin, E. (1995). Ad libitum food intake on a "cafeteria diet" in Native American women: Relations between body composition and 24-h energy expenditure. *American Journal of Clinical Nutrition, 62*, 911–917.

Lattimore, P., & Caswell, N. (2004). Differential effects of active and passive stress on food intake in restrained and unrestrained eaters. *Appetite, 42*, 167–173.

Laurier, D., Guiguet, M., Chau, N. P., Well, J. A., & Valleron, A. J. (1992). Prevalence of obesity: A comparative survey in France, the United Kingdom, and the United States. *International Journal of Obesity, 16*, 565–572.

Lee, C. D., Blair, S. N., & Jackson, A. S. (1999). Cardiorespiratory fitness, body composition, and all cause and cardiovascular disease mortality in men. *American Journal of Clinical Nutrition, 69*, 375–380.

Lee, I., & Paffenbarger, R. S. (1996). Is weight loss hazardous? *Nutrition Reviews, 54*(Suppl.), S116–S124.

LeGeoff, D. B., & Spigelman, M. N. (1987). Salivary response to olfactory food stimuli as a function of dietary restraint and body weight. *Appetite, 8*, 29–35.

Levine, J. A., Eberhardt, N. L., & Jensen, M. D. (1999, January 8). Role of nonexercise activity thermogenesis in resistance to fat gain in humans. *Science, 283,* 212–214.

Levine, J. A., Lanningham-Foster, L. M., McCrady, S. K., Krizan, A. C., Olson, P. H., Kane, P. H., et al. (2005, January 28). Interindividual variation in posture allocation: Possible role in human obesity. *Science, 307,* 584–586.

Levine, J. A., Vander Weg, M. W., & Klesges, R. C. (2006, August). Increasing Non-Exercise Activity Thermogenesis: A NEAT way to increase energy expenditure in your patients. *Obesity Management,* 146–151.

Levitsky, D. A. (2005). The non-regulation of food intake in humans: Hope for reversing the epidemic of obesity. *Physiology and Behavior, 86,* 623–632.

Levitsky, D. A., Halbmeyer, C. A., & Mrdjenovic, T. (2004). The freshman weight gain: A model for the study of epidemic obesity. *International Journal of Obesity, 28,* 1435–1442.

Levy, A. S., & Heaton, A. W. (1993). Weight control practices of U.S. adults trying to lose weight. *Annuals of Internal Medicine, 119,* 661–666.

Lightfood, L. (2007, July 12). "Jamie may have spelled end of school meals." *Daily Telegraph.* Retrieved October 31, 2007, from http://www.telegraph.co.uk/news/main.jhtml?xml=/news/2007/07/12/nfood112.xml

Lissner, L., & Heitmann, B. L. (1995). Dietary fat and obesity: Evidence from epidemiology. *European Journal of Clinical Nutrition, 49,* 79–90.

Lissner, L., Levitsky, D. A., Strupp, B. J., Kalkwarf, H. J., & Roe, D. A. (1987). Dietary fat and the regulation of energy intake in human subjects. *American Journal of Clinical Nutrition, 46,* 886–892.

Louis-Sylvestre, J., Tournier, A., Verger, P., Chabert, M., Delorme, B., & Hossenlopp, J. (1989). Learned caloric adjustment of human intake. *Appetite, 12,* 95–103.

Lowe, M. R. (1984). Dietary concern, weight fluctuation and weight status: Further explorations of the Restraint Scale. *Behaviour Research and Therapy, 22,* 243–248.

Lowe, M. R. (1993). The effects of dieting on eating behavior: A three-factor model. *Psychological Bulletin, 114,* 100–121.

Lowe, M. R. (1995). Restrained eating and dieting: Replication of their divergent effects on eating regulation. *Appetite, 25,* 115–118.

Lowe, M. R., & Butryn, M. L. (2007). Hedonic hunger: A new dimension of appetite. *Physiology and Behavior, 91,* 432–439.

Lowe, M. R., Foster, G. D., Kerzhnerman, I., Swain, R. M., & Wadden, T. A. (2001). Restrictive dieting vs. "undieting": Effects on eating regulation in obese clinic attenders. *Addictive Behaviors, 26,* 253–266.

Lowe, M. R., & Kleifield, E. (1988). Cognitive restraint, weight suppression, and the regulation of eating. *Appetite, 10,* 159–168.

Lowe, M. R., & Kral, T. V. E. (2006). Stress-induced eating in restrained eaters may not be caused by stress or restraint. *Appetite, 46,* 16–21.

Lowe, M. R., & Maycock, B. (1988). Restraint, disinhibition, hunger and negative affect eating. *Addictive Behaviors, 13,* 369–377.

Lowe, M. R., Miller-Kovach, K., & Phelan, S. (2001). Weight-loss maintenance in overweight individuals one to five years following successful completion of a commercial weight loss program. *International Journal of Obesity, 25,* 325–331.

Lowe, M. R., Whitlow, J. W., & Bellwoar, V. (1991). Eating regulation: The role of restraint, dieting, and weight. *International Journal of Eating Disorders, 10,* 461–471.

MacLeod, C., Mathews, A., & Tata, P. (1986). Attentional bias in emotional disorders. *Journal of Abnormal Psychology, 95,* 15–20.

Maes, H. H. M., Neale, M. C., & Eaves, L. J. (1997). Genetic and environmental factors in relative body weight and human adiposity. *Behavior Genetics, 27,* 325–351.

Major, G. C., Doucet, E., Trayhurn, P., Astrup, A., & Tremblay, A. (2007). Clinical significance of adaptive thermogenesis. *International Journal of Obesity, 31,* 204–212.

Malik, V. S., Schulze, M. B., & Hu, F. B. (2006). Intake of sugar-sweetened beverages and weight gain: A systematic review. *American Journal of Clinical Nutrition, 84,* 274–288.

Manios, Y., Panagiotakos, D. B., Pitsavos, C., Polychronopoulos, E., & Stefanidis, C. (2005). Implication of socio-economic status on the prevalence of overweight and obesity in Greek adults: The ATTICA study. *Health Policy, 74,* 224–232.

Mann, T. A., Tomiyama, J., Westling, E., Lew, A.-M., Samuels, B., & Chatman, J. (2007). Medicare's search for effective obesity treatments: Diets are not the answer. *American Psychologist, 62,* 220–233.

Manson, J. E., Willett, W. C., Stampfer, M. J., Colditz, G. A., Hunter, D. J., Hankinson, S. E., et al. (1995). Body weight and mortality among women. *New England Journal of Medicine, 333,* 677–685.

Marlatt, G. A. (1985). Relapse prevention: Theoretical rationale and overview of the model. In G. A. Marlatt & J. R. Gordon (Eds.), *Relapse prevention* (pp. 3–70). New York: Guilford Press.

Marmonier, C., Chapelot, D., Fantino, M., & Louis-Sylvestre, J. (2001). Snacks consumed in nonhungry state have poor satiating efficiency: Influence of snack composition on substrate utilization and hunger. *American Journal of Clinical Nutrition, 76,* 518–528.

Matheson, D. M., Killen, J. D., Wang, Y., Varady, A., & Robinson, T. N. (2004). Children's food consumption during television viewing. *American Journal of Clinical Nutrition, 79,* 1088–1099.

Mattes, R. D. (1996). Dietary compensation by humans for supplemental energy provided as ethanol or carbohydrate in fluids. *Physiology and Behavior, 59,* 179–187.

McArthur, L. Z., & Burstein, B. (1975). Field dependent eating and perception as a function of weight and sex. *Journal of Personality, 43,* 402–420.

McCann, K. L., Perri, M. G., Nezu, A. M., & Lowe, M. R. (1992). An investigation of counterregulatory eating in obese clinic attenders. *International Journal of Eating Disorders, 12,* 161–169.

McCrory, M. A., Fuss, P. J., Hays, N. P., Vinken, A. G., Greenberg, A. S., & Roberts, S. B. (1999). Overeating in America: Association between restaurant food consumption and body fatness in healthy adult men and women aged 19 to 80. *Obesity Research, 7,* 564–571.

McCrory, M. A., Fuss, P. J., McCallum J. E., Yao, M., Vinken, A. G., Hays, N. P., & Roberts, S. B. (1999). Dietary variety within food groups: Association with energy intake and body fatness in men and women. *American Journal of Clinical Nutrition, 69,* 440–447.

McDonald's. (2007, November 1). Retrieved November 5, 2007, from Wikipedia.com: http://en.wikipedia.org/wiki/Mcdonald%27s and from German Wikipedia.com: http://de.wikipedia.org/wiki/McDonald%E2%80%99s#International

McGee, D. L. (2005). Body mass index and mortality: A meta-analysis based on person-level data from twenty-six observational studies. *Annals of Epidemiology, 15,* 87–97.

McGuire, M. T., Wing, R. R., & Hill, J. O. (1999). The prevalence of weight loss maintenance among American adults. *International Journal of Obesity, 23,* 1314–1319.

McGuire, M. T., Wing, R. R., Klem, M. L., Lang, W., & Hill, J. O. (1999). What predicts weight regain in a group of successful weight losers? *Journal of Consulting and Clinical Psychology, 67,* 177–185.

McKenna, R. J. (1975). Some effects of anxiety level and food cues on the eating behavior of obese and normal subjects: A comparison of the Schachterian and psychosomatic concepts. *Journal of Personality and Social Psychology, 22,* 311–319.

McKoon, G., & Ratcliff, R. (1986). Inferences about predictable events. *Journal of Experimental Psychology: Learning, Memory and Cognition, 12,* 82–91.

Mela, D. J. (1995). Understanding fat preferences and consumption: Applications of behavioural sciences to a nutritional problem. *Proceedings of the Nutrition Society, 54,* 453–464.

Mela, D. J., & Rogers, P. J. (1998). *Food, eating and obesity.* London: Chapman & Hall.

Mensink, W. (2005). *Why dieting fails: Testing a goal conflict model of eating behavior.* Unpublished doctoral dissertation, Utrecht University, Utrecht, the Netherlands.

Mensink, W., Stroebe, W., Schut, H., & Aarts, H. (2003). Waarom lijnen niet lukt: Het conflict tussen lekker eten and lijnen [Why dieting fails: The conflict between eating enjoyment and weight control]. In E. van Dijk, E. Kluwer, & D. Wigboldus (Eds.), *Jaarboek Sociale Psychologie 2002* (pp. 219–226). Delft, the Netherlands: Eburon.

Metcalfe, J., & Mischel, W. (1999). A hot/cool-system analysis of delay of gratification: Dynamics of willpower. *Psychological Review, 106,* 3–19.

Metropolitan Life Insurance Company. (1959, November–December). New weight standards for men and women. *Statistical Bulletin of the Metropolitan Life Insurance Company, 40,* 1–11.

Michaud, D. S., Liu, S., Giovannucci, E., Willett, W. C., Colditz, G. A., & Fuchs, C. S. (2002). Dietary sugar, glycemic load, and pancreatic cancer risk in a prospective study. *Journal of the National Cancer Institute, 94,* 1293–1300.

Miles, A., Rapoport, L., Wardle, J., Afuape, T., Duman, M. (2001). Using the mass-media to target obesity: An analysis of the characteristics and reported behaviour change of participants in the BBC's "Fighting Fat, Fighting Fit" campaigns. *Health Education Research, 16,* 357–372.

Miller, C. T., & Downey, K. T. (1999). A meta-analysis of heavyweight and self-esteem. *Personality and Social Psychology Review, 3,* 68–84.

Miller, W. C., & Wadden, T. A. (2004). Exercise as a treatment for obesity. In G. A. Bray & C. Bouchard (Eds.), *Handbook of obesity: Clinical applications* (2nd ed., pp. 169–183). New York: Dekker.

Mischel, W., & Ayduk, O. (2004). Willpower in a cognitive-affective processing system. In R. F. Baumeister & K. D. Vohs (Eds.), *Handbook of self-regulation* (pp. 99–29). New York: Guilford Press.

Mischel, W., & Moore, B. (1973). Effects of attention to symbolically presented rewards on self-control. *Journal of Personality and Social Psychology, 28,* 172–179.

Mischel, W., Shoda, Y., & Rodriguez, M. L. (1989, May 26). Delay of gratification in children. *Science, 244,* 933–938.

Mitchell, S. L., & Epstein, L. H. (1996). Changes in taste and satiety in dietary-restrained women following stress. *Physiology & Behavior, 60,* 495–499.

Monteiro, C. A., Moura, E. C., Conde, W. L., & Popkin, B. M. (2004). Socioeconomic status and obesity in adult populations of developing countries: A review. *Bulletin of the World Health Organization, 82,* 940–946.

Morgan, K. J., Johnson, S. R., & Stampley, G. L. (1983). Children's frequency of eating, total sugar intake and weight/height stature. *Nutrition Research, 3,* 635–652.

Morgan, P. J., & Jeffrey, D. B. (1999). Restraint, weight suppression, and self-report reliability: How much do you really weigh? *Addictive Behaviors, 24,* 679–682.

Moskowitz, G. B., Li, P., & Kirk, E. R. (2004). The implicit volition model: On the preconscious regulation of adopted goals. In M. Zanna (Ed.), *Advances in experimental social psychology* (Vol. 36, pp. 317–414). San Diego, CA: Academic Press.

"Mums in burger backlash over healthy eating." (2006, September 15). *The Star.* Retrieved October 28, 2007, from http://www.thestar.co.uk/news/Mums-in-burger-backlash-over.1771824.jp

Muraven, M., Tice, D. T., & Baumeister, R. F. (1998). Self-control is a limited resource: Regulatory depletion patterns. *Journal of Personality and Social Psychology, 74,* 774–789.

Murphy, T. K., Calle, E. E., Rodriguez, C., Kahn, H. S., & Thun, M. J. (2000). Body mass index and colon cancer mortality in a large prospective study. *American Journal of Epidemiology, 152,* 847–854.

Narayan, K. M. V., Boyle, J. P., Thompson, T. J., Gregg, E. W., & Williamson, D. F. (2007). Effect of BMI on lifetime risk for diabetes in the U.S. *Diabetes Care, 30,* 1562–1566.

National Center for Health Statistics. (2003).*Table 68 (page 1 of 4). Overweight, obesity, and healthy weight among persons 20 years of age and over, according to sex, age, race, and Hispanic origin: United States, 1960–62, 1971–74, 1976–80, 1988–94, and 1999–2000.* Retrieved September 28, 2007, from http://www.cdc.gov/nchs/data/hus/tables/2003/03hus068.pdf

National Center for Health Statistics. (2006). *Prevalence of overweight among children and adolescents: United States, 1999–2002.* Retrieved November 28, 2006, from http://www.cdc.gov/nchs/products/pubs/pubd/hestats/overwght99.htm#Table%201

National Heart, Lung, and Blood Institute. (1998). Clinical guidelines on the identification, evaluation, and treatment of overweight and obesity in adults: The evidence report. *Obesity Research, 6*(Suppl. 2), S51–S210.

National Heart, Heart, Lung, and Blood Institute. (n.d.). *Body mass index table.* Retrieved October 2, 2007, from http://www.nhlbi.nih.gov/guidelines/obesity/bmi_tbl.pdf

National Task Force on the Prevention and Treatment of Obesity. (2000a). Overweight, obesity, and health risk. *Archives of Internal Medicine, 160,* 898–904.

National Task Force on the Prevention and Treatment of Obesity. (2000b). Dieting and the development of eating disorders in overweight and obese adults. *Archives of Internal Medicine, 160,* 2581–2589.

Neel, J. V. (1962). Diabetes mellitus: A "thrifty" genotype rendered detrimental by "progress"? *American Journal of Human Genetics, 14,* 353–362.

Neely, J. (1991). Semantic priming effects in visual word recognition: A selective review of current findings and theories. In D. Besner & G. Humphreys (Eds.), *Basic processes in reading: Visual word recognition* (pp. 264–336). Hillsdale, NJ: Erlbaum.

Nestle, M. (2002). *Food politics.* Berkeley: University of California Press.

Neumarkt-Sztainer, D., Wall, M., Guo, J., Story, M., Hines, J., & Eisenberg, M. (2006). Obesity, disordered eating, and eating disorders in a longitudinal study of adolescents: How do dieters fare 5 years later? *Journal of the American Dietetic Association, 106,* 559–568.

Neville, L., Thomas, M., & Bauman, A. (2005). Food advertising on Australian television: The extent of children's exposure. *Health Promotion International, 20,* 105–112.

Nielsen, S. J., & Popkin, B. M. (2003). Patterns and trends in food portion sizes, 1977–1998. *Journal of the American Medical Society, 289,* 450–453.

Nielsen, S. J., Siega-Riz, A. M., & Popkin, B. M. (2002). Trends in energy intake in U.S. between 1977 and 1996: Similar shifts seen across age groups. *Obesity Research, 10,* 370–378.

Nisbett, R. E. (1968). Taste, deprivation and weight determinants of eating behavior. *Journal of Personality and Social Psychology, 10,* 107–116.

Nisbett, R. E. (1972). Hunger, obesity, and the ventromedial hypothalamus. *Psychological Review, 79,* 433–453.

Norman, D. A., &a Shallice, T. (1986). Attention and action: Willed and automatic control of behavior. In R. J. Davidson, G. E. Schwartz, & D. Shapiro (Eds.), *Consciousness and self-regulation: Advances in research and theory* (Vol. 4, pp. 1–18). New York: Plenum Press.

Norris, J., Harnack, L., Carmicheal, S., Puane, T., Wikimoto, P., & Block, G. (1997). US trends in nutrient intake: The 1987 and 1992 National Health Interview Survey. *American Journal of Public Health, 87,* 740–746.

Ogden, C. L., Carroll, M. D., Curtin, L. R., McDowell, M. A., Tabak, C. J., & Flegal, K. M. (2006). Prevalence of overweight and obesity in the United States, 1999–2004. *Journal of the American Medical Association, 295,* 1549–1555.

Ogden, J., & Wardle, J. (1991). Cognitive and emotional responses to food. *International Journal of Eating Disorders, 10,* 297–311.

Oliver, G., Wardle, J., & Gibson, L. E. (2000). Stress and food choice: A laboratory study. *Psychosomatic Medicine, 62,* 853–865.

Onyike, C. U., Crum, R. M., Lee, H. B., Lyketsos, C. G., & Eaton, W. W. (2003). Is obesity associated with major depression? Results from the third National Health and Nutrition Examination Survey. *American Journal of Epidemiology, 158,* 1139–1147.

Ouwens, M. (2005). *The disinhibition effect.* Unpublished doctoral dissertation, Radboud University of Nijmegen, Nijmegen, the Netherlands.

Oxford American dictionary (2nd ed.). (2005). New York: Oxford University Press.

Papies, E., Stroebe, W., & Aarts, H. (2005). Is pizza eten altijd smullen? De role von lijnen by hedonisch gevolgstrekken [Is eating pizza always a feast? The role of restrained eating in drawing hedonic inferences]. In L. W. Albers, A. Dijksterhuis, M. van Rhoon, & M. Rotteveel (Eds.), *Jaarboek Sociaal Psychologie 2004* (pp. 313–320). Amsterdam: ASPO Press.

Papies, E., Stroebe, W., & Aarts, H. (2007a). *The allure of palatable food: Biased selective attention among restrained eaters.* Unpublished manuscript.

Papies, E., Stroebe, W., & Aarts, H. (2007b). *Healthy cognitions: Processes of self-regulatory success in restrained eaters.* Unpublished manuscript.

Papies, E., Stroebe, W., & Aarts, H. (2007c). Pleasure in the mind: Food imagery of restrained and unrestrained eaters. *Journal of Experimental Social Psychology, 43,* 810–817.

Patton, G. C., Selzer, R., Coffey, C., Carlin, J. B., & Wolfe, R. (1999). Onset of adolescent eating disorders: Population based cohort study over 3 years. *British Medical Journal, 318,* 765–768.

Peake, P., Hebl, M., & Mischel, W. (2002). Strategic attention deployment in waiting and working situations. *Developmental Psychology, 38,* 313–326.

Pereira, M. A., Kartashov, A. I., Ebeeling, C. B., Van Horn, L., Slattery, M. L., Jacobs, Jr., D. R., et al. (2005). Fast-food habits, weight gain, and insulin resistance (the CARDIA study): 15-year prospective analysis. *Lancet, 365,* 36–42.

Perri, M. G., Martin, A. D., Leermakers, E. A., Sears, S. F., & Notelovitz, M. (1997). Effects of group- versus home-based exercise in the treatment of obesity. *Journal of Consulting and Clinical Psychology, 65*, 278–285.

Petersen, L., Schnohr, P., & Sorensen, T. I. A. (2004). Longitudinal study of the long-term relation between physical activity and obesity in adults. *International Journal of Obesity, 28*, 105–112.

Phelan, S., Hill, J. O., Lang, W., Dibello, J. R., & Wing, R. R. (2003). Recovery from relapse among successful weight maintainers. *American Journal of Clinical Nutrition, 78*, 1079–1084.

Phillips, S. M., Bandini, L. G., Naumova, E. N., Cyr, H., Colclough, S., Dietz, W. H., & Must, A. (2004). Energy-dense snack food intake in adolescence: Longitudinal relationship to weight and fatness. *Obesity Research, 12*, 461–472.

Pine, C. J. (1985). Anxiety and eating behavior in obese and nonobese American Indians and white Americans. *Journal of Personality and Social Psychology, 49*, 774–780.

Pinel, J. P. J., Assanand, S., & Lehman, D. R. (2000). Hunger, eating, and ill health. *American Psychologist, 55*, 1105–1116.

Pi-Sunyer, F. X. (2002). Medical complications of obesity in adults. In C. G. Fairburn & K. D. Brownell (Eds.), *Eating disorders and obesity* (2nd ed., pp. 467–472). New York: Guilford Press.

Polivy, J. (1976). Perception of calories and regulation of intake in restrained and unrestrained subjects. *Addictive Behavior, 1*, 237–243.

Polivy, J., Heatherton, T. F., & Herman, C. P. (1988). Self-esteem, restraint, and eating behavior. *Journal of Abnormal Psychology, 97*, 354–356.

Polivy, J., & Herman, C. P. (1992). Undieting: A program to help people stop dieting. *International Journal of Eating Disorders, 11*, 261–268.

Polivy, J., & Herman, C. P. (1999). Distress and eating: Why do dieters overeat? *International Journal of Eating Disorders, 26*, 153–164.

Polivy, J., Herman, C. P., Hackett, R., & Kuleshnyk, I. (1986). The effects of self-attention and public attention on eating in restrained and unrestrained eaters. *Journal of Personality and Social Psychology, 50*, 1253–1260.

Polivy, J., Herman, C. P., & McFarlane, T. (1994). Effects of anxiety on eating: Does palatability moderate stress-induced overeating in dieters? *Journal of Abnormal Psychology, 103*, 505–510.

Porrini, M., Santangelo, S., Crovetti, R., Riso, P., Testolin, G., & Blundell, J. E. (1997). Weight, protein, fat, and timing of preloads affect food intake. *Physiology & Behavior, 62*, 563–570.

Powell, L. H., Calvin III, J. E., & Calvin, J. E., Jr. (2007). Effective obesity treatments. *American Psychologist, 62*, 234–246.

Powell, L. M., Szczypka, B. A., & Chaloupka, F. J. (2007). Exposure to food advertising on television among US Children. *Archives of Pediatrics and Adolescent Medicine, 161*, 553–560.

Prentice, A. (1999a). Aetiology of obesity IV: Metabolic factors. In British Nutrition Foundation (Ed.), *Obesity* (pp. 61–68). Oxford, England: Blackwell Science.

Prentice, A. (1999b). Aetiology of obesity V: Macronutrient balance. In British Nutrition Foundation (Ed.), *Obesity* (pp. 69–71). Oxford, England: Blackwell Science.

Prentice, A., & Jebb, S. (1999). Aetiology of obesity IX: Dietary factors. In British Nutrition Foundation (Ed.), *Obesity* (pp. 91–100). Oxford, England: Blackwell Science.

Presnell, K., & Stice, E. (2003). An experimental test of the effect of weight-loss dieting on bulimic pathology: Tipping the scales in a different direction. *Journal of Abnormal Psychology, 112*, 166–170.

Proctor, M. H., Moore, L. L., Gao, D., Cupples, L. A., Bradlee, M. L., Hood, M. Y., & Ellison, R. C. (2003). Television viewing and change in body fat from preschool to early adolescence: The Framingham children's study. *International Journal of Obesity, 27*, 827–833.

Puhl, R. M., & Latner, J. D. (2007). Stigma, obesity, and the health of the nation's children. *Psychological Bulletin, 133*, 557–580.

Quetelet, M. A. (1842). *A treatise on man and the development of his faculties*. New York: Franklin.

Raben, A., Agerholme-Larsen, L., Flint, A., Holst, J. J., & Astrup, A. (2003). Meals with similar energy densities but rich in protein, fat, carbohydrate, or alcohol have different effects on energy expenditure and substrate metabolism but not on appetite and energy intake. *American Journal of Clinical Nutrition, 77*, 91–100.

Raben, A., Vassilareas, T. H., Moller, A. C., & Astrup, A. (2002). Sucrose compared with artificial sweeteners: Different effects on ad libitum food intake and body weight after 10 wk of supplementation in overweight subjects. *American Journal of Clinical Nutrition, 76*, 721–729.

Rankinen, T., & Bouchard, C. (2006). Genetics of food intake and eating behavior phenotypes in humans. *Annual Review of Nutrition, 26*, 413–434.

Ransley, J. R., Donnelly, J. K., Botham, H., Khara, T. N., Greenwood, D. C., & Cade, J. E. (2003). Use of supermarket receipts to estimate energy fat content of food purchased by lean and overweight families. *Appetite, 41*, 141–148.

Rapoport, L., Clark, M., & Wardle, J. (2000). Evaluation of a modified cognitive behavioural programme for weight management. *International Journal of Obesity, 24*, 1726–1737.

Ravussin, E. (2002). Energy expenditure and body weight. In C. G. Fairburn and K. D. Brownell (Eds.), *Eating disorders and obesity* (2nd ed., pp. 55–61). New York: Guilford Press.

Ravussin, E., Burnand, B., Schutz, Y., & Jéquier, E. (1985). Energy expenditure before and during energy restriction in obese patients. *American Journal of Clinical Nutrition, 41*, 753–759.

Ravussin, E., Lillioja, S., Knowler, W. C., Christin, L., Freymond, D., Abbott, W. G., et al. (1988). Reduced rate of energy expenditure as a risk factor for body weight gain. *New England Journal of Medicine, 318*, 467–472.

Ravussin, E., Valencia, M. E., Esparza, J., Bennett, P. H., & Schulz, L. O. (1994). Effects of a traditional lifestyle on obesity in Pima Indians. *Diabetes Care, 17,* 1067–1074.

Raynor, H. A., & Epstein, L. H. (2003). The relative-reinforcing value of food under differing levels of food deprivation and restriction. *Appetite, 40,* 15–24.

Register, C. A., & Williams, D. R. (1990). Wage effects of obesity among young workers. *Social Science Quarterly, 71,* 131–141.

Rennie, K. L., & Jebb, S. A. (2005). National prevalence of obesity: Prevalence of obesity in Great Britain. *Obesity Reviews, 6,* 11–12.

Rexrode, K. M., Hennekens, C. H., Willett, W. C., Colditz, G. A., Stampfer, M. J., Rich-Edwards, J., et al. (1997). A prospective study of body mass index, weight change, and risk of stroke in women. *Journal of the American Medical Association, 227,* 1539–1545.

Reynolds, K., Gu, D., Whelton, P. K., Wu, X., Duan, X., Mo, J., & He, J. (2007). Prevalence of risk factors of overweight and obesity in china. *Obesity, 15,* 10–18.

Reznick, H., & Balch, P. (1977). The effect of anxiety and response cost manipulations on eating behavior of obese and normal weight subjects. *Addictive Behaviors, 2,* 219–225.

Ridgeway, P. S., & Jeffrey, D. B. (1998). A comparison of the Three-Factor Eating Questionnaire and the Restraint Scale and consideration of Lowe's three-factor model. *Addictive Behaviors, 23,* 115–118.

Rijksinstituut voor Volksgezondheid en Milieu. (2004). *Ons eten gemeten* [Our food measured]. Bilthoven, the Netherlands: RIVM.

Rippe, J. M., Price, J. M., Hess, S. A., Kline, G., DeMers, K. A., Damitz, S., et al. (1998). Improved psychological well-being, quality of life, and health practice in moderately overweight women participating in a 12-week structured weight loss program. *Obesity, 6,* 208–218.

Robert Koch-Institut. (2005). Übergewicht [Overweight]. *Gesundheitsberichterstattung des Bundes, Heft 16.*

Roberts, R. E., Kaplan, G. E., Shema, S. J., & Strawbridge, W. J. (2000). Are the obese at greater risk for depression? *American Journal of Epidemiology, 152,* 163–170.

Robinson, T. E., & Berridge, K. C. (2000). The psychology and neurobiology of addiction: An incentive sensitization view. *Addiction, 95*(Suppl. 2), S91–S117.

Robinson, T. N. (1999). Reducing children's television viewing to prevent obesity. *Journal of the American Medical Association, 282,* 1561–1567.

Robinson, T. N., Hammer, L., Killen, J. D., Kramer, H. C., Wilson, D. M., Hayward, C., & Taylor, C. B. (2001). Does television viewing increase obesity and reduce physical activity? Cross-sectional and longitudinal analyses among adolescent girls. *Pediatrics, 91,* 273–280.

Rock, C. L., Pakiz, B., Flatt, S. W., & Quintana, E. L. (2007). Randomized trial of a multifaceted commercial weight loss program. *Obesity, 15,* 939–949.

Rodin, J. (1981). Current status of the internal-external hypothesis of obesity: What went wrong? *American Psychologist, 36,* 361–372.

Rodin, J., Elman, D., & Schachter, S. (1974). Emotionality and obesity. In S. Schachter & J. Rodin (Eds.), *Obese humans and rats* (p. 15–20). Potomac, MD: Erlbaum.

Rodin, J., Herman, C., & Schachter, S. (1974). Obesity and various tests of external sensitivity. In S. Schachter & J. Rodin (Eds.), *Obese humans and rats* (pp. 89–96). Potomac, MD: Erlbaum.

Rodin, J., Slochower, J., & Fleming, B. (1977). Effects of degree of obesity, age of onset, and weight loss on responsiveness to sensory external stimuli. *Journal of Comparative and Physiological Psychology, 91*, 586–597.

Roefs, A., Herman, C. P., MacLeod, C. M., Smulders, F. T. Y., & Jansen, A. (2005). At first sight: How do restrained eaters evaluate high-fat palatable foods? *Appetite, 44*, 103–114.

Roefs, A., & Jansen, A. (2002). Implicit and explicit attitudes towards high-fat foods in obesity. *Journal of Abnormal Psychology, 111*, 517–521.

Roehling, M. (1999). Weight-based discrimination in employment: Psychological and legal aspects. *Personnel Psychology, 52*, 969–1016.

Rogers, P. J., & Blundell, J. E. (1980). Investigation of food selection and meal parameters during the development of dietary induced obesity [Abstract]. *Appetite, 1*, 85.

Rolls, B. (2000). The role of energy density in the overconsumption of fat. *Journal of Nutrition, 23*, 268S–271S.

Rolls, B. J., Morris, E. L., & Roe, L. (2002). Portion size of food affects energy intake in normal-weight and overweight men and women. *American Journal of Clinical Nutrition, 76*, 1207–1213.

Rolls, B. J., Roe, L. S., Kral, T. V. E., Meengs, J. S., & Wall, D. E. (2004). Increasing the portion size of packaged snack increases energy intake in men and women. *Appetite, 42*, 63–69.

Rosenbloom, A. L., Joe, J. R., Young, R. S., & Winter, N. E. (1999). Emerging epidemic of type 2 diabetes in youth. *Diabetes Care, 22*, 345–354.

Ross, L. (1974). Effects of manipulating salience of food upon consumption by obese and normal eaters. In S. Schachter & J. Rodin (Eds.), *Obese humans and rats* (pp. 43–52). Potomac, MD: Erlbaum.

Ross, R., Dagnone, D., Jones, P. J. H., Smith, H., Paddags, A., Hudson, R., & Janssen, I. (2000). Reduction in obesity and related comorbid conditions after diet-induced weight loss or exercise-induced weight loss in men: A randomized controlled trial. *Annals of Internal Medicine, 133*, 92–103.

Rotenberg, K. J., & Flood, D. (1999). Loneliness, dysphoria, dietary restraint, and eating behavior. *International Journal of Eating Disorders, 25*, 55–64.

Rotenberg, K. J., & Flood, D. (2000). Dietary restraint, attributional styles for eating, and preloading effects. *Eating Behaviors, 1*, 63–78.

Rothacker, D. Q. (2000). Five-year self-management of weight using meal replacements: Comparison with matched controls in rural Wisconsin. *Nutrition, 16*, 344–348.

Ruderman, A. J. (1983). Obesity, anxiety and food consumption. *Addictive Behaviors*, *8*, 235–242.

Ruderman, A. J. (1985). Dysphoric mood and overeating: A test of restraint theory's disinhibition hypothesis. *Journal of Abnormal Psychology*, *94*, 78–85.

Ruderman, A. J., Belzer, L. J., & Halperin, A. (1985). Restraint, anticipated consumption, and overeating. *Journal of Abnormal Psychology*, *94*, 547–555.

Ruderman, A. J., & Christensen, H. (1983). Restraint theory and its applicability to overweight individuals. *Journal of Abnormal Psychology*, *92*, 210–215.

Ruderman, A. J., & Wilson, G. T. (1979). Weight, restraint, cognitions and counterregulation. *Behavior Research and Therapy*, *17*, 581–590.

Rutledge, T., & Linden, W. (1998). To eat or not to eat: Affective and physiological mechanisms in the stress-eating relationship. *Journal of Behavioral Medicine*, *21*, 221–240.

Ruxton, C. H. S., Kirk, T. R., & Belton, N. R. (1996). The contribution of specific dietary patterns to energy and nutrient intakes in 7–8-year-old Scottish school children: III. Snacking habits. *Journal of Human Nutrition and Dietetics*, *9*, 23–31.

Saelens, B. E., & Epstein, L. H. (1996). Reinforcing value of food in obese and nonobese women. *Appetite*, *27*, 41–50.

Saelens, B. E., Sallis, J. F., & Frank, L. D. (2003). Environmental correlates of walking and cycling: Findings from the transportation, urban design, and planning literatures. *Annals of Behavioral Medicine*, *25*, 80–91.

Sbrocco, T., Nedegaard, R. C., Stone, J. M., & Lewis, E. L. (1999). Behavioral choice treatment promotes continuing weight loss: Preliminary results of a cognitive–behavioral decision-based treatment for obesity. *Journal of Consulting and Clinical Psychology*, *67*, 260–266.

Schachter, S. (1971). *Emotion, obesity, and crime*. New York: Academic Press.

Schachter, S. (1982). Recidivism and self-cure of smoking and obesity. *American Psychologist*, *37*, 436–444.

Schachter, S., & Friedman, L. N. (1974). The effects of work and cue prominence on eating behavior. In S. Schachter & J. Rodin (Eds.), *Obese humans and rats* (pp. 11–14). Potomac, MD: Erlbaum.

Schachter, S., Goldman, R., & Gordon, A. (1968). Effects of fear, food deprivation, and obesity on eating. *Journal of Personality and Social Psychology*, *10*, 91–97.

Schachter, S., & Gross, R. (1968). Manipulated time and eating behavior. *Journal of Personality and Social Psychology*, *10*, 98–106.

Schachter, S., & Rodin, J. (Eds.). (1974). *Obese humans and rats*. Potomac, MD: Erlbaum.

Schlosser, E. (2002). *Fast food nation*. London: Penguin Books.

Schmitz, K. H., Jacobs, D. R., Jr., Leon, A. S., Schreiner, P. J., & Sternfeld, B. (2000). Physical activity and body weight: Associations over ten years in the CARDIA study. *International Journal of Obesity*, *24*, 1475–1487.

Schmitz, K. H., & Jeffery, R. W. (2002). Prevention of obesity. In T. A. Wadden & A. J. Stunkard (Eds.), *Handbook of obesity treatment* (pp. 556–593). New York: Guilford Press.

Schotte, D. E. (1992). On the special status of "ego threats": Comment on Heatherton, Herman, and Polivy (1991). *Journal of Personality and Social Psychology, 62,* 798–800.

Schotte, D. E., Cools, J., & McNally, R. J. (1990). Induced anxiety triggering overeating in restrained eaters. *Journal of Abnormal Psychology, 99,* 317–320.

Schulz, L. O., & Schoeller, D. A. (1994). A compilation of total daily energy expenditure and body weights in healthy adults. *American Journal of Clinical Nutrition, 60,* 676–681.

Schutz, Y., & Jéquier, E. (2004). Resting energy expenditure, thermic effect of food, and total energy expenditure. In G. A. Bray & C. Bouchard (Eds.), *Handbook of obesity: Etiology and pathophysiology* (pp. 615–630). New York: Dekker.

Segal, N. L., & Allison, D. B. (2002). Twins and virtual twins: Bases of relative body weight revisited. *International Journal of Obesity, 26,* 437–441.

Seibt, B., Häfner, M., & Deutsch, R. (2007). Prepared to eat: How immediate affective and motivational response to food cues are influenced by food deprivation. *European Journal of Social Psychology, 37,* 359–379.

Seidell, J. C. (1998). Dietary fat and obesity: An epidemiological perspective. *American Journal of Clinical Nutrition, 67*(Suppl. 3), 546S–500S.

Seidell, J. C., Muller, D. C., Sorkin, J. D., & Andres, R. (1992). Fasting respiratory exchange ratio and resting metabolic rate as predictors of weight gain: The Baltimore Longitudinal Study on Ageing. *International Journal of Obesity, 16,* 667–674.

Select Committee on Health, UK Parliament. (2004). *Health—Third report.* Retrieved September 28, 2005, from http://www.publications.parliament.uk/pa/cm200304/cmselect/cmhealth/23/2302.htm

Serdula, M. K., Mokdad, A. H., Williamson, D. F., Galuska, D. A., Mendlein, J. M., & Heath, G. W. (1999). Prevalence of attempting weight loss and strategies for controlling weight. *Journal of the American Medical Association, 282,* 1353–1358.

Shah, J. Y., Friedman, R., & Kruglanski, A. W. (2002). Forgetting all else: On the antecedents and consequences of goal shielding. *Journal of Personality and Social Psychology, 83,* 1261–1280.

Shah, J. Y., & Kruglanski, A. W. (2002). Priming against your will: How accessible alternatives affect goal pursuit. *Journal of Experimental Social Psychology, 38,* 384–396.

Shallice, T. (1972). Dual function of consciousness. *Psychological Review, 79,* 383–393.

Sheppard-Sawyer, C. L., McNally, R. J., & Harnden Fischer, J. (2000). Film-induced sadness as a trigger for disinhibited eating. *International Journal of Eating Disorders, 28,* 215–220.

Silventoinen, K., Sans, S., Tolonen, H., Monterde, D., Kuulasmaa, K., Kesteloot, H., et al. (2004). Trends in obesity and energy supply in the WHO MONICA Project. *International Journal of Obesity, 28,* 710–718.

Simkin-Silverman, L., Wing, R. R., Boraz, M. A., Meilahn, E. N., & Kuller, L. H. (1998). Maintenance of cardiovascular risk factor changes among middle-aged women in a lifestyle intervention trial. *Women's Health, 4,* 255–271.

Simopoulos, A. P. (1986). Obesity and body weight standards. *Annual Review of Public Health, 7,* 475–492.

Sjöström, C. D., Peltonen, M., Wedel, H., & Sjöström, L. (2000). Differential long-term effects of intentional weight loss on diabetes and hypertension. *Hypertension, 36,* 20–25.

Skinner, B. F. (1953). *Science of human behavior.* New York: Macmillan.

Slochower, J. A. (1983). *Excessive eating: The role of emotions and the environment.* New York: Human Sciences Press.

Sobal, J., & Stunkard, A. J. (1989). Socioeconomic status and obesity: A review of the literature. *Psychological Bulletin, 105,* 260–275.

Sonko, B. J., Prentice, A. M., Murgatroyd, P. R., Goldberg, G. R., van de Ven, M., & Coward, W. A. (1994). Effects of alcohol on postmeal fat storage. *American Journal of Clinical Nutrition, 59,* 619–625.

Sopko, G., Leon, A. S., Jacobs, D. R., Foster, N., Moy, J., Kuba, K., et al. (1985). The effects of exercise and weight loss on plasma lipids in young obese men. *Metabolism, 34,* 227–233.

Spencer, J. A., & Fremouw, W. J. (1979). Binge eating as a function of restraint and weight classification. *Journal of Abnormal Psychology, 88,* 262–267.

Stephens, G., Prentice-Dunn, S., & Spruill, J. C. (1994). Public self-awareness and success-failure feedback as disinhibitors of restrained eating. *Basic and Applied Social Psychology, 15,* 509–522.

Stevens, J., Cai, J., Evenson, K. R., & Thomas, R. (2002). Fitness and fatness as predictors of mortality from all causes and from cardiovascular disease in men and women in the Lipid Research Clinics Study. *American Journal of Epidemiology, 156,* 832–841.

Stevens, J., Cai, J., Pamuk, E. R., Williamson, D. F., Thun, M. J., & Wood, J. L. (1998). The effect of age on the association between body-mass index and mortality. *New England Journal of Medicine, 338,* 1–7.

Stice, E. (2002). Risk and maintenance factors for eating pathology: A meta-analytic review. *Psychological Bulletin, 128,* 825–848.

Stice, E., Cameron, R. P., Killen, J. D., Hayward, C., & Taylor, C. B. (1999). Naturalistic weight-reduction efforts prospectively predict growth in relative weight and onset of obesity among female adolescents. *Journal of Consulting and Clinical Psychology, 67,* 967–974.

Stice, E., Fisher, M., & Lowe, M. R. (2004). Are dietary restraint scales valid measures of acute dietary restriction? Unobtrusive observational data suggest not. *Psychological Assessment, 16,* 51–59.

Stice, E., Presnell, K., Groesz, L., & Shaw, H. (2005). Effects of a weight maintenance diet on bulimic symptoms in adolescent girls: An experimental test of the dietary restraint theory. *Health Psychology, 24,* 402–412.

Stice, E., Presnell, K., Shaw, H., & Rhode, P. (2005). Psychological and behavioral risk factors for obesity onset in adolescent girls: A prospective study. *Journal of Consulting and Clinical Psychology, 73,* 195–2002.

Stice, E., Presnell, K., & Spangler, D. (2002). Risk factors for binge eating onset in adolescent girls: A 2-year prospective investigation. *Health Psychology, 21,* 131–138.

Stice, E., & Shaw, H. (2004). Eating disorder prevention programs: A meta-analytic review. *Psychological Bulletin, 130,* 206–227.

Stice, E., Shaw, H., & Marti, C. N. (2006). A meta-analytic review of obesity prevention programs for children and adolescents: The skinny on interventions that work. *Psychological Bulletin, 132,* 667–691.

Stoneman, Z., & Brody, G. H. (1982). The indirect impact of child-oriented advertisements on mother-child interaction. *Journal of Applied Developmental Psychology, 2,* 369–376.

Story, M., & Faulkner, P. (1990). The prime time diet: A content analysis of eating behavior and food messages in television program content and commercials. *American Journal of Public Health, 80,* 738–740.

Story, M., Kaphingst, K. M., & French, S. (2006). The role of school in obesity prevention. *The Future of Children, 16,* 109–142.

Strack, F., & Deutsch, R. (2004). Reflective and impulsive determinants of social behavior. *Personality and Social Psychology Review, 8,* 220–247.

Stroebe, W. (2000). *Social psychology and health* (2nd ed.). Buckingham, England: Open University Press.

Stroebe, W. (2002). Übergewicht als Schicksal? Die kognitive Steuerung des Essverhaltens [Obesity as fate: The cognitive regulation of eating behaviour]. *Psychologische Rundschau, 53,* 14–22.

Stroebe, W., Insko, C. A., Thompson, V. D., & Layton, B. D. (1971). Effects of physical attractiveness, attitude similarity, and sex on various aspects of interpersonal attraction. *Journal of Personality and Social Psychology, 18,* 79–91.

Stroebe, W., Mensink, W., Aarts, H., Schut, H., & Kruglanski, A. W. (2008). Why dieters fail: Testing the goal conflict model of eating. *Journal of Experimental Social Psychology, 44,* 26–36.

Stroebele, N., & de Castro, J. (2004). Television viewing is associated with an increase in meal frequency in humans. *Appetite, 42,* 111–113.

Stubbs, R. J., Harbron, C. G., Murgatroyd, P. R., & Prentice, A. M. (1995). Covert manipulation of the dietary fat and energy density of food intake on and substrate flux in men feeding ad libitum. *American Journal of Clinical Nutrition, 62,* 316–329.

Stunkard, A. J., Foch, T. T., & Hrubec, Z. (1986). A twin study of human obesity. *Journal of the American Medical Association, 256,* 51–54.

Stunkard, A. J., Harris, J. R., Pedersen, N. L., & McClearn, G. E. (1990). The body-mass index of twins who have been reared apart. *New England Journal of Medicine, 322,* 1483–1487.

Stunkard, A. J., & Koch, C. (1964). The interpretation of gastric motility: I. Apparent bias in the reports of hunger by obese persons. *Archives of Genetic Psychiatry, 11,* 74–82.

Stunkard, A. J., & Messick, S. (1985). The three-factor eating questionnaire to measure dietary restraint, disinhibition and hunger. *Journal of Psychosomatic Research, 29,* 71–83.

Stunkard, A. J., & Sobal, J. (1995). Psychosocial consequences of obesity. In K. D. Brownell & C. G. Fairburn (Eds.), *Eating disorders and obesity* (pp. 417–421). New York: Guilford Press.

Stunkard, A. J., & Stellar, E. (Eds.). (1984). *Eating and its disorders.* New York: Raven Press.

Tanco, S., Linden, W., & Earle, T. (1998). Well-being and morbid obesity in women: A controlled therapy evaluation. *International Journal of Eating Disorders, 23,* 325–339.

Tanofsky-Kraff, M., Wilfley, D. E., & Spurrell, E. (2000). Impact of interpersonal and ego-related stress on restrained eaters. *International Journal of Eating Disorders, 27,* 411–418.

Taras, H. L., & Gage, M. (1995). Advertised foods on children's television. *Archives of Pediatrics and Adolescent Medicine, 149,* 649–652.

Tataranni, P. A., Larson, D. E., Snitker, S., & Ravussin, E. (1995). Thermic effect of food in humans. Methods and results from use of a respiratory chamber. *American Journal of Clinical Nutrition, 61,* 1013–1019.

Tataranni, P. A., & Ravussin, E. (2002). Energy metabolism and obesity. In T. A. Wadden & A. J. Stunkard (Eds.), *Handbook of obesity treatment* (pp. 42–72). New York: Guilford Press.

Taveras, E. M., Berkey, C. S., Rifas-Shiman, S. L., Ludwig, D. S., Rockett, H. R. H., Field, A. E., et al. (2005). Association of consumption of fried food away from home with body mass index and diet quality in older children and adolescents. *Pediatrics, 116,* 518–524.

Tepper, B. J. (1992). Dietary restraint and responsiveness to sensory-based food cues as measured by cephalic phase salivation and sensory specific satiety. *Psychopharmacology, 157,* 67–74.

Thompson, M. M., Zanna, M. P., & Griffin, D. W. (1995). Let's not be indifferent about (attitudinal) ambivalence. In R. E. Petty & J. A. Krosnick (Eds.), *Attitude strength: Antecedents and consequences* (pp. 361–386). Mahwah, NJ: Erlbaum.

Thompson, O. M., Ballew, C., Resnicow, K., Must, A., Bandini, L. G., Cyr, H., & Dietz, W. H. (2004). Food purchased away from home as a predictor of change in BMI z-score among girls. *International Journal of Obesity, 28,* 282–289.

Tillotson, J. E. (2004). America's obesity: Conflicting public policies, industrial economic development, and unintended human consequences. *Annual Review of Nutrition, 24*, 617–643.

Tjepkema, M. (2006). *Measured obesity: Adult obesity in Canada: Measured height and weight.* Retrieved November 6, 2007, from http://www.statcan.ca/english/research/82-620-MIE/2005001/pdf/aobesity.pdf

Tom, G., & Rucker, M. (1975). Fat, full, and happy. *Journal of Personality and Social Psychology, 32*, 761–766.

Tomarken, A. J., & Kirschenbaum, D. S. (1984). Effects of plans for future meals on counterregulatory eating by restrained and unrestrained eaters. *Journal of Abnormal Psychology, 93*, 458–472.

Tordoff, M. G., & Alleva, A. M. (1990). Effects of drinking soda sweetened with aspartame or high-fructose corn syrup on food intake and body weight. *American Journal of Clinical Nutrition, 51*, 963–969.

Tremblay, M. S., Katzmarzyk, P. T., & Willms, J. D. (2002). Temporal trends in overweight and obesity in Canada 1981–1996. *International Journal of Obesity, 26*, 358–343.

Tremblay, M. S., & Willms, J. D. (2002). Is the Canadian childhood obesity epidemic related to physical inactivity? *International Journal of Obesity, 27*, 1100–1105.

Tremblay, A., Wouters, E., Wenker, M., St-Pierre, S., Bouchard, C., & Déspres, J.-P. (1995). Alcohol and a high-fat diet: A combination favoring overfeeding. *American Journal of Clinical Nutrition, 62*, 639–644.

Troiano, R. P., Frongillo, E. A., Sobal, J., & Levitsky, D. A. (1996). The relationship between body weight and mortality: A quantitative analysis of combined information from existing studies. *International Journal of Obesity, 20*, 63–75.

Trope, Y., & Fishbach, A. (2000). Counteractive self-control in overcoming temptation. *Journal of Personality and Social Psychology, 79*, 493–506.

Truby, H., Baic, S., deLooy, A., Fox, K. R., Livingstone, M. B. E., Logan, C. M., et al. (2006). Randomised controlled trial of four commercial weight loss programmes in the UK: Initial findings from the BBC "diet trials." *British Medical Journal, 332*, 1309–1311.

Tsai, A. G., & Wadden, T. A. (2006). The evolution of very-low-calorie-diets: An update and meta-analysis. *Obesity, 14*, 1283–1293.

Tuomilehto, J., Lindström, J., Eriksson, J. G., Valle, T. T., Hämäläinen, H., Ilanne-Parikka, P., et al. (2001). Prevention of type 2 diabetes mellitus by changing lifestyle among subjects with impaired glucose tolerance. *New England Journal of Medicine, 344*, 1343–1350.

Tuschen, B., Florin, I., & Baucke, R. (1993). Beeinflusst die Stimmung den Appetit? [Does mood influence appetite?]. *Zeitschrift für Klinische Psychologie, 12*, 315–321.

U.S. Department of Agriculture. (2000). Major trends in U.S. food supply, 1909–99. *FoodReview, 23*(1), 8–15.

U.S. Department of Agriculture Economic Research Service. (2005). *The price is right: Economics and the rise in obesity*. Retrieved June 29, 2007, from http://www.ers.usda.gov/amberwaves/february05/features/thepriceisright.htm

U.S. Department of Health and Human Services. (1996). *Physical activity and health: A report of the Surgeon General*. Washington, DC: International Medical Publishing.

U.S. Department of Health and Human Services and the Department of Agriculture. (1990). *Dietary guidelines for Americans* (Publication No. 1990-261-463/20444). Washington, DC: Government Printing Office.

U.S. Department of Health and Human Services and the Department of Agriculture. (1995). *Dietary guidelines for Americans* (Publication No. 1996-402-519). Washington, DC: Government Printing Office.

Utz, R. L. (2004). *Obesity in America 1960–2000*. Unpublished doctoral dissertation, University of Michigan, Ann Arbor.

Vander Wal, J. S., & Thelen, M. H. (2000). Predictors of body image dissatisfaction in elementary-age school girls. *Eating Behaviors, 1*, 105–122.

van Strien, T., Cleven, A., & Schippers, G. (2000). Restraint, tendency toward overeating and ice cream consumption. *International Journal of Eating Disorders, 28*, 333–338.

van Strien, T., Frijters, J. E., Bergers, G. P., & Defares, P. B. (1986). Dutch Eating Behavior Questionnaire for the assessment of restrained, emotional, and external eating behavior. *International Journal of Eating Disorders, 5*, 295–315.

Viner, R. M., & Cole, T. J. (2006). Who changes body mass between adolescence and adulthood? Factors predicting change in BMI between 16 years and 30 years in the British Birth Cohort. *International Journal of Obesity, 30*, 1368–1374.

Voorrips, L. E., Meijers, J. H. H., Sol, P., Seidell, J. C., & van Staveren, W. A. (1992). History of body weight and physical activity of elderly women differing in current physical activity. *International Journal of Obesity, 16*, 199–205.

Vreke, J., Donder, J. L., Langers, F., Salverda, I. E., & Veeneklaas, F. R. (2006). *Potentie van groen!* [The potential of green!] (Alterra-Rapport 1356). Retrieved September 28, 2007, from http://www2.alterra.wur.nl/webdocs/pdffiles/Alterra Rapporten/AlterraRapport1356.pdf

Wadden, T. A., Foster, G. D., Sarwer, D. B., Anderson, D. A., Gladis, M., Sanderson, R. S., et al. (2004). Dieting and the development of eating disorders in obese women: Results of a randomized controlled trial. *American Journal of Clinical Nutrition, 80*, 560–568.

Wallis, D. J., & Hetherington, M. M. (2004). Stress and eating: The effects of ego-threat and cognitive demand on food intake in restrained and emotional eaters. *Appetite, 43*, 39–46.

Wannamethee, S. G., Shaper, A. G., & Lennon, L. (2005). Reasons for intentional weight loss, unintentional weight loss, and mortality in older men. *Archives of Internal Medicine, 165*, 1035–1040.

Wansink, B. (2004). Environmental factors that increase the food intake and consumption volume of unknowing consumers. *Annual Review of Nutrition, 24,* 455–479.

Wansink, B., & Chandon, P. (2006). Meal size, not boy size, explains errors in estimating the calorie content of meals. *Annals of Internal Medicine, 145,* 326–333.

Wansink, B., & Kim, J. (2005). Bad popcorn in big buckets: Portion size can influence intake as much as taste. *Journal of Nutrition Education and Behavior, 37,* 242–245.

Wansink, B., & van Ittersum, K. (2007). Portion size me: Downsizing our consumption norms. *Journal of the American Dietetic Association, 107,* 1103–1106.

Ward, A., & Mann, T. (2000). Don't mind if I do: Disinhibited eating under cognitive load. *Journal of Personality and Social Psychology, 78,* 753–763.

Wardle, J., & Beales, S. (1987). Restraint and food intake: An experimental study of eating pattern in the laboratory and in normal life. *Behavior Research and Therapy, 25,* 179–185.

Wardle, J., & Beales, S. (1988). Control and loss of control over eating: An experimental investigation. *Journal of Abnormal Psychology, 97,* 35–40.

Wardle, J., & Griffith, J. (2001). Socioeconomic status and weight control practices in British adults. *Journal of Epidemiology and Community Health, 55,* 185–190.

Wardle, J., Griffith, J., Johnson, F., & Rapoport, L. (1999). Intentional weight control and food choice habits in a national representative sample of adults in the UK. *International Journal of Obesity, 24,* 534–540.

Webster's encyclopedic unabridged dictionary of the English language. (1989). New York: Portland House.

Weinsier, R. L., Hunter, G. R., Heini, A. F., Goran, M. I., & Sell, S. M. (1998). The etiology of obesity: Relative contribution of metabolic factors, diet, and physical activity. *American Journal of Medicine, 105,* 145–150.

Weinsier, R. L., Hunter, G. R., Zuckerman, P. A., & Darnell, B. E. (2003). Low resting and sleeping energy expenditure and fat use does not contribute to obesity in women. *Obesity Research, 11,* 937–944.

Weinsier, R. L., Nagy, T. R., Hunter, G. R., Darnell, B. E., Hensrud, D. D., & Weiss, H. L. (2000). Do adaptive changes in metabolic rate favor weight regain in weight-reduced individuals? An examination of set-point theory. *American Journal of Clinical Nutrition, 72,* 1088–1094.

Weinsier, R. L., Nelson, K. M., Hensrud, D. D., Darnell, B. E., Hunter, G. R., & Schutz, Y. (1995). Metabolic predictors of obesity. *Journal of Clinical Investigations, 95,* 980–985.

Weinsier, R. L., Wilson, L. J., & Lee, J. (1995). Medically safe rate of weight loss for treatment of obesity: A guideline based on risk of gallstone formation. *American Journal of Medicine, 98,* 115–117.

Weinstein, A. R., Sesso, H. D., Lee, I. M., Cook, N. R., Manson, J. E., Buring, J. E., & Gaziano, J. M. (2004). Relationship of physical activity vs. body mass index with type 2 diabetes in women. *Journal of the American Medical Association, 292,* 1188–1194.

Wen, L. M., Orr, N., Millett, C., & Rissel, C. (2005). Driving to work and overweight and obesity: Findings from the 2003 New South Wales Health Survey, Australia. *International Journal of Obesity, 30,* 782–786.

Wessel, T. R., Arant, C. B., Olson, M. B., Johnson, B. D., Reis, S. E., & Sharaf, B. L. (2004). Relationship of physical fitness vs. body mass index with coronary artery disease and cardiovascular events in women. *Journal of the American Medical Association, 292,* 1179–1187.

Westenhoefer, J., Broeckmann, P., Munch, A.-K., & Pudel, V. (1994). Cognitive control of eating behaviour and the disinhibition effect. *Appetite, 23,* 27–41.

Westenhoefer, J., Stunkard, A. J., & Pudel, V. (1999). Validation of the flexible and rigid control dimensions of dietary restraint. *International Journal of Eating Disorders, 26,* 53–64.

Westenhoefer, J., von Falck, B., Stellfeldt, A., & Fintelmann, S. (2004). Behavioural correlates of successful weight reduction over 3 y. results from the lean habits study. *International Journal of Obesity, 28,* 334–335.

Westerterp-Platenga, M. S., Saris, W. H. M., Hukshorn, C. J., & Campfield, L. A. (2001). Effects of weekly administration of pegylated recombinant human OB protein on appetite profile and energy metabolism in obese men. *American Journal of Clinical Nutrition, 74,* 426–434.

Westerterp-Platenga, M. S., & Verwegen, C. (1999). The appetizing effect of an aperitif in overweight and normal weight humans. *American Journal of Clinical Nutrition, 69,* 205–212.

Whybrow, S., Mayer, C., Kirk, T. R., Mazlan, N., & Stubbs, R. J. (2007). Effects of two weeks' mandatory snack consumption on energy intake and energy balance. *Obesity, 15,* 673–685.

Willett, W. C. (1998). Is dietary fat a major determinant of body fat? *American Journal of Clinical Nutrition, 67*(Suppl. 3), 556S–562S.

Willett, W. C., Manson, J. E., Stampfer, M. J., Colditz, G. A., Rosner, B., Speizer, F. E., & Hennekens, C. H. (1995). Weight, weight change, and coronary heart disease in women. Risk within the "normal" weight range. *Journal of the American Medical Association, 273,* 461–465.

Williamson, D. F. (1991). Epidemiological analysis of weight gain in U.S. adults. *Nutrition, 7,* 285–286.

Williamson, D. F., Madans, J., Anda, R. F., Kleinman, J. C., Kahn, H. S., & Byers, T. (1993). Recreational physical activity and 10-year weight change in a US national cohort. *International Journal of Obesity, 17,* 279–286.

Williamson, D. F., Serdula, M. K., Anda, R. F., Levy, A., & Byers, T. (1992). Weight loss attempts in adults: Goals, duration, and rate of weight loss. *American Journal of Public Health, 82,* 1251–1257.

Wilson, J. M. B., Tripp, D. A., & Boland, F. J. (2005). The relative contribution of subjective and objective measures of body shape and size to body image and disordered eating in women. *Body Image, 2,* 233–247.

Wing, R. R. (2004). Behavioral approaches to the treatment of obesity. In G. A. Bray & C. Bouchard (Eds.), *Handbook of obesity: Clinical applications* (2nd ed., pp. 147–167). New York: Dekker.

Wing, R. R., & Hill, J. O. (2001). Successful weight loss maintenance. *Annual Review of Nutrition, 21*, 323–341.

Wing, R. R., Jeffery, R. W., Hellerstedt, W. L., & Burton, L. R. (1996). Effects of frequent phone contact and optional food provision on maintenance of weight loss. *Annals of Behavioral Medicine, 18*, 172–176.

Wing, R. R., & Phelan, S. (2005). Long-term weight loss maintenance. *American Journal of Clinical Nutrition, 82*(Suppl. 11), 222S–225S.

Wintour, P. (2003, November 28). Blame obesity on bad diets, say food chiefs. *The Guardian*, p. 7.

Witkin, H. A., Lewis, H. B., Hertzman, M., Machover, K., Meissner, P. B., & Wapner, S. (1954). *Personality through perception*. New York: Harper & Brothers.

Wittenbrink, B., Judd, C. M., & Park, B. (1997). Evidence for racial prejudice at the implicit level and its relationship with questionnaire measures. *Journal of Personality and Social Psychology, 72*, 262–274.

Womble, L. G., Wadden, T. A., McGuckin, B. G., Sargent, S. L., Rothman, R. A., & Krauthamer-Ewing, E. S. (2004). A randomized controlled trial of a commercial Internet weight loss program. *Obesity Research, 12*, 1011–1018.

Womble, L. G., Wang, S. S., & Wadden, T. A. (2002). Commercial and self help weight loss programs. In T. A. Wadden & A. J. Stunkard (Eds.), *Handbook of obesity treatment* (pp. 395–415). New York: Guilford Press.

Woody, E. Z., Costanzo, P. R., Liefer, H., & Conger, J. (1981). The effects of taste and caloric perceptions on the eating behavior of restrained and unrestrained subjects. *Cognitive Therapy and Research, 5*, 381–390.

World Health Organization. (2000). *Obesity: Preventing and managing the global epidemic*. Geneva, Switzerland: WHO.

World Health Organization. (2005). *World Health Statistics 2005*. Geneva, Switzerland: WHO.

Wyatt, H. R., Grunwald, G. K., Seagle, H. M., Klem, M. L., McGuire, M. T., Wing, R. R., & Hill, J. O. (1999). Resting energy expenditure in reduced-obese subjects in the National Weight Control Registry. *American Journal of Clinical Nutrition, 69*, 1189–1193.

Yeomans, M. R., Blundell, J. E., & Leshem, M. (2004). Palatability: Response to nutritional need or need-free stimulation of appetite? *British Journal of Nutrition, 92*(Suppl. 1), S3–S14.

Young, L. R., & Nestle, M. (2002). The contribution of expanding portion sizes to the US obesity epidemic. *American Journal of Public Health, 92*, 246–249.

Zhang, Y., & Scarpace, P. J., (2006). The role of leptin in leptin resistance and obesity. *Physiology and Behavior, 88*, 249–256.

Zhang, Q., & Wang, Y. (2004). Trends in the association between obesity and socioeconomic status in U.S. adults: 1971 to 2000. *Obesity Research, 12*, 1622–1632.

Zizza, C., Siega-Riz, A. M., & Popkin, B. M. (2001). Significant increase in young adults' snacking between 1977–1978 and 1994–1996 represents a cause for concern! *Preventive Medicine, 32*, 303–310.

Zurlo, F., Lillioja, S., Esposito-Del Puente, A., Nyomba, B. L., Baz, I., Saad, M. F., et al. (1990). Low ratio of fat to carbohydrate oxidation as a predictor of weight gain: Study of 24-h RQ. *American Journal of Physiology, 259*, E650–E657.

AUTHOR INDEX

Bartholow, B. D., 144
Bartlett, S. J., 77
Basdevant, A., 72
Batterham, R. L., 39, 40
Batty, G. D., 21
Baucke, R., 123
Baucom, D. H., 123, 125, 128
Bauman, A., 76
Baumeister, R. F., 121, 123, 136, 154, 188, 200
Baxter, J. E., 202
Beales, S., 123–125, 128, 130
Beecher, M. D., 173
Bell, A. C., 86
Bellwoar, V., 130
Belton, N. R., 72
Belzer, L. J., 133
Bendixen, H., 14, 184
Benecke, A., 15, 16, 18, 82
Bengtsson, C., 12
Benjamin, A. J., Jr., 144
Bennett, P. H., 60
Bergers, G. P., 117, 163
Berkowitz, L., 144
Berridge, K. C., 151–154, 157
Bertéus Forslund, H., 72
Bes-Rastrollo, M., 67
Bessenoff, G. R., 19
Beuman, B., 53
Biernat, M., 19
Biing-Hwan, L., 65
Birch, L. L., 80
Bish, C. L., 167, 183
Black, A. E., 41
Blair, S. N., 25, 31
Blanchard, F. A., 123
Blane, D., 21
Blass, E. M., 79
Bleau, R., 123, 125, 126
Blix, G., 78
Blundell, J. E., 40n3, 95, 138
Bohr, Y., 124
Boland, F. J., 23, 132, 133
Bolger, N., 61, 128n4
Boon, B., 79, 122, 123, 127, 136, 158–160
Booth, D. A., 72

Boraz, M. A., 200
Bordi, P. L., 68
Borten, O., 184
Bouchard, C., 3, 10, 44, 45, 47–50, 52, 57, 78, 92, 136
Boutelle, K. N., 63
Bowman, S. A., 66
Boxer, A., 84, 85
Boyce, W. F., 78
Boyle, J. P., 29
Braam, L. A. J. L., 41, 62
Bratslavsky, E., 188
Bray, G. A., 10, 15, 40n2, 52
Brenner, M., 127
Briefel, R. R., 61
Brody, G. H., 80
Broeckmann, P., 130
Broemer, P., 145
Brown, L. B., 132n5
Brown, V., 80
Brownell, K. D., 3, 6, 19, 24, 59, 75, 76, 82, 168, 182
Brozek, J., 55
Bruch, H., ix, x, 93, 95, 103
Brunstrom, J. M., 155
Buchan, I., 18
Bueno-de-Mesquita, B., 41, 62
Bulik, C. M., 58
Bundred, P., 18
Burchiviel, C. M., 27
Burley, V. J., 40n3
Burnand, B., 51
Burr, H., 23
Burstein, B., 104, 107, 110
Burton, L. R., 175, 176
Butryn, M. L., 136, 138, 196, 197
Byers, T., 167

Cai, J., 25, 31
Calle, E. E., 25, 26, 28, 30
Calvin, J. E., III, 171
Calvin, J. E., Jr., 171
Cameron, R. P., 195
Campbell, S. M., 15
Campfield, L. A., 54
Canning, H., 20
Carlin, J. B., 195
Caro, J. F., 53

SUBJECT INDEX

Body image, 124n2
Body mass index (BMI), 10–13
    classification, 11–13
    and energy-intake trends, 62
    limitations of, 12
    and mortality, 25–27
    and snacking, 73
    trends in U.S. of, 18
    for weight/height, 12, 13
Body weight
    genetic factors influencing, xi, 48–58
    overconcern with, 196
    and RMR, 36
    set point for, 55–57
Body-weight standards, 10–13
Boundary model of eating, 6–7,
        119–121
    and eating restraint, 116, 136–137
    and goal conflict, 142
    goal conflict theory vs., 164
    and motivation, 137–138
    and palatability, 137
    and "what-the-hell" effect, 138–139
Boys
    fast-food consumption by, 67
    snacking by, 73, 74
    television viewing by, 77
Breast cancer, 30
BRFSS. *See* Behavioral Risk Factor Sur-
        veillance System
British Broadcasting Corporation
        (BBC), 66, 201
Brownell, K. D., 59, 182
Bruch, H., 95
Bulimia nervosa, 115, 119, 196, 197
Burger King, 76

Calorie intake. *See also* Energy intake;
        Food intake
    long-term trends in, 61–64
    perceived, 131–132
Calorie restriction, 184
Canada
    fast-food consumption and obesity
        in, 66
    obesity rates in, 14
    obesity trends in, 18

physical inactivity in, 88
    television viewing in, 78
Cancer, 30
Cancer Prevention studies, 28
Carbohydrates
    energy content of, 39
    food sources of, 39–40
    storage of, 43
Cardiac arrest, 194
Cardiac arrhythmias, 194
CARDIA Study, 67
Cardiorespiratory fitness, 31
Cardiovascular mortality, 32
Car use and weight gain, 86, 88–89
CDC (U.S. Centers for Disease Con-
        trol), 82
Changing Individuals' Purchases of
        Snacks Study, 203
Channel One, 81
Children
    with adult-onset diabetes, 29
    behavioral treatment approaches for,
        196–197
    behavioral treatment for obesity in,
        172–173
    BMI for, 11
    discretionary income of, 81
    health education programs for,
        198–200
    obesity trends for, 18
    physical activity levels for, 90
    physical inactivity of, 88
    snacking by, 70
    and television advertisements, 76,
        80–81
    walking/biking by, 87
    weight discrimination in, 19
    weight-loss programs for, 198
Cholesterol, 30
Chronic dieters. *See* Restrained eaters
Coca-Cola, 74, 76
Cognitive accessibility, 143, 145, 171
Cognitive investment hypothesis, 127,
        165
Cognitive representation, of palatable
        food, 155–157

Cognitive resources, 122, 127, 161
Cognitive restructuring, 170–171
Cognitive salience of food cues, 107–109
College admissions process, 20
Colon cancer, 30
Comfort hypothesis, 94–97, 103, 121
Commercial weight-loss programs
    effectiveness of, 178–182
    Jenny Craig, 181
    Rosemary Conley, 180, 181
    Weight Watchers International, 179–180, 182
Compensatory behavior
    bulimia nervosa as, 115n1
    and fast-food consumption, 67–68
    and snacking, 69, 73–74
    and soft drinks, 75
Computer games, 78
Concern-for-dieting factor, 117, 146
Conscious goal pursuit, 142
Consequences, of overweight and obesity, 18–31
    morbidity, 28–31
    mortality, 25–28
    psychological, 23–25
    social, 19–23
Container sizes, 74, 88
Convenience food, 65
Coronary Artery Risk Development in Young Adults (CARDIA) Study, 67
Coronary heart disease, 28–29
Cost, of food, 204
Counterregulation, 130, 131, 134–135
Craving, 151, 157
Cue salience, 101, 107–108
Cycle travel, 85

Daily caloric intake, 118
Dancing, 38
DEBQ. *See* Dutch Eating Behavior Questionnaire
Deep freezing, 65
Delay gratification, 154, 155, 157, 158
Denmark, 14, 22, 23, 62–63, 184
Depression, 24–25, 186, 195

Diabetes, 29–30, 192
    Adult-onset diabetes, 29
    Non-insulin-dependent diabetes, 29
    Type 1 diabetes, 29
    Type 2 diabetes, 29–30
Diagnostic and Statistical Manual of Mental Disorders (3rd ed.), 24
Diagnostic Interview Schedule, 24
Dietary Guidelines for Americans, 27
Dietary recommendations, 39
Dietary violations, 128–136
    and anticipation of future consumption, 133
    and equivalence hypothesis, 133–136
    and perceived calorie content, 131–132
Diet books, 180, 182
Diet boundaries, 116, 128
Dieting, 168–185
    behavioral treatment approaches to, 168–178
    with commercial weight-loss programs, 178–182
    defined, 4
    improving effectiveness of, 173–176
    and physical health, 191–194
    and psychological health, 194–198
    restrained eating vs., 168
    without professional help, 182–185
Dieting goal, 144
Dieting rules, 7, 120, 184
Diet pills, 184, 194
Diets, popular
    Atkins diet, 180, 181
    Ornish diet, 180
    Zone diet, 180
Differential sensitivity hypothesis, 93–96, 103
Digestive tract, 36
Discretionary income, of children and adolescents, 81
Discrimination, weight, 3, 19–23
    among children, 19
    in the educational system, 20–21
    in the job market, 22–23
    and partner choice, 20

Disinhibition, 119, 133, 190
Distancing, 154, 171
Distraction, 127, 154
Diuretics, 196
Diversion, 155
Dizygotic (DZ) twins, 45
Domestic activities, 86
Dopamine antagonists, 152
Dopaminergic system, 152
Dot probe paradigm, 159
Dr. Atkins' New Diet Revolution
    (R. Atkins), 181
Drug craving, 158
Dutch Eating Behavior Questionnaire
    (DEBQ), 117–118
Dyslipidemia, 30

East Germany, former, 14, 82–83
Eating disorder prevention programs,
    201
Eating disorders, 195–198
Eating Disorders Inventory (EDI), 118
Eating enjoyment
    dieting thoughts and priming of,
        147–149
    as goal, x, 144–145
Eating out, 65
Eating pathology, 186–187
Eating-related external stimuli, 93. *See
    also* External food-relevant cues
Eating restraint, 116–137. *See also*
    Restrained eating, dieting vs.
    and attentional bias, 157–161
    boundary model of, 119–121
    and cognitive representation of
        palatable food, 155–157
    defined, 116
    and eating disorders, 196, 197
    and evaluation of palatability,
        149–151
    measurement scales for, 116–119
    and priming for eating enjoyment,
        147–149
    and television viewing, 79
EDI (Eating Disorders Inventory), 118
Educational attainment and weight dis-
    crimination, 21–22

Educational system, antifat prejudice in,
    21
Effort to obtain food, 107, 110, 111, 190
Ego depletion theory, 200
Ego threats, 122–127
Emotional distress, 124n2, 125
Emotional eating, 94–103, 121–128
Emotional well-being, 185
Emotion hypothesis, 121–128
Employment and weight discrimination,
    22–23
"Empty calories," 43
Endometrial cancer, 30
Energy balance, 35–58
    energy expenditure components in,
        36–39
    energy intake components in, 39–44
    genetic influence on, 44–48
    and risk factors for weight gain,
        48–57
Energy density, 204
Energy expenditure, 36–39
    genetic influence on, 49, 50, 52
    and physical activity, 37–38
    and resting metabolic rate, 36
    and thermic effect of food, 37
    and weight gain/loss, 38–39
Energy intake, 39–44, 60–83
    alcohol, 40
    behavioral measures of, 42
    carbohydrates, 39–40
    ecological measures of, 63–64
    and energy storage, 43–44
    and environment, 60–83
    and fast food, 64–68
    fats, 40–42
    genetic influence on, 49
    long-term trends in, 61–64
    marketing effects on, 75–82
    measurement of, 40–42, 61–64
    and portion sizes, 68–70
    proteins, 40
    self-report measures of, 62–63
    and snacking, 70–74
    and soft drink consumption, 74–75
    underreporting of, 41
Energy-saving mode, 57

and unintentional weight loss,
192–194
Motivation, 121, 137–138
and dieting, 170
of self-control, 189
Multinational Monitoring of Trends
and Determinants in Cardiovas-
cular Disease (MONICA), 63
Multiple health behaviors, 200
"Mums in Burger Backlash Over
Healthy Eating," 66
Muscles, 36, 39
Muscular persons, 12
Musculoskeletal disease, 30–31

Naltrexone, 151
National Center for Health Statistics
(NCHS), 10, 16
National Food Survey, 61
National Health and Nutrition Exam-
ination Surveys III (NHANES
III), 24, 77
National Health and Nutrition Exam-
ination Surveys (NHANES), 16
National Health Interview Survey
(NHIS), 183
National Heart, Lung, and Blood Insti-
tute, 12
National Institutes of Health, 12
National Task Force on the Prevention
and Treatment of Obesity, 4, 27,
28, 195
National Travel Survey, 85
National Weight Control Registry
(NWCR), 188, 190, 191, 195,
204
NCHS. *See* National Center for Health
Statistics
NEAT. *See* Nonexercise activity
thermogenesis
Negative emotions, 123–124
Netherlands, 13
fast food restaurants in, 64
obesity rates for, 17
obesity rates in, 14
obesity trends in, 18
public transport in, 87–88

Next-in-line effect, 127
NHANES I Epidemiologic Follow-up
Study, 28, 88
NHANES III. *See* National Health
and Nutrition Examination
Surveys III
NHANES (National Health and Nutri-
tion Examination Surveys), 16
NHIS Mortality Follow-up Study, 28
Nisbett, R. E., 105–106
Nonconscious goal pursuit, 142–143
Nondieting treatment programs,
185–187
Nonexercise activity thermogenesis
(NEAT), 49–50
Normative pressure (to be slim), 15
Nuclear family studies, 46
Nurses' Health Study, 25–30, 32, 49, 55
Nutrition education, 169–170
NWCR. *See* National Weight Control
Registry

Obesity
and anxiety, 95–100, 108
and body dissatisfaction, 23
and cancer, 30
consequences of, 18–31
and coronary heart disease, 28–29
defined, 95n1
and depression, 24–25
and diabetes, 29–30
and discrimination, 3, 19–23
and dyslipidemia, 30
and educational attainment, 21
and effort, 107
and emotional eating, 94–103,
127–128
environmental causes of, 59–92
epidemiology of, 13–18
and ethnicity/race, 16–17
and external food-relevant cues,
104–111
and gender, 15
genetic influence on, 3–4, 44–48
long-term trends in, 61–64
and mortality, 25–27
and musculoskeletal disease, 30–31

Priming
 affective, 150–151
 and attentional bias, 160–161
 definition, 143
 for eating enjoyment, 147–149
 goal, 143–144
 and salience, 108
 and successful retrained eaters, 162
Priming task, 19–20
Probe recognition paradigm, 155
Problem diagnosis, 169
Protein
 energy content of, 39
 food sources of, 40
 storage/processing of, 43–44
Psychological consequences, of overweight and obesity, 23–25
Psychological health, 194–198
 depression, 195
 eating disorders, 195–198
Psychosomatic theory of weight regulation, 94–103
 comfort hypothesis, 94–97
 differential sensitivity hypothesis,
  93–96
Psychotropic medicine, 60
Public transport system, 87–88
Purchasing behavior, 77, 80

Quetelet, Adolphe, 10

Race
 epidemiology of overweight/obesity
  by, 16–17
 and weight recommendations, 27–28
Raking leaves, energy costs of, 38
Reasoned action, theory of, 142
Regular sustained activity, 82
Regular vigorous activity, 82
Relapse process theory, 171
Respiratory disease, 31
Respiratory fitness, 31–32
Respiratory quotient, 52–53
Restaurants, 65
Resting metabolic rate (RMR), 36
 low, 50–52
 and ongoing fasting, 56
 and weight loss, 57

Restrained eaters (chronic dieters). *See*
  also Eating restraint
 and availability of palatable food, 7
 and dietary violations, 128–136
 and diet boundaries, 120
 and emotional distress, 121–128
 flexible vs. rigid, 189–190
 and motivation, 121
 successful, 161–163
Restrained eating, dieting vs., 168
Restraint Scale (RS), 116–117, 119, 135
Restraint theory, 115
Rewards, 178
Rigid restrained eaters, 189, 190
Risk factors, for weight gain, 48–57
 food-induced thermogenesis, 52
 high food intake, 49
 high set point for body weight,
  55–57
 low fat oxidation, 52–53
 low leptin, 53–55
 low physical activity, 49–50
 low resting metabolic rate, 50–52
RMR. *See* Resting metabolic rate
Rodin, J., 111–112
Rosemary Conley program, 180, 181
RS. *See* Restraint Scale
Running, energy costs of, 38

Salience, of food, 100–102
 cognitive, 107–109
 and effort, 110
Salty snacks, 68
Satiation, 40n2, 95–96, 121
Satiety, 54, 120, 137
Satiety center, 112
Schachter, S., 104–105, 111–112
Schlosser, E., 64
School-based programs, 199–200
Schools
 fast food offerings in, 64–66
 food advertising in, 81–82
 Jamie's School Dinners and, 65
 locations of, 87
Sedentary adults
 energy expenditure in, 37
 RMR in, 36
Self-awareness, 121–127

Self-control, 186, 189
Self-esteem, 23–24, 122
Self-image, 123
Self-labeled dieting, 196
Self-monitoring, 169, 188
Self-regulation, 4, 162
Self-reporting
    of food intake, 62–63
    inaccuracy of, 118
    of television viewing, 78
Self-worth, 124
Sensitivity to external cues, 111–113
SES. *See* Socioeconomic status
Set-point theory, 55–57, 137, 195
Shared-environment effects, 46
Shopping habits, 88
Sickness absences, 23
Skills acquisition in weight control,
    169–170
Slim, normative pressure to be, 15
Slim-Fast, 180–181
Slochower, J. A., 98–103
Smelling food, 138–139, 149
Smokers and smoking
    attempts to quit, 187
    awareness of effects of, 198
    mortality rate of, 25–27
    rates of, 60
    and weight gain, 64
Snack food, 70–74
    package size of, 69
    taxing, 202
    and television viewing, 79, 80
Snacking, 70–74
Social consequences of overweight and
    obesity, 19–23
Social dancing, energy costs of, 38
Social pressures
    for eating full portion, 69
    for healthier eating, 62
Socioeconomic status (SES)
    and energy density of food, 204
    epidemiology of overweight/obesity
        by, 15–16
    and obesity stereotypes, 20
    and psychological consequences of
        obesity, 23–24

Soft drinks, 39, 56
    consumption of, 74–75, 82
    increased consumption of, 60–61
    portion sizes of, 68
    school pouring rights for, 81–82
    and snacks, 71
    taxing, 202
Starches, 39
Starvation, 36
Stereotypes about obese individuals,
    19–23
Stimulus control, 170
Stress. *See* Anxiety
Strokes, 28–29
Stroop task, 158–159
Structural ambivalence, 145, 146
Subliminal priming, 147, 148
Sugars, 39
Supraliminal priming, 147
Surgically treated patients, 192
Swedish Obese Subjects Study, 192

Table tennis playing, energy costs of, 38
Taxing soft drinks and fast food, 202
TEF. *See* Thermic effect of food
Television
    advertising on, 76, 80–81
    food behavior modeled on, 76
Television viewing, 75–80
    and consumption of unhealthy food,
        79
    during meals, 79–80
    and obesity in adolescents, 77
    reduction in, 199
    and snacking, 79, 80
TFEQ (Three Factor Eating Question-
    naire), 117
Thermic effect of food (TEF), 37, 52
Thermodynamics, first law of, 36
Thin idealization, 201
Three Factor Eating Questionnaire
    (TFEQ), 117
"Thrifty gene" hypothesis, 48
Training, diet, 169–170
Treatment(s), 167–198, 203–205
    dieting, 168–185
    harmful effects of, 191–198

Weight control
  and energy expenditure, 38–39
  as goal, x
  physical attractiveness as motivator
    of, 23
  successful, 161–163
  in United States, 203–204
Weight-control behaviors. *See* Weight-
    loss practices
Weight cycling, 56, 192, 195
Weight discrimination, 3, 19–23
Weight-fluctuation factor, 117, 119, 146
Weight gain
  and age, 172
  and physical inactivity, 88–91
  risk factors for, 48–57
Weight loss
  effectiveness of, 3
  and longevity, 192–194
  and mortality, 194
Weight-loss practices, 5, 183, 184, 194,
    196, 197
  effectiveness of, 5, 184, 197
Weight Loss Practices Survey (WLPS),
    183, 184
Weight recommendations
  by age, 27
  by race, 27–28
Weight regulation, 93–113
  determinants of, 93–113
  externality theory of, 103–113
  psychosomatic theory of, 94–103
Weight Watchers International,
    179–180, 182
Western culture, 19–23, 59–60
Western diet, 39
"What-the-hell" effect, 129, 138–139,
    142

White girls, physical activity levels for,
    90
White men, obesity rates for, 17
White women
  obesity rates for, 16
  weight discrimination in, 19
WHO. *See* World Health Organization
WLPS. *See* Weight Loss Practices
    Survey
Women
  and discrimination in college admis-
    sions, 20
  eating disorders in, 201
  and employment discrimination, 22
  and exercise programs, 177
  fast-food consumption by, 67
  health education programs for, 201
  ischemic strokes in, 29
  obesity rates for, 15
  obesity trends for, 17, 18
  physical activity levels for, 84
  and physical-attractiveness stereo-
    type, 20
  and social class, 15, 16
  social consequences for, 19
  television viewing by, 78
  and weight loss, 194
  and Weight Watchers program, 180
  in workforce, 65
Women's Health Study, 29
Women's Healthy Lifestyle Project, 201
Work-related physical activity, 37, 86,
    90
World Health Organization (WHO), ix,
    9, 11, 14, 63, 76

Zone diet, 180